THE ENCYCLOPEDIA OF
PREGNANCY
AND BIRTH

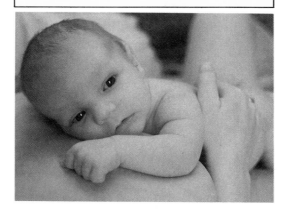

A **Macdonald Illustrated** BOOK

© Macdonald & Co (Publishers) Ltd 1987, 1989
© Text Janet Balaskas and Yehudi Gordon, 1987, 1989
© Photographs Anthea Sieveking, 1987, 1989

First published in Great Britain in 1987
Reprinted in 1989 by Macdonald & Co (Publishers) Ltd
London & Sydney
Second Reprint 1990

A member of Maxwell Macmillan Pergamon Publishing
Corporation

British Library Cataloguing in Publication Data

Balaskas, Janet
  Pregnancy birth and infancy.
  1. Pregnancy   2. Childbirth   3. Parenthood
  I. Title   II. Gordon, Yehudi
  618.2   RG525

    ISBN 0-356-10685-3

    ISBN 0-356-15323-1   (Pbk)

Filmset by Bookworm Typesetting, Manchester
Printed in Great Britain by
BPCC Paulton Books Limited

Editors: Sarah Chapman, Nancy Duin,
Jonathan Elphick, Sybil del Strother
Designer: Anne Braybon
Art Director: Linda Cole

Illustrations: Lucy Su

Macdonald & Co (Publishers) Ltd
Orbit House
1 New Fetter Lane
London EC4A 1AR

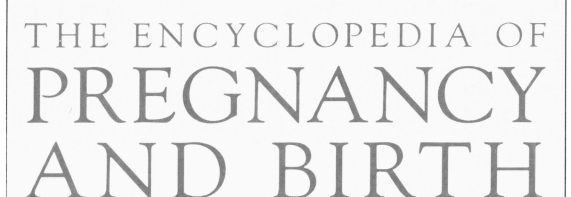

THE ENCYCLOPEDIA OF
PREGNANCY AND BIRTH

JANET BALASKAS
YEHUDI GORDON

PHOTOGRAPHS BY ANTHEA SIEVEKING

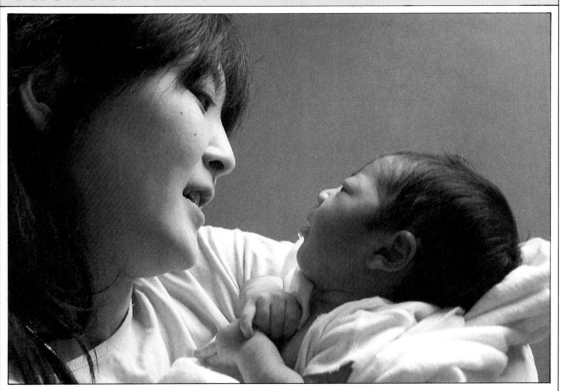

Macdonald Illustrated

CONTENTS

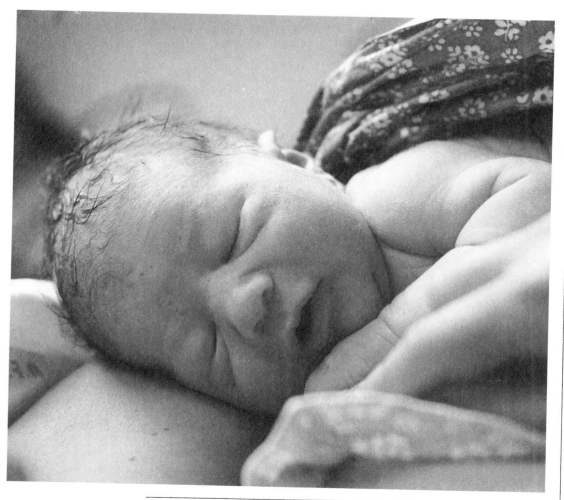

INTRODUCTION

I am pleased and proud to have had the opportunity of writing this book with my friend and colleague Janet Balaskas. Our work together began in 1978 and since then the Active Birth Movement has evolved, birth practices have altered throughout Britain and there are more choices and greater mobility for women in labour.

The Encyclopedia of Pregnancy and Birth has had a long gestation, during which we were involved in many discussions about the philosophy and the practical aspects of the vital first year of life – the twelve months from conception onwards. It is a synthesis of our views, which sometimes differ in detail, but remain similar on all the major issues.

Birth is an adventure for everyone involved and is probably the most important 'rite of passage' in the life cycle of any individual. The miraculous journey re-traces the path of evolution from fertilized egg through to the emergence of a fully formed human being. It is the most intense experience many of us ever undergo. The needs and emotions of the baby are important and these are highlighted throughout the book.

The passage from adult to parent, from woman to mother, man to father and parents to grandparents is filled with wonder, excitement and emotion. The emotions range from elation and euphoria to fear, anxiety and depression. We have not confined our attention to the rosy aspects of parenthood, but try to deal realistically with the problems which sometimes complicate pregnancy. It is a time when human support is often needed; a time for caring and being cared for; a time of both dependence and independence.

New technological advances have made birth less hazardous for mother and baby. However, the improvement in safety ceases at a certain point and thereafter the excessive use of machines or drugs creates problems and complications by interfering with the normal physiology of mother and baby. Birth is an intricate and finely balanced process which has evolved over hundreds of thousands of years, whereas the new technology is often crude in comparison and frequently promises more than it can deliver. The basic tenet of this book is that active birth and baby care is normal and attainable for the vast majority of women and babies. Technology is useful for the minority and should be present in the background and used when indicated in individual cases.

Throughout the world, an increasing number of people welcome the opportunity to take responsibility for themselves and their loved ones. Our aim is to inform and assist parents to make the optimal use of their own resources. This book is a guide to help prepare for parenthood. We intend it to be comprehensive, friendly, easy to understand and to use, as well as offering sound practical advice on all aspects of the subject.

I have had the experience of being a research scientist, obstetrician and a father, present at the births of my three children. I am always suprised at the mystery and the emotion which accompany birth. It is a sacred, profound and moving event, filled with the adventure of a new life, the joy of welcoming a new person and the responsibility of new parenthood.

Parents often relive their own past experiences and many long forgotten emotions emerge at this time. I hope this book will encourage understanding, warmth, contact, kindness and love, because the way we are born and nurtured has a profound effect on the way we live our lives.

Dedication

I dedicate this book to my wife Wendy and our children Gabi, Nicky and Tanya, who have supported and helped me in the long process of its creation, and taught me so much along the way.

YEHUDI GORDON, LONDON, JUNE 1987

I first met Yehudi Gordon, with whom I have had the privilege of writing this book, when I asked him to read the manuscript of my first book, *New Life*, in 1978. *New Life* is a book which broke new ground at the time it was published, by focusing on the physiological events of labour and birth and demonstrating how a woman's body is ideally designed to give birth in an upright position, rather than semi-reclining like a stranded beetle. It clearly described the advantages of the squatting position and suggested a programme of yoga-based exercises a woman could practise throughout her pregnancy in order to prepare herself for the birth.

At the time *New Life* was written, these ideas were revolutionary. The prevalent use of the reclining position denied the help of gravity, so that the woman in labour was a passive patient rather than an active participant in the birth. Ante-natal classes were mainly informative and were attended in the last weeks of pregnancy. Practising yoga throughout pregnancy is a less 'cerebral' way of preparing for birth, which increases the pregnant woman's enjoyment and awareness of her body and enables her to discover her instinctive potential. It gives her a sense of her own autonomy, power and inner strength during pregnancy, which continues naturally into the labour itself and on into motherhood.

When I was pregnant with my second child in the late 1970s, I began to hold yoga classes for pregnant women and encouraged them to attend throughout pregnancy. Many of them found that the yoga positions felt more comfortable during labour than the conventional lying-down position, and chose to give birth kneeling or squatting. By following the inner logic of their bodies, these women were unwittingly making history in the annals of childbirth. They were among a growing number of women throughout the world, who were taking control and responsibility for their own labours for the first time in three hundred years, since forceps were invented in 17th-century France. The phrase 'Active Birth', originally intended as a pun on the active management of labour, soon became a popular way of expressing the change of consciousness about childbirth that was taking place among these women.

In an active birth, the mother has complete freedom to follow her own instincts in an atmosphere of security, peace and privacy. Research has shown that when this is the case, the labour is likely to progress better, the safety of the baby is enhanced and a spontaneous vaginal birth is more likely. Complications occur less frequently and the mother's experience is usually more satisfying. For the baby, the birth is more likely to be gentle and untraumatic and good psychological 'bonding' between parents and baby after birth is made easier.

My two youngest children were born at home, where it is easiest to establish the perfect conditions for a natural, active birth. When Yehudi Gordon encouraged the pregnant women he met to practise the yoga-based exercises, we discovered that it was also possible for a completely active, instinctive birth to take place in hospital.

For this to occur – whether at home or in hospital – a profound change of attitude is necessary. The woman giving birth needs to learn to trust her body and its potential. The midwives and doctors who take care of her need to be able to resist the temptation to control, stepping in only when their expertise is specifically needed.

We are now approaching a new era in childbirth. For the first time in history it is becoming widely possible for normal, physiological birth to take place, with the safety net of modern obstetrics in the background. Starting from the standpoint of trust in a woman's own potential to carry, give birth, nurture and mother her children, a sensible perspective can be gained on the appropriate use of medical back-up. *The Encyclopedia of Pregnancy and Birth* is unusual in that it combines the views of a woman with those of an obstetrician. We deliberately decided not to write individually on our own specialities, but instead we have, as far as possible, reflected both our views throughout this book.

The result is a book neither of us could have written alone. I believe it is therefore a book which may be especially useful at this time, when the advances of modern obstetrics are happening alongside a new understanding of the physiological event and psychological changes that occur when a baby is born.

Dedication

I dedicate this book to my children Nina, Kassandra and Iasonas, without whom this book would not exist. It is also for my husband Keith, whose constant support enabled me to devote so much time to the project.

JANET BALASKAS, LONDON, JUNE 1987

Acknowledgements

We would like to thank the mothers, fathers and babies whose births have been both an inspiration and a source of knowledge to us. We also thank the midwives for their loyalty and devotion and all our other colleagues whose support has been essential.

We owe special thanks to Stephen Russell, who introduced us to Taoist philosophy and massage, and to Carole Elliott, Sheila Kitzinger, Frederick Leboyer, Ronald Laing and Michel Odent for their inspiration. Our special thanks also go to Anthea Sieveking and the families she photographed so beautifully, for their invaluable contribution to the content of the book, and to Lucy Su for her clear illustrations.

Finally, we must thank all those at the publishers, Macdonald & Co., who helped to bring this book to birth, including Anne Braybon, Sarah Chapman, Clare Chatel, Linda Cole, Rachel Duffield, Nancy Duin, Jonathan Elphick and Sybil de Strother.

PART I

PREPARING FOR PREGNANCY

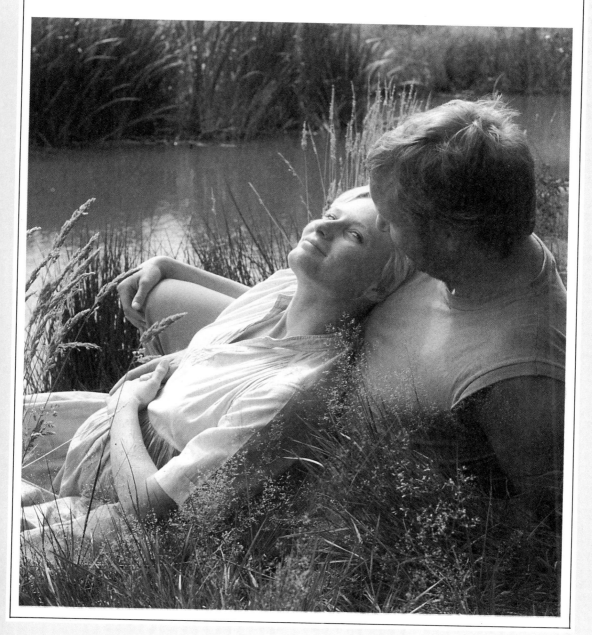

CHAPTER 1

FERTILITY AND CONCEPTION

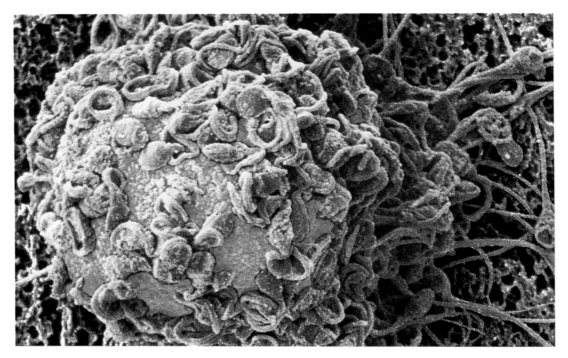

Microphotograph of sperm (pale brown) surrounding and attached to an egg (pale pink). During fertilization, only one sperm succeeds in penetrating the egg's wall.

Deciding to have a baby is the first step in a chain of events which are likely to be among the richest and most rewarding of a lifetime. The urge to conceive and give birth to a child is a strong, primitive biological drive common to every living species, which ensures the continuity of life on earth and is almost as powerful as the need to eat and breathe.

Once you have decided to have a child, the weeks and months leading to conception may be full of anticipation, as you contemplate the challenges and choices that lie ahead and begin to explore the responsibilities involved in starting a family. Perhaps you will wait a long time for conception to take place, or on the other hand you may conceive quickly. Sometimes conception is unplanned, and this is bound to involve considerable adjustment and the need to consider carefully the implications of accepting responsibility for a new life.

Whether or not the pregnancy is intentional, it is bound to generate great change in your life and open up a new world, as you gradually become aware of your child's life taking root inside you and the adventure of being pregnant and becoming a parent begins.

Planning for parenthood

Prior to conception, many couples choose to pay a visit to their doctor or to a pre-conceptual clinic so that they can benefit from a general health examination as well as counselling about fertility, conception, ante-natal care and different aspects of birth and parenthood, about which they may need information or which may be causing anxiety. The types of questions you are likely to be asked and the topics discussed are very similar to those that you will encounter at your first visit to an ante-natal clinic when you become pregnant (*see* p. 81).

Another very good reason for seeing your doctor before trying to conceive is to have a blood test to see if you are immune to rubella (German measles). This illness, so mild in adults and children, can have devastating effects on the unborn child during the first 12 or so weeks after conception (*see* p. 334). If it is found that you are not already immune, you should be vaccinated against rubella and then avoid conception for at least three months afterwards.

Attending a pre-conceptual clinic will not guarantee fertility or a trouble-free pregnancy, but it is a preventive and holistic approach to your health care in pregnancy, which will help promote your well-being and that of your baby both during and after pregnancy.

Your health and fitness

Your health and nutrition *before* conception will affect the well-being of your child and the successful outcome of the birth, and this is the ideal time to take positive steps towards achieving a good nutritional balance. The months preceding pregnancy are the most important in this respect, so that your body can provide the necessary nutrients for the crucial first ten weeks of pregnancy, when your baby's organs are forming and developing.

To check your diet, follow the advice on foods to eat during pregnancy in Chapter 7. It is unwise to try to lose weight if you are trying to conceive as this may alter the vitamin and mineral balance in your body.

There is also no better time to begin working on your body. Before conception, practising yoga regularly will be very beneficial — as will some form of daily exercise such as swimming, jogging, dancing, playing tennis or going for brisk walks in the fresh air.

It is advisable to discontinue taking the contraceptive pill or to have an IUD ('coil') removed so that three menstrual cycles can occur before conception is attempted, to allow your body time to recover. Menstruation is often erratic after a woman has been taking the Pill, and it may take some months before cycles become regular. You will be able to establish the date of conception much more accurately if your cycles have returned to their natural rhythm. There is usually no problem if conception occurs while an IUD is still in place or within three months of having one removed. However, there is a slight increase in the risk of miscarriage (*see* p. 323) or ectopic pregnancy (*see* p. 309).

Your emotional well-being

It is extremely valuable, if circumstances allow, to have time to prepare yourself emotionally for parenthood. Pregnancy is a time of great transformation for both parents, and has great value and potential in terms of your personal development and maturation.

Becoming a parent will present new dimensions within your relationship with your partner and/or immediate family, so it is important to become open to change and exploration, to allow for the new emotional challenges that inevitably come with having a baby. This is an appropriate time to consider your own early life and parenting – starting with your birth and infancy – and to try to resolve any residual conflicts or confusions.

However, very few people approach parenthood in ideal circumstances. A further problem is that there is usually much more emphasis placed on the physical or medical aspects of pregnancy, while the emotional side is often neglected. If there are difficulties that cannot be sorted out with your partner, family or friends, you may need the help of a therapist or counsellor; or your ante-natal teacher, doctor or midwife may be able to advise you.

Practical matters

Getting pregnant and having a baby are bound to involve considerable new demands on your finances. If you have been working, you may have to cope with the loss of a regular income, and your partner may have to shoulder most of the financial responsibilities for a while. This may be further complicated by the necessity of moving to a larger flat or house, compatible with an increased family. It is very helpful if you can plan your finances in advance of starting a family, to avoid unnecessary stress during this time.

If you need to and can move house, try to choose an area which offers suitable health care for pregnant women as well as the right facilities for the birth and infancy of your child. It may be important for you to live close to family and friends with whom you can share the joys and trials of parenthood. It is also worthwhile to look ahead and consider what is available in terms of pre-school activities and playgroups, primary schools and facilities for young children.

The female reproductive organs

The miracle of conception takes place deep within a woman's body as part of a finely tuned and orchestrated physiological process. The moment new life begins, the rhythmic ebb and flow of the menstrual cycle alters, and a series of changes are set in motion which prepare your body for pregnancy, childbirth and breastfeeding. A woman's body is perfectly designed to produce and nurture a child, and it is both fascinating and helpful to understand how the female reproductive system works.

The uterus

The uterus, or womb, is the principal organ involved in pregnancy and childbirth. It is similar in size and shape to an upside-down pear, and is capable of enormous expansion to accommodate your growing baby during pregnancy. Before pregnancy, the uterus lies in the pelvis between the bladder (in front) and the rectum (behind), but by the time you are full-term, it will have expanded into the abdominal cavity to reach just below your lower ribs.

The lower part of, or entrance to, the uterus is known as the *cervix* – commonly called the 'neck of the womb'. Above that is the main part of the uterus, known as the *uterine body*; the top part is called the *fundus*.

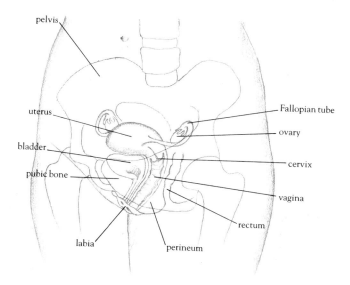

The female reproductive organs within the pelvic cavity.

The cervix This is a hollow passage about 4 cm (1½ in) long at the base of the uterus, which leads from the vagina to the uterine cavity. It consists of a circle, or *sphincter*, of fibrous, elastic and smooth muscle tissue, and it carries out a variety of important functions.

The glands in the lining of the cervix secrete mucus and are very active through adult life. The nature of the mucus varies during the menstrual cycle, being thin and watery around the time of ovulation to assist sperm mobility, and thick and viscous before and after menstruation to discourage sperm from entering the uterus. During pregnancy, the mucous glands produce a thick plug which seals the opening to the cervix and, together with the membranes which enclose the amniotic fluid that surrounds the foetus, acts as a barrier to prevent bacteria from reaching the baby.

The cervical canal is closed during most of the menstruation cycle, opening about 1 cm (⅖ in) at ovulation and again at menstruation to allow the passage of sperm and menstrual blood. During pregnancy, the cervix remains tightly shut to protect and contain the growing baby, until the last ten weeks when the muscular action of the uterus causes the sphincter to thin and shorten as it stretches, and then it begins to open (i.e. dilate) gradually when labour starts.

The uterine body This comprises the upper two-thirds of the uterus, above the cervix. Most of the muscle tissue of the uterus is contained in the walls of the uterine body, and its power during labour derives from the rhythmic contractions of the muscle fibres. They are made of smooth muscle, which acts involuntarily like the muscle in your blood vessels and intestines and does not come under your conscious control.

The uterine body is made up of three layers. The outer layer, or cover, is a strong, smooth membrane called the *peritoneum*. The muscular middle layer is called the *myometrium*, which consists of three layers of muscle fibres which run vertically, horizontally and diagonally. The inside of this muscular wall is lined with an inner layer: the *endometrium*.

The uterine muscle contracts and relaxes constantly throughout a

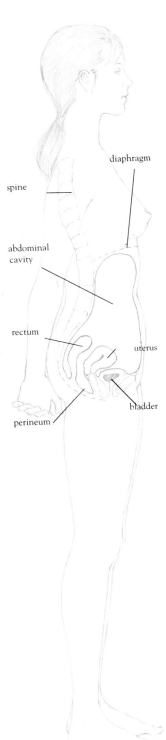

spine

diaphragm

abdominal
cavity

rectum

uterus

perineum

bladder

woman's life, but you will only be aware of any contractions before and during menstruation and during pregnancy and childbirth. During pregnancy, the muscle fibres of the uterus increase massively in size but do not increase in number, and by the time the baby is ready to be born, the upper portion of the uterine wall – that is, the fundus – will have expanded from a thickness of 1 cm (2/5 in) to 5 cm (2 in). As well as being able to contract and relax, the uterine muscle can also retract – that is, it can shorten and remain shortened. An example of this is when the uterus shrinks by two-thirds within minutes after the baby is born and the placenta separates.

The hollow centre of the uterus is called the uterine, or endometrial, cavity. This is connected below to the vagina via the cervix and to the two Fallopian tubes above, thereby providing a pathway for sperm to travel up to meet an egg in one of the Fallopian tubes and to fertilize it.

The endometrium This mucous membrane which lines the inner cavity of the uterus is richly supplied with blood vessels. During the menstrual cycle, it builds up, ready to nourish a fertilized egg. However, if none arrives, the superficial layer is shed during menstruation and then builds up again from the deeper layer of the endometrium during the menstrual cycle. The thickened endometrium is also shed after childbirth.

If an egg is fertilized, the resulting embryo will become implanted within the endometrium, and the placenta will be embedded in its deeper layers throughout pregnancy.

Blood supply and supporting structures The uterus is supplied with blood from the ovarian artery above and the uterine artery below, and their branches pierce the muscle. This double blood supply ensures adequate nourishment to the placenta and the baby. During menstruation and after childbirth, the muscle of the uterus contracts and retracts, and the pressure exerted on the blood vessels constricts them, arresting the flow of blood and thus providing a mechanism for stopping bleeding at these times.

The uterus has two main supports: the levator muscles in the lower part of the pelvis (commonly called the 'pelvic-floor muscles'); and ligaments which run from the sides of the lower half of the uterus to the front, sides and back of the pelvis. These ligaments are not rigid and allow the uterus to move up, down and sideways by as much as 2.5 cm (1 in). This facility allows the uterus to move when your bladder or rectum fill, and during sexual intercourse.

The Fallopian tubes

The two Fallopian tubes (also called *uterine tubes*) curve out from either side of the top of the uterus and end in numerous frond-like projections, called *fimbriae*, which surround the two ovaries. The tubes themselves are thin, hollow, muscular canals lined with mucous glands containing cells from which project microscopic hair-like structures called *cilia*.

The Fallopian tubes have two main functions: to transport the egg to the uterus; and to nourish the egg and sperm. At ovulation – when an egg is released from an ovary – the delicate fimbriae envelop the ovary like an anemone, thus coaxing the egg into the tube. The egg is then wafted towards the uterus by the rhythmic contractions of the tubal muscle and also by the wave-like motion of the cilia, which beat rhythmically towards the uterus. The sperm, meanwhile, are swimming up the Fallopian tube against the current. Both they and the egg are sustained by fluid secreted by the tubal cells, which contains oxygen and food. Fertilization takes place in the tube about two-thirds of the way to the ovary, and the fertilized egg then needs about seven days to reach the uterine cavity.

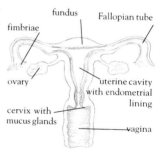

Cross-section of the female reproductive organs showing the uterine lining and the glands of the cervix.

The ovaries

The two ovaries are each the size of an almond, and are located on either side of the uterus, near the end of each Fallopian tube. They are situated deep in the pelvis and are thus protected from injury.

The ovaries have two functions: they produce eggs (or *ova*); and also produce the hormones *oestrogen* and *progesterone* which are responsible for female body hair and contours and for the menstrual cycle.

In the developing female embryo, the ovaries contain four to five million eggs, but by the time a woman begins to menstruate, only about half a million immature eggs remain. Each one is surrounded by a shimmering, translucent membrane called the *zona pellucida*, and underlying this tough outer layer is a finer membrane which covers the egg. The nucleus in the centre of the egg contains genetic information in the form of 23 chromosomes, which are waiting to be mingled with the 23 chromosomes of the sperm at fertilization.

During every menstrual cycle, between 10 and 100 eggs begin to ripen, but usually only one of these reaches full maturity on the day of ovulation and is then capable of being fertilized. As the egg ripens, the ovarian cells which surround it secrete fluid containing oestrogen, which then enters the bloodstream and affects the whole body. The fluid increases and, with hundreds of surrounding cells, forms a grape-like *follicle* on the surface of the ovary which may become as large as 2 cm (¾ in) across. The oestrogen that is then secreted by the follicle triggers the release of hormones from the pituitary gland, which in turn causes the follicle to rupture and release the egg. This is then drawn into the Fallopian tube where fertilization can take place.

The empty follicle now becomes the *corpus luteum*, or 'yellow body', which produces the hormones needed to maintain pregnancy for the next 6–10 weeks, until the placenta takes over.

The vagina

The vagina is the passage that extends from the cervix to the external genitals. It is approximately 10 cm (4 in) in length, and extends upward and backward, so that the lower portion is close to the pubic bone and the upper portion lies near the sacrum (tailbone). It is supported by ligaments attached to the side and back walls of the pelvis, and by the levator (or 'pelvic floor') muscles at the bottom of the pelvis. These supports, shared with the uterus, are flexible to enable the vagina to move.

The vaginal walls are composed of muscle and elastic tissue; these are lined with skin that is very folded, or pleated, and capable of stretching both during sexual intercourse and during childbirth. The walls normally touch one another, and this, combined with the contraction of the muscles surrounding the vaginal entrance, ensures that the vagina is usually closed and thus protected. The skin at the vaginal entrance forms a fold called the *hymen*, which has an opening to allow the flow of menstrual blood. This is usually broken with the first sexual intercourse.

Facing page: side view of the pelvic organs within the abdominal cavity. During pregnancy the uterus will expand to fill most of the abdominal cavity.

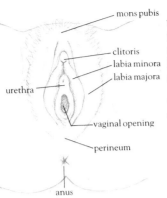

mons pubis

clitoris
labia minora
labia majora

urethra

vaginal opening

perineum

anus

The external genital
organs.

The vagina is normally moist and well lubricated, due to secretions from the cervix and from the two Bartholin's glands, located on either side of the outer end of the vagina, and to fluid from underlying blood vessels. In the middle of the menstrual cycle, when ovulation occurs, the vaginal lubrication is increased by mucus released from the cervix; this aids the sperm in their journey to meet the egg.

The vulva

The outer part of the female reproductive system is called the *vulva*, and consists of the *labia majora* (outer lips), *labia minora* (inner lips) and the *clitoris*. The labia majora contain fat and are covered by skin with hair and sweat glands. The labia minora, on the other hand, comprise folds of delicate and sensitive skin, meeting at the front to form a protective hood over the clitoris, and surround and protect the opening to the vagina.

The clitoris is the female equivalent of the male penis. Covered with skin, it consists of tissue richly supplied with nerves, which becomes engorged with blood and erect when the woman is aroused, thus making it one of the most erotically sensitive parts of a woman's body. Only the outer part, or *glans*, is visible when the woman is not sexually excited.

In front of the vulva is the *mons pubis*, – a thick pad of fatty tissue which covers the pubic bone.

The perineum

This is the fleshy area between the vagina and the anus, and it is here that the muscles surrounding the vaginal entrance and anus meet muscles running from the side walls of the pelvis. These help to keep the vaginal entrance closed as well as providing additional support and strength for the pelvic floor. During childbirth, the tissues of the perineum are capable of an enormous amount of expansion as the baby's head emerges.

The menstrual cycle

A woman has approximately 500 menstrual cycles during her lifetime. Each one usually lasts about 28 days – day one being the first day of menstruation – but a variation of between 21 and 35 days is quite normal. The events which occur during each cycle are delicately controlled by the secretions of hormones – the chemical messengers which, among many other functions, ensure a continuous cycle of fertility.

Hormones are produced by *endocrine glands*, and are then transported around the body in the bloodstream. There are four major endocrine glands involved in the menstrual cycle: the thyroid gland in the neck; the hypothalamus and pituitary gland deep in the brain; and the ovaries. Each cycle is directly affected by hormones from the pituitary gland and the ovaries, with the thyroid hormones controlling the flow of energy around the body and providing an essential background for the normal function of other hormones. In particular, the pituitary gland is known as the 'conductor of the endocrine orchestra' that stimulates the menstrual cycle.

There is an intimate feedback system between the ovaries, the hypothalamus and the pituitary gland, which maintains the rhythm of the cycle. In addition, because the hypothalamus is connected to other areas of the brain, emotional factors may affect the menstral cycle.

A menstrual cycle has three phases:

1 *The follicular phase* The first hormones of the cycle are secreted by the pituitary gland: *follicle-stimulating hormone* (FSH) and *luteinizing hormone* (LH). These travel to one of the ovaries via the bloodstream and stimulate the development of between ten and a hundred follicles. The latter, in turn, begin to produce increasing amounts of the female hormone *oestrogen*, which affects many parts of the body. (Usually each of the ovaries is stimulated during alternate cycles; however, if one of the ovaries is not able to function, the remaining one is capable of continuing the work alone with no loss of fertility.)

The pituitary gland also secretes another hormone, *prolactin*. Low levels of this are essential for ovulation, and it is produced continuously throughout the cycle. It reaches high levels during breastfeeding, when it inhibits ovulation and fertility.

The oestrogen produced by the ovary also acts on the hypothalamus in the brain to stimulate the production of releasing hormones which will then act on the pituitary gland. This is called a feedback system, whereby the pituitary hormones initiate the development of follicles in an ovary, and they in turn produce oestrogen which acts on the hypothalamus to stimulate the production of more pituitary hormones.

About halfway through the cycle, when there is a high level of oestrogen in the bloodstream, the pituitary releases a surge of LH and FSH. This causes one egg (and sometimes more than one) to rise to the surface of a follicle, ready for ovulation. The other stimulated follicles gradually disappear during the next 14 days.

Meanwhile, oestrogen has been causing the endometrium (the lining of

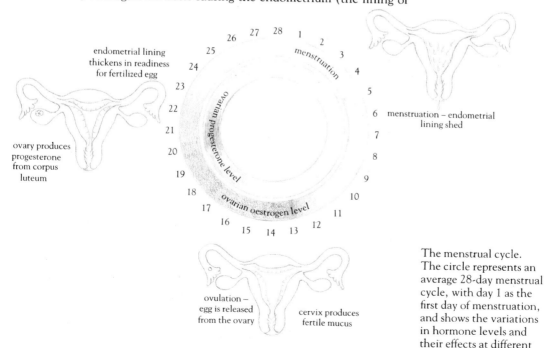

endometrial lining thickens in readiness for fertilized egg

ovary produces progesterone from corpus luteum

menstruation

menstruation – endometrial lining shed

ovarian progesterone level

ovarian oestrogen level

ovulation – egg is released from the ovary

cervix produces fertile mucus

The menstrual cycle. The circle represents an average 28-day menstrual cycle, with day 1 as the first day of menstruation, and shows the variations in hormone levels and their effects at different phases of the cycle.

the uterus) to thicken in readiness to receive the fertilized egg. In addition, the hormone stimulates the lining of the cervix to release watery mucus which will encourage sperm penetration.

2 *Ovulation* About 32 hours after the surge of LH and FSH, the follicle surrounding the egg ruptures, and the egg, surrounded and protected by follicular cells, bursts out of the ovary and is wafted by the frond-like fimbriae into a Fallopian tube, where it is nourished and available for fertilization by a sperm for between 12 and 36 hours, the follicular cells having fallen away. If fertilization does not occur, the egg disintegrates and is absorbed.

3 *The luteal phase* The ruptured follicle on the ovary now begins to take up fatty cholesterol, which turns it yellow – hence its new name: *corpus luteum*, which is Latin for 'yellow body'. It continues to produce oestrogen, but to this is now added another hormone – *progesterone*. Progesterone alters the mucus secreted by the cervix, making it too thick for sperm to swim through, and also causes the glands in the Fallopian tubes and uterus to produce a fluid which will nourish the egg, creating conditions for fertilization in the tube and implantation of the egg in the uterine wall.

If fertilization does not occur, the corpus luteum disintegrates and levels of both progesterone and oestrogen fall over a period of about ten days. Since these two hormones no longer stimulate the lining of the uterus, this is now shed and menstruation occurs. The cycle is now complete, and a new cycle begins.

If the egg is fertilized, some of its cells (which will eventually become the placenta) will produce *human chorionic gonadotrophin* (HCG); pregnancy tests detect the presence or absence of this. HCG will maintain the corpus luteum so that it can continue to produce progesterone to keep the endometrium nourished; this function of the corpus luteum is essential during the first ten weeks of pregnancy, until the placenta can take over.

Menstruation

On the first day of the menstrual flow – i.e. the first day of a period – the lining of the uterus is twice as thick as it will be after menstruation. If fertilization has not occurred and the levels of oestrogen and progesterone decline, the blood vessels of the uterine lining shrink and the spongy glands contained within it become detached, along with droplets of blood from the underlying blood vessels. The average blood loss is 40-60ml – that is, 2½-4 tablespoons – but the variation in the amount is very wide.

Menstruation usually lasts between three and five days, depending on the rate at which the lining is shed. It ceases when the top part of the lining (the superficial lining) is completely shed and the deeper layer comprising glands and blood vessels begins to grow and a new cycle starts.

The male reproductive organs

The male reproductive system fulfils three functions: the manufacture of sperm in the testicles; the transport of sperm through the penis during love-making; and the production of male sex hormones, the principal one of which is *testosterone*, responsible for such male characteristics as body hair distribution, a masculine build and a deep voice.

The hormonal feedback system of the menstrual cycle. FSH and LH, produced in the pituitary, stimulate an ovarian follicle to ripen and at the same time to make oestrogen and then progesterone which are released into the bloodstream and feed back to the pituitary to control the output of FSH and LH. This ensures that the FSH, LH peak which causes ovulation occurs when the ovarian follicle is ripe.

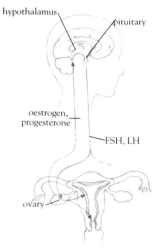

hypothalamus

pituitary

oestrogen, progesterone

FSH, LH

ovary

The testicles

The two testicles – each about 4 cm (1½ in) in length and 2.5 cm (1 in) wide – lie suspended in the scrotum, a bag of skin attached to the perineum at the base of the penis on the outside of the body. During the development of the male embryo, the testicles are formed deep in the abdominal cavity, to descend later through the abdominal wall into the scrotum.

Each testicle contains *seminiferous tubules*, where sperm are produced, and *interstitial* cells, where male hormones are made. At the back of the testicle, in the scrotum, lies a comma-shaped structure called the *epididymis*, where sperm are collected in tiny tubules to complete their maturation. These tubules come together to form one relatively large tube called the *vas deferens*, which carries the sperm to the prostate gland and seminal vesicles at the base of the bladder deep in the pelvis.

Sperm production is optimal when the testicles are 1–2 °C (1.8–3.6°F) below body temperature. In hot weather, the temperature inside the scrotum is reduced by the activity of sweat glands in the skin, whereas in cold weather, the cremasteric muscle which surrounds the vas deferens draws the testicle up closer to the body for warmth.

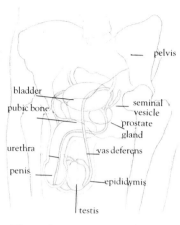

The male reproductive organs within the pelvic cavity.

The seminal vesicles and prostate gland

The vas deferens travels up from a testicle until it loops down over the pubic bone to lie alongside the base of the bladder deep in the pelvis. It ends by branching to form one of the two seminal vesicles which secrete a fluid which will make up part of the semen. Hereafter, the vas deferens is called an ejaculatory duct, and it now runs through the prostate gland, where a milky fluid will be added to the duct's contents. In the prostate, the duct joins with the urethra, which carries urine from the bladder. The final ingredient for the semen is secreted by the two Cowper's glands at the base of the penis.

Semen is necessary for the transport and nourishment of sperm. These are forced up from the epididymis by muscular contraction when the man is sexually aroused and, joined by the various components of the semen, are ejaculated through the penis during orgasm.

The penis

This is suspended from the pubic bone and consists of skin and erectile tissue, with the urethra running down through the middle. At the tip of the penis is the *glans*, a particularly sensitive part that is well endowed with nerve endings; in uncircumsized men, it is protected by the foreskin.

When a man is not aroused, the penis hangs down limply, its skin covering wrinkled and loose. However, during love-making, the erectile tissue becomes engorged with blood, and the penis as a whole distends, stiffens and, the skin stretched tightly over it, increases its length from 7.5–10 cm (3–4 in) to 15–18 cm (6–7 in). The urethra, which carries the sperm and semen, also carries urine from the bladder, but just before orgasm, the urinary entrance is sealed by muscular contraction, thus protecting the delicate sperm from contact with urine.

Sperm production and ejaculation

The pituitary gland in a man's brain produces the hormones FSH and LH, which are identical to those produced by a woman, and there is also a similar feedback system. However, the production of male hormones is a continuous process rather than a cyclical one as it is in women.

Sperm (also called *spermatozoa*) are produced throughout a man's adult life; unlike a woman, whose ovaries will cease to produce eggs when she is in her late 40s or 50s, a man will be relatively fertile for many years beyond that age. Sperm are produced continuously – several hundred million a day – by specialized cells in the seminiferous tubules within each testicle. This process, which includes the maturing of the sperm in the epididymis, takes seven weeks and is known as *spermatogenesis*.

A mature sperm is microscopic in size – only 1/20 of a millimetre – and looks like a tadpole, with a head, body and tail. The *head* contains genetic material in the form of 23 chromosomes which will enter and fertilize the egg, as well as special enzymes which will make it possible for it to penetrate the egg's protective covering, the zona pellucida. The *body* comprises special structures called mitochondria, which provide the energy the sperm needs to swim to meet the egg. The *tail* is a long, thin structure which propels the sperm forward by moving rapidly from side to side. In relative terms, the distance covered by a sperm from the cervix to a Fallopian tube is equivalent to a person swimming across the Atlantic!

Every ejaculation produces about 3–5 millilitres (approximately 1/2–1 teaspoon) of semen, which contains between 150 and 750 million sperm. At orgasm, rhythmic muscular contractions of the genital area cause the man to ejaculate the sperm through his penis into the vagina and on to the opening of the cervix. The mucus secreted by the cervix forms a mesh that is impenetrable to sperm except for three or four days in the middle of the woman's cycle, around the time of ovulation. The sperm will not live for more than 24 hours unless they are protected and nourished by this watery mucus, and they can live within it for several days.

When sperm are examined under the microscope, it is normal to find that up to 20 per cent are not perfectly formed: either they do not move properly or their heads are too large or their tails too small. These abnormal forms usually cannot swim far enough to reach a Fallopian tube, but if they do, they are usually unable to fertilize an egg.

Fertility awareness

For a woman, it is very helpful if she wishes to conceive – or to avoid conception – that she becomes aware of the pattern of her fertility cycle. The possibility of conceiving a baby in any menstrual cycle is limited to about five days: whereas a woman's egg will survive for only 12 to 36 hours in a Fallopian tube unless it is fertilized, it is thought that a man's sperm can live for up to five days in that environment. However, fertilization usually occurs within 24 hours after sexual intercourse.

The crucial time for a woman is about 14 days before her next period. During the lives of most women, menstrual cycles usually have a regular rhythm. However, irregularity is common in adolescence, middle age and after giving birth. It can also be caused by emotional stress, travel, illness and malnutrition, and the periods of some fertile women quite commonly follow an irregular pattern or are simply infrequent. However, if you keep a record of the events of your menstrual cycle, after a time you will probably observe a discernible pattern, and you can maximize the chances of conception by timing sexual intercourse to coincide with ovulation.

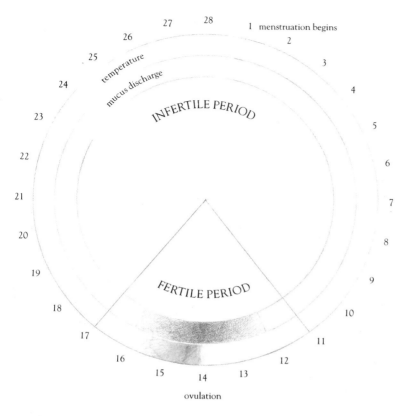

The pattern of fertility in a 28-day cycle. The changes in cervical mucus begin on about day 12, peak at the time of ovulation on day 14 and end on day 16. Body temperature rises after ovulation. Ovulation always occurs about 14 days before menstruation; if the cycle is longer than 28 days the onset of the mucus changes is delayed and the fertile period is later.

Signs of fertility in women

There are a number of things you can look for to determine whether or not — and when — you are ovulating. These include: cycle length, from period to period; changes in your cervical mucus and in the cervix itself; changes in your body temperature before rising in the morning; and general physical changes.

The length of menstrual cycles This varies from woman to woman, but the average cycle lasts between 21 and 35 days. You should be ovulating on about the 14th day before your next period, so if you have discovered that your menstrual cycles have a pattern of lasting between, say 27 and 34 days, you could possibly be fertile any time between day 13 and day 20 of each cycle.

Changes in cervical mucus The oestrogen produced by the ovaries in increasing amounts before ovulation also activates the cervix to secrete a wet, slippery, sticky, clear or whitish mucus — similar to raw egg white — which will appear outside the vagina. This filters out damaged sperm, provides nourishment for healthy sperm and guides and channels them as they move through the cervix and the uterus and into the Fallopian tubes. The number of days when the fertile-type mucus is present varies, but if you keep a record, you will see that you have your own individual and recognizable pattern.

This change in the cervical mucus indicates that you are fertile. If you wish to avoid getting pregnant at this time, you need to refrain from sexual intercourse or genital-to-genital contact, or else use an effective method of contraception. If, however, you do wish to conceive, you will be at your most fertile on the last two days that this type of mucus is present. This *fertile peak* usually occurs within a day of ovulation.

After ovulation, the cervix produces very thick mucus which forms a plug, allowing little or no mucus to descend through the vagina; thus, the vaginal entrance will be dry or only slightly sticky, and will remain so until a few days before the next ovulation. During this time, the cervix is closed, and the vaginal environment is acidic and hostile to sperm. Once the dryness has been obvious for three consecutive days, you can assume that ovulation has taken place and that the egg is no longer viable. (However, this cannot be entirely depended upon as a method of avoiding pregnancy: all women can ovulate suddenly out of sequence, and it is even known – though rare – for women to get pregnant during their periods. See pages 304-5 for information on the various methods of contraception that are currently available.)

Changes in the cervix   The cervix rises up the vagina by about 2.5 cm (1 in) at midcycle, and the external opening softens and becomes slightly open. This corresponds to the alteration in cervical mucus, and provides additional information about your body. The cervix is easy to feel if you squat and insert one finger into the vagina; if you do this frequently during a few cycles, you will learn to recognize the changes.

Changes in body temperature   Another indication of fertility is the changes in your temperature around the time of ovulation. Your temperature may drop slightly when the egg is released – i.e. at ovulation – and then rise to a higher level immediately afterwards, although this does not happen to everyone.

Because these changes in temperature are so slight, it is best if you use a special thermometer to measure them. You should mark each result on a chart, and these plus the special fertility thermometers are available from family doctors and family planning clinics. For these measurements to be meaningful, you must take your temperature by mouth immediately on waking, before you get up or eat or drink anything. The measurements should be taken every day.

General physical changes   There may be other changes in your body during your menstrual cycle, due to the variation in the amounts of the hormones oestrogen and progesterone in your bloodstream. These may include the following:

   A general feeling of tenderness, or a twinge or a sharp pain on one side of the abdomen; the latter is called *mittelschmerz* and generally occurs at or very near the time of ovulation.
   Very slight bleeding which colours the cervical mucus pink or a brownish colour.
   After ovulation, some or all of the symptoms of pre-menstrual syndrome may occur: irritability, headache, backache, general aches and pains, breast discomfort, swelling of the abdomen, a bloated feeling, weight gain and skin disorders.

Love-making

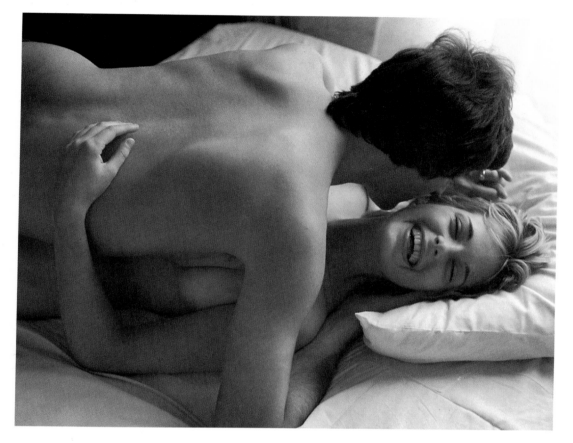

Making love takes on a special significance when you consciously decide to conceive a child.

On a purely physical level, love-making involves a spontaneous surrender to the flow of biological energy between man and woman, starting with mutual attraction, stimulation and excitation, and culminating in a peak, or *orgasm*, which is satisfying to both partners. A man must ejaculate sperm to conceive a child, and this occurs at orgasm; however, in women, conception can happen without orgasm.

For a truly satisfactory sexual life, it is important that both men and women experience orgasm, although the way this is achieved is variable and it is not necessary to reach orgasm every time you make love. Although simultaneous orgasm can be very pleasurable for a couple, it should never be a goal to strive for on every occasion. In practice, each partner's rhythms should be respected and nurtured, and orgasms at different times should give both mutual satisfaction. Such sexual satisfaction plays an important part in our health and happiness, and any difficulties in this area may be helped by professional counselling or therapy.

Equally important is the emotional side of love-making. In making love, you enter into a deep intimacy with your partner, in which you are both open and responsive to each other. Deep-seated emotions surface, and both partners find themselves needing or giving at the same or different times. Sex is both loving and aggressive, and can be serious or playful, soft and tender or strong and powerful. All of this is healthy and normal. The vital thing is for both partners to tune in to the other's needs and desires, both physical and emotional, and to be willing to adapt and compromise.

There are many subtle messages given during love-making – transmitted via noises, facial and body expressions, speech or silence – and it is good for both partners to show or tell the other candidly what they need and what satisfies them. It may not be easy to tell your partner that a particular act is unappealing, but provided this is done with love, it is an essential part of building a solid relationship.

Sexual intercourse

This can be divided into two phases – the voluntary and the involuntary – and is usually preceded by foreplay.

1 *Voluntary excitation phase* The man experiences erection and develops an urge to penetrate the woman. The woman is aroused, and her outer genitals swell and become engorged with blood. The walls of her vagina produce secretions which moisten it, and its inner diameter increases. Excitation increases in both partners with penetration of the penis.

This is followed by mutual, slow, spontaneous and effortless movements of both the man and the woman, which stimulate the glans at the tip of the man's penis and the woman's clitoris and vagina. In both partners the skin flushes, nipples become erect and the heart rate increases.

The consciousness of both partners is concentrated on perception of pleasurable sensations, and changes in position or method enhance this pleasure. Slow, gentle movements tend to intensify the sensations as well as the feeling of harmony between both partners. Resting for short periods may increase the depth of the flow of energy.

This phase can continue for as long as the couple choose. Gradually, with continuing friction, the excitation level increases and spreads from the genitals throughout the body. While this is happening the vaginal opening swells and grips the penis more tightly, the uterus is elevated and the upper vagina widens as the clitoris draws up.

2 *The involuntary phase* In this, voluntary control of the course of excitation is no longer possible. Body movements are speeded up, the heartbeat increases, and breathing becomes deeper. Physical excitation becomes concentrated in the genital area, and a 'melting' sensation sets in which seems to radiate from the genitals to other parts of the body. Involuntary spasmodic contractions of the penis, seminal vesicles and prostate in the man bring about ejaculation, and in the woman, waves of contractions occur in the clitoris and of the vagina and anus, the uterus contracts and the cervix opens. This is orgasm. Accompanying it, there is a very pleasant clouding of consciousness as orgasmic excitation takes hold of the whole body.

This is followed by a decrease in tension, and energy flows back from the genitals to the rest of the body. There is then pleasant physical and mental relaxation, usually accompanied by a strong desire for sleep as well as a tender, grateful feeling between the partners.

Conception

During a woman's fertile period, the sperm enter the uterus through the cervix, guided by the fertile mucus. In the meantime, the egg is drawn into the entrance of the Fallopian tube. At this stage, it is surrounded by cells from the follicle which form the *corona radiata* – the 'radiant crown'. These cells are gradually washed away by secretions from the Fallopian tube until only a gelatinous outer membrane remains; this protects the egg as it awaits the arrival of the sperm. Each egg is 100 times bigger than a sperm as, within the outer membrane, it contains nutrients to nourish the *conceptus* (fertilized egg) until it comprises more than 32 cells.

Fertilization

Within about an hour, the sperm have reached the Fallopian tube. Thousands surround the egg, and the first sperm to touch the outer membrane begins to penetrate inward. The membrane immediately undergoes a change which prevents any more sperm from entering, while the successful one burrows further inward with the help of a special digestive enzyme contained within its head. It then breaches a second, thinner membrane to arrive inside the body of the egg. When it reaches the egg's central nucleus, fertilization – involving the fusion of the nuclei of the two cells – takes place, and they unite to form a single cell that is smaller than a pinpoint. From this dynamic and vital event, the first cell of your baby's body is formed.

Heredity and the determination of sex

Each new baby is a unique individual made up of a combined heritage from both mother and father. At the moment of conception, when the egg and sperm meet, the parent cells unite into a single cell and the genetic structure of the future child is determined.

This genetic material is contained in the nucleus of each cell in our bodies, in tiny, rod-like structures called *chromosomes*. All human cells, except sperm and eggs, have 23 pairs of chromosomes – i.e. 46 in all. Sperm and eggs, on the other hand, each only have a total of 23.

Each chromosome consists of tens of thousands of minute units called *genes*, which are composed of a remarkable substance known as DNA (deoxyribonucleic acid). This takes the form of the famous double helix – two spiral strands twisted round one another – and this DNA in the

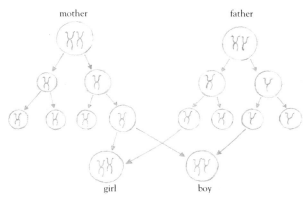

mother   father

girl   boy

The sex of your baby is determined by two of its 46 chromosomes, 23 of which come from the mother and 23 from the father. The sex chromosome of each egg is always an X (female), while a sperm contains either an X or a Y. If an X sperm fertilizes the egg the baby is a girl, if a Y sperm fertilizes it the baby is a boy.

chromosomes comprises the chemical formulae for the complete design of every cell of the new baby.

When a normal body cell (i.e. not an egg or sperm) divides, its chromosomes split so that there are two identical sets – one for each of the two newly formed cells – and this process occurs in the body millions of times every day. This ingenious mechanism ensures that the same set of genes is handed over from generation to generation of new cells in the same person. Each of us remains the same individual throughout life, although most of our body cells are continually replaced.

During conception, the process is different. As the nuclei of egg and sperm unite, the 23 chromosomes of each join up to form the 23 pairs found in the body cells. Within one hour, all the characteristics of a new human being have been decided – for example, the sex, the colour of the eyes, hair and skin, and the physical features of the face and body. In addition, the inherited constitutional tendencies to be short or tall, fat or thin, as well as ultimate longevity, health, temperament and intelligence, have all been determined for a lifetime.

A chromosome also determines the sex of the baby. In the body cells of all women, each of which contain 23 pairs of chromosomes, the sex chromosome pair is known as XX, whereas in men, it is XY. In eggs and sperm, however, there are only a total of 23 chromosomes in each. This means that, while the woman will always contribute an X chromosome, the man's sperm could contain either an X chromosome or a Y chromosome. If it is the former, the child will have an XX sex chromosome pair and will be a girl; if it is the latter, the child will be XY and, therefore, a boy. Thus, it is the male chromosome that will determine which sex the child will be.

These earliest beginnings take place deep inside your body, and the first feelings of having created a new human being are very private, unique and special. In the days and weeks that lie ahead, your awareness of the pregnancy will increase as your body changes to protect and nourish the tiny embryo growing inside it. Gradually the reality that you are to be a parent will dawn as the presence of the child you are carrying becomes more evident.

PART II
PREGNANCY

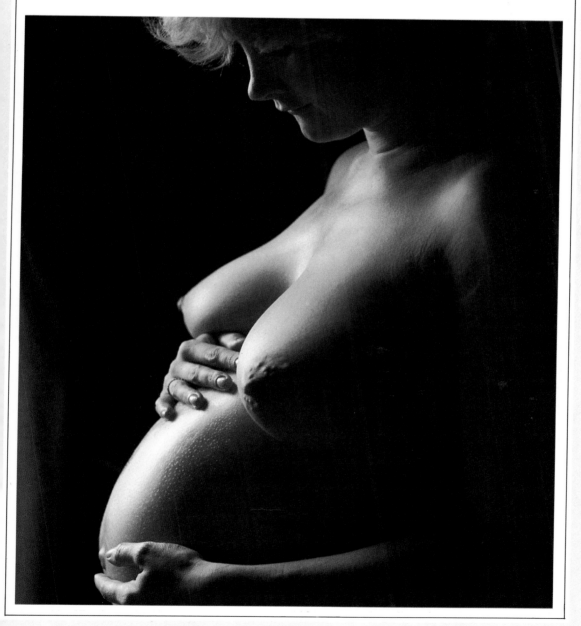

CHAPTER 2

CONFIRMING PREGNANCY

Many women are aware that they are pregnant from the moment of conception, while others may not notice for several months. The majority observe the first sign of pregnancy within two weeks after conception, when a period is missed. A few women continue to bleed slightly around the times of their periods even though conception has taken place; this bleeding may be scantier than usual and is unlikely to disturb the pregnancy. However, bleeding which continues may be a sign of a threatened miscarriage (*see* p.323). In some women, there are no marked changes at first. Others experience within days physical and emotional changes indicating pregnancy has begun. These include a missed period, maybe accompanied by breast swelling, tenderness or tingling, unusual fatigue, nausea and/or vomiting and increased or decreased appetite. The sense of taste may alter, and there are often unusual food cravings or an inability to tolerate certain foods. Emotional changes are frequent, with mood swings and intensified feelings similar to the ones that can occur before menstruation.

When you suspect you are pregnant, you may wish to go to your doctor for confirmation of the pregnancy. Alternatively, you might want to organize a test to confirm it. If this is positive, you can begin to make plans for the rest of the pregnancy, for the birth and for the first few months of caring for your baby.

Pregnancy tests

When an egg is fertilized, it starts to grow by cell division, and two parts are quickly established: the embryo itself and the placenta. After the embryo implants in the wall of the uterus, the placental cells secrete the hormone HCG – human chorionic gonadotrophin – into the woman's bloodstream and urine; this will help maintain the pregnancy by stimulating the ovary to produce oestrogen and progesterone. All pregnancy tests detect the presence or absence of HCG.

Pregnancy tests can be carried out by your doctor and health clinic, and by family planning organizations; in addition, most chemists offer a pregnancy testing service. These laboratory tests are accurate in 95 per cent of cases when done on or after the 40th day after the first day of your last period – that is, when your period is about 13 days late. There is also a newly developed blood test that can ascertain whether or not you are pregnant on the day your period is due, only 14 days after conception.

In addition, there are do-it-yourself kits, which are available from most chemists. These are not as accurate as the laboratory tests, giving the right answer in 85–90 per cent of cases.

Urine tests

There are two types of these: the slide test and the tube test. For both you will have to collect a urine sample: using a clean jar (or the container supplied to you in a kit or by your doctor), collect a small amount – a few tablespoons or so will do – of urine as you pass water first thing in the morning.

The slide test is the fastest, easiest and least expensive pregnancy test, and will be accurate for most women within two weeks of the first missed period. The tube test, also the basis of the DIY kits, may be accurate a day or two earlier.

Blood tests

Recently developed tests – called *immunoassay tests* – are supersensitive to traces of HCG in the blood or urine. They may be accurate as early as 14 days after conception – i.e. two weeks earlier than the slide or tube tests – but require a sophisticated laboratory with expensive equipment. They are useful for testing women with infertility problems or with suspected ectopic pregnancies.

The test result

This can be positive, negative or inconclusive. A positive result nearly always means that you are pregnant; a false positive is rare. A negative test may mean that you are not pregnant, but false negatives are fairly common. These may occur if a urine test is carried out at too early a stage in the pregnancy, when the amounts of HCG in the urine are too small to be measured. Even the blood test can give a false result, although this is less likely.

If you do have a negative result after having a pregnancy test and yet you still have what seem to be signs of pregnancy – or if you just simply *feel* that you are pregnant – you should consult your doctor. He or she will usually arrange for you to have another test. This is especially important if you have previously used a do-it-yourself kit, as it may have shown the wrong result.

Other tests

Pelvic examination To check and confirm the results of a pregnancy test, a pelvic examination can be done at around six weeks after the last menstrual period.

If you are pregnant, the doctor or midwife will be able to feel that the tip of the cervix has softened and may have changed from a pink to a bluish colour because of increased blood circulation. The uterus itself will feel softer and enlarged.

Ultrasound testing This is discussed in detail on pages 340-1. When this is expertly done, pregnancy can be confirmed as early as three weeks after the first missed menstrual period, or even earlier, before clinical tests are effective if the most sophisticated equipment is used. The baby's well-being can also be checked at this early stage; its heart can already be seen pumping rhythmically.

It is, however, only advisable to have an ultrasound test in early pregnancy if you have a problem such as bleeding or pain, and then only after careful consideration.

Establishing the length of pregnancy

During the nine months of pregnancy, a human being develops from a single cell to become a highly complex organism with millions of cells. At no other time in the life cycle will he or she go through such rapid growth in such a short span of time.

As soon as your pregnancy is confirmed, the time of your child's birth will be estimated. This is called the 'due date' or the 'estimated date of delivery' (EDD).

Embryologists calculate the length of pregnancy from conception onward, whereas most doctors, midwives and hospitals begin their calculations from the first day of a pregnant woman's last menstrual period. These two ways of estimating how long a pregnancy will last are simply used for convenience. In fact, the length of any pregnancy can vary considerably, just as the length of the menstrual cycle does in different women. Here, to avoid confusion, we will be using the last menstrual period for all calculations.

By this system, every woman is presumed to have a four-week menstrual cycle, and thus will have ovulated (and thus conceived) 14 days after her last period. Pregnancy lasts approximately 280 days – that is, 40 weeks (or nine months and one week) – from the first day of the last period, and 38 weeks from ovulation and conception.

To calculate your own due date, take the first day of your last period and add nine months and one week. For example, if the first day of the period was 1 January, adding nine months will give you 1 October and a further week will make your due date 8 October.

However, it is highly likely that the birth will happen at any time within approximately two weeks before or after this date. This is because the length of any pregnancy depends on the maturity of the baby (some need a shorter incubation time than others), and also on the length of a woman's menstrual cycle; those with cycles shorter than four weeks will have ovulated earlier; those with longer cycles will have ovulated later. For example:

3-week cycle: 280-day pregnancy minus 1 week = 39 weeks
4-week cycle: 280-day pregnancy   = 40 weeks
5-week cycle: 280-day pregnancy plus 1 week   = 41 weeks

Women with irregular menstrual cycles or who do not know the date of their last period may require additional help in calculating the duration of their pregnancies, for example, by pelvic examination or an ultrasound scan which are other ways of estimating a due date. The accuracy of both is highest early in pregnancy; after 20 weeks, the estimate will be very unreliable. Examination by your doctor during the first 16 weeks should be able to establish the due date within two weeks; it cannot be exactly pinpointed because of variations in the size and shape of the uterus and the size of the baby. Measuring the baby directly using ultrasound in the first 12 weeks will give a due date that is generally reliable to within one week. However, ultrasound dating should be reserved for problem pregnancies; it is unnecessary for the majority.

It is important to bear in mind, while reading the following chapters, that quite a wide variation is possible and that your own pregnancy may vary in length from the 40 weeks described.

C H A P T E R 3

YOUR PREGNANT BODY

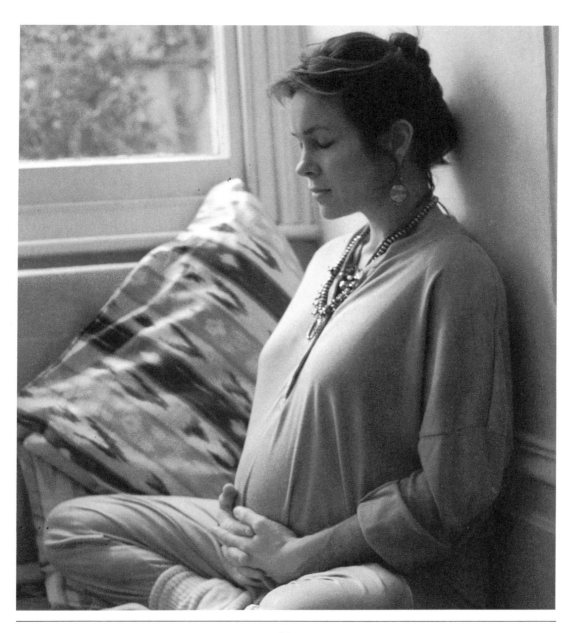

Long before the fact that you are carrying a baby becomes visibly apparent, you may become aware of the tremendous changes that are taking place within your body. From the moment the embryo implants in the wall of the womb, your body begins an amazing hormonal and physiological adaptation as it begins to fulfil its potential to nurture and produce a child.

In the first 12 weeks, the changes happen internally and may not show on the outside of your body. Then your abdomen will begin to enlarge, and soon after – somewhere between 16 and 20 weeks – the first fluttering movements of the baby will be felt. In the next few months, as your baby grows, your uterus will expand into the abdominal cavity and your pregnant belly will increase in size, and all your vital life systems will adapt to sustain the growing needs of the child within your womb.

By the last few weeks, your body will be full and majestic as both you and your baby become ready for the day of the birth.

Hormonal changes

As we have seen, hormones are chemical messengers produced by various endocrine glands (including the ovaries) and by the placenta. They act as signals which, in coordination with your nervous system, ensure the smooth functioning of all your organs. In women, hormones are also responsible for triggering all the phases of the menstrual cycle, maintaining pregnancy and regulating labour, birth and breastfeeding. Many of the physical changes that you will experience during pregnancy are caused by the secretion of various hormones.

Oestrogen and progesterone Immediately after ovulation, the corpus luteum on the ovary begins to secrete oestrogen and progesterone, and subsequently they are produced by the placenta and the foetus. The amount of each in the circulation during pregnancy is hundreds of times higher than in a non-pregnant woman.

During pregnancy, they relax the smooth muscle of the uterus, bladder, intestines and veins and thus, as we shall see later, help to adapt your body to its increased needs during pregnancy. In particular, they help the uterus to accommodate the pregnancy, as well as contributing to such common side-effects as constipation and varicose veins. They are also partly responsible for the fluid retention that is often a feature of pregnancy.

After the birth, the levels of oestrogen and progesterone in the body drop within minutes, and by the second day they are very low. This assists the return of the tissues to the pre-pregnant state, and may account for some of the mood changes which can occur after childbirth.

Relaxin This hormone is produced by the placenta, and causes the soft connective tissues and ligaments in the body to become more elastic and softer. This allows the body joints of the spine and pelvis to become flexible in preparation for the birth, and the ligaments supporting the uterus to expand during labour.

Prolactin This is the pituitary hormone that is essential for normal ovulation and for preparing the breasts for feeding. In combination with oestrogen and progesterone, it also plays an important role in stimulating the production of breastmilk. Prolactin levels rise throughout pregnancy and peak after the birth during breastfeeding.

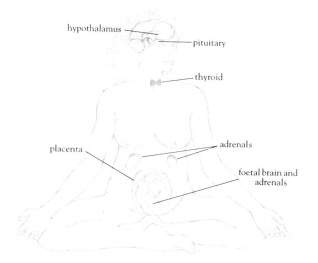

hypothalamus

pituitary

thyroid

placenta

adrenals

foetal brain and
adrenals

The hormones produced
by the endocrine glands,
as well as by the placenta
and foetus, are
responsible for
maintaining pregnancy
and regulating labour,
birth and breastfeeding.

Other hormones   Levels of *cortisone*, produced by the adrenal glands
situated above each kidney, increase during pregnancy. This is part of the
reason why allergic disorders such as asthma and eczema often improve
during pregnancy.

Adrenalin and *noradrenalin* (two adrenal hormones) and *endorphins* (a
group of brain hormones) are all part of the complex autonomic nervous
system which ensures that the involuntary functions of the body are
maintained. They alter heart rate, breathing, the working of the intestines
and the activity of the uterus, and also have important effects on mood and
the psyche.

During pregnancy, many women notice a change in their moods, and
much of this is related to variations in hormone and endorphin levels. The
adrenalin system is the body's 'fight or flight' mechanism designed to
protect us from danger. Fear and anxiety will increase the secretion of
adrenalin. On the other hand, increased adrenalin is useful in stimulating
energy and the expulsive reflex at the end of labour.

In addition to their other functions, endorphins also have a major effect
on the perception of pain and feelings of well-being – in fact, they are the
body's natural painkillers and tranquillizers. The levels of endorphins in
the body increase throughout pregnancy, reaching a peak during labour.

Fluid balance

Some of the hormones released during pregnancy affect the circulatory and
fluid systems in your body by relaxing the muscular walls of blood and
lymph vessels. This results in an enormous increase in the fluid content of
your blood and within your body tissues and cells.

In fact your body acquires an extra 7 litres (about 12 pints) of water by
the end of pregnancy, half of which is concentrated in the uterus, in the
uterine muscle, the amniotic fluid and the baby. The rest is distributed in
your bloodstream, muscles, soft tissues and organs. This essential fluid gain
performs a number of functions:

- The amniotic fluid supports and protects the baby.
- Increased blood flow to the placenta nourishes the baby.

Weight gain

Every woman should gain weight during pregnancy. This increase arises from a number of different sources:

	Approximate weight
Baby, placenta and amniotic fluid	4.5 kg (10 lb)
Increased size of uterus	1.0 kg (2¼ lb)
Increased size of breasts	0.4 kg (1 lb)
Fluid retention	3.0 kg (6⅝ lb)
Increase in fat and protein stores	3.0 kg (6⅝ lb)
Total	11.9 kg (26½ lb)

The above weights are approximate as each of the components can vary – in particular, the weight of the baby and the amount of fluid retention. However, a gain of over 15 kg (34 lb) is the upper limit of the normal range, and anything in excess of this will probably result in fat that will have to be lost after the birth (see Weight gain in pregnancy, p.346).

You can help yourself to avoid excessive weight gain by paying attention to what you eat (see Chapter 7) and by making sure that you have enough exercise. It is neither appropriate nor safe to diet to lose weight during pregnancy.

Additional fluid in the muscles and soft tissues allows them to become more pliable so that your body is more able to accommodate your growing child; this will also prepare your pelvic joints and tissues to open during labour and childbirth.

Over half of the normal weight gain in pregnancy (see left) results from this increase in body fluid. Some of this excess tends to collect in the lower parts of the body, so a certain amount of swelling – called oedema (see pp. 325-6) – in the feet, ankles and fingers is common. This is normal and no cause for concern unless it is accompanied by high blood pressure and protein in the urine (see High blood pressure and pre-eclampsia, p.315). Oedema is more likely to occur if weight gain is excessive.

Exercise, good nutrition and certain homoeopathic remedies are all helpful in reducing excessive fluid retention.

The circulatory system

The blood The volume of blood in your circulation increases during pregnancy from about 4 litres (7 pints) to 4.5 litres (7¾ pints) at 20 weeks and 5.2 litres (just over 9 pints) at 40 weeks. This ensures that there is an adequate supply for both the baby and for your own vital organs.

The increase is mainly in the fluid component of the blood, but the number of red blood cells also rises. These contain haemoglobin which carries oxygen from the lungs to all the cells of the body, thereby providing one of the essential components for life. Although the total amount of haemoglobin in your red blood cells is increased in pregnancy, the extra fluid dilutes this, and therefore the actual haemoglobin concentration in the blood drops by about 20 per cent. This is known as the *physiological anaemia of pregnancy* and is quite normal. Despite this reduction in concentration, the rise in the number of red blood cells does mean that there is an overall increase in the oxygen-carrying capacity of the blood.

One essential ingredient of haemoglobin is iron, which a foetus requires to build up its own body stores. One-third of a pregnant woman's iron reserves passes over to her baby, and this loss must be replaced by a diet containing adequate amounts of iron-containing foods (see page 99) or by iron supplements, obtainable on prescription. If your iron stores fall, there will be a decline in the amount of haemoglobin in your blood (and thus a drop in the amount of oxygen available to the body) to below 10 g per decilitre – a condition called *iron-deficiency anaemia* (see p. 292). Blood checks are made during pregnancy to determine the level of haemoglobin in your blood.

Your heart and blood vessels The heart pumps oxygenated blood rhythmically through the arteries, which carry it to all the cells in the body. In the cells, waste products are exchanged for oxygen and nutrients, and the now de-oxygenated blood flows back via the veins to the heart, where the blood is first sent to the lungs to pick up more oxygen before being sent off through the arteries to the entire body.

During pregnancy, the pumping power of your heart increases so that, at every beat, more blood is ejected into the circulation, while the actual heart rate remains about the same. This begins within weeks of the first missed period. The heart's output increases throughout pregnancy, reaching a plateau just before labour, and a peak immediately after the birth, when the placenta separates. This accounts for the breathlessness commonly found in pregnancy.

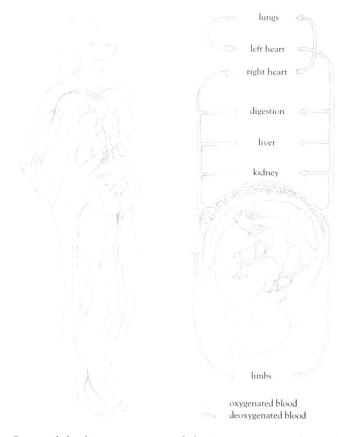

lungs

left heart

right heart

digestion

liver

kidney

limbs

oxygenated blood
deoxygenated blood

Far left: During pregnancy the growing baby and placenta act as an extra organ, requiring 25 per cent of the mother's cardiac output. The extra output is achieved by an increase in the volume of blood and by faster cycling of the blood through the mother's body. The mother's vital organs also require additional blood to meet the demands of pregnancy.

Left: This simplified diagram of the mother's circulation shows the blood supply to the placenta and uterus. This blood provides the baby with oxygen and nutrients and carries carbon dioxide and waste products back into the mother's circulation.

Some of the hormones secreted during pregnancy relax and widen the muscular walls of the blood vessels, thus ensuring that your blood circulates around your body more quickly to transport oxygen and nutrients to your baby via the placenta. Hormones also cause the valves in the larger veins to soften, possibly leading to the development of varicose veins in the legs, vulva and anus (*see* p. 344).

'Blood pressure' is the term used to describe the pressure exerted by the blood on the walls of the arteries. It remains fairly constant throughout pregnancy, except that it tends to drop somewhat in the second trimester (when the vessel walls are relaxed) and then rises back up to normal towards the end.

The largest artery in the body is the aorta, through which blood from the heart first flows, and the largest vein is the inferior vena cava, which returns blood to the heart from the lower part of the body. Both of these run along the inside of the spine, and you may find that, if you lie down in late pregnancy and during labour, the weight of your heavy uterus can cause pressure on these great blood vessels, thus reducing the blood flow to your uterus and back to your heart. This will decrease the oxygen supply to your baby and may cause your blood pressure to drop, resulting in a feeling of faintness. If you stand for prolonged periods, especially in hot weather, blood may pool in the veins of your legs, likewise causing a feeling of lightheadedness or faintness. (*See* Low blood pressure, p. 322.)

While the heart has the power to send blood to all the tissues, it does not provide energy to return it. The return of de-oxygenated blood through the veins in the lower part of the body to the heart and lungs is stimulated by breathing movements: the alternating negative and positive pressures in your chest and abdominal cavity both sucks and pushes blood up through your trunk. The muscles in your legs when you move also pump blood upwards towards the heart. This is why exercise and breathing practice help to ensure good circulation (see Part V).

Breathing

The increased blood circulation that occurs during pregnancy creates a demand for an increased oxygen flow through the lungs. Your body will automatically adapt to this with improved lung expansion, and you will probably not be aware of this as your breathing rate does not rise. As the pregnancy advances, however, you may be able to see evidence of this increased lung expansion by the flaring of your ribs to the front and sides.

Breathlessness in pregnancy is usually caused by the increased demands on the blood flow to the uterus and vital organs. In late pregnancy, this is exaggerated by the expanding uterus pressing up on the diaphragm into the chest cavity, thus decreasing the amount of lung expansion that is possible. This can cause occasional pain in the lower ribs, especially if the baby's limbs are under this area. It may help if you avoid lying on your back.

Regular practice of the deep-breathing exercises on pages 246-59 will help you to provide plenty of oxygen to your baby as well as efficiently eliminating carbon dioxide, during both pregnancy and labour.

The pelvic nerves

The genitals and pelvis are richly supplied with nerves which come from two different parts of the spinal cord.

The nerves of the body of the uterus originate in the middle section of the spine (i.e. the thoracic spine) at the back of the chest. These are involved in the transmission of sensation when the uterus contracts during the course of labour.

The nerves that supply the vagina and the external genitals stem from the sacral area at the bottom of the spinal cord. They come into action in the second stage of labour.

The digestive tract

As we have seen, the hormones released by the placenta have the effect of relaxing muscle all over the body. This is also true of the smooth muscle which forms part of the wall of the digestive tract, from the oesophagus (gullet), through the stomach and the small and large intestines to the rectum. Because of this, muscle tone is reduced, and activity along its entire length is slowed down.

This lessened activity means that the stomach tends to empty more slowly, causing you to feel full a relatively long time after you have eaten. In addition, the muscular valve at the entrance to the stomach may also relax so that acid may leak back up into the oesophagus, causing a burning sensation just behind the breastbone, which is commonly known as heartburn (see p. 314).

The slower emptying of the large intestine (large bowel) may be a cause of constipation (see p. 303), which may result from the increased pressure

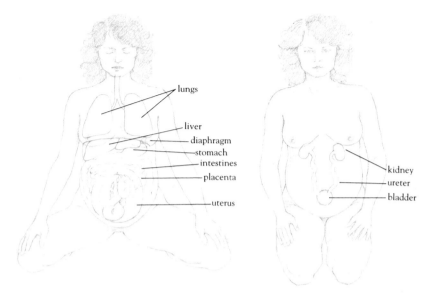

lungs
liver
diaphragm
stomach
intestines
placenta
uterus

kidney
ureter
bladder

The lungs, digestive and urinary systems in pregnancy. As the uterus expands it presses the intestines and other abdominal organs up against the diaphragm into the chest cavity. The increased demands for oxygen cause the lungs to expand and as a result the ribs flare out. The rise in kidney blood flow causes an increase in urine production, as more water is filtered out of the blood, and the ureters which transport the urine to the bladder become dilated and slightly convoluted.

on the bowel from the uterus. An altered diet and iron supplements can cause stools to become hard, making them more difficult to pass.

The nausea and vomiting of early pregnancy – commonly called 'morning sickness' even though it may occur at any time of day – is a phenomenon that only some women experience (*see* Vomiting in pregnancy, p 345). It may be the earliest sign of pregnancy, and certainly a change in food tastes (*see* p. 97) and appetite may occur as early as your first missed period.

The urinary system

The kidneys are responsible for filtering fluid waste products from the blood, to be excreted as urine from the body. During pregnancy, they handle an increased load derived both from the baby who excretes via the placenta into your blood and also from the increased activity of your own organs and tissues. However, because of the increase in the flow of blood through your kidneys, their function is much improved and they can cope.

This rise in kidney blood flow causes an increase in urine production. You will therefore have to pass urine more frequently, an effect accentuated in early pregnancy by the pressure of the enlarging uterus on the base of the bladder. When the uterus rises out of your pelvis into the abdomen at around 12 weeks, the bladder pressure is reduced until, at 34 weeks, your baby's head begins to press on it. In addition, in late pregnancy, fluid that has accumulated in your tissues during the day is absorbed into your bloodstream when you are in bed asleep and causes a rise in urine output at night. Urinary frequency that is combined with a burning sensation may be caused by an infection (*see* Urinary tract and kidney problems in the mother, p. 342).

The increased kidney function during pregnancy often allows small amounts of glucose to spill into the urine. This may not be a sign of diabetes (*see* p. 307), which is associated with high glucose levels in the blood. However, if sugar is detected in your urine, you may need to have a blood test to make sure that diabetes is not the cause.

The growth of the uterus during pregnancy causes the dynamics of the spine to change, to compensate for the altered centre of gravity caused by the extra weight.

non-pregnant

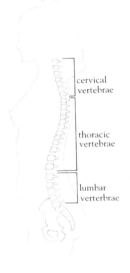

cervical vertebrae

thoracic vertebrae

lumbar verterbrae

pregnant

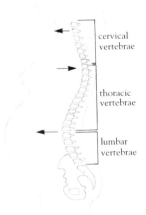

cervical vertebrae

thoracic vertebrae

lumbar vertebrae

Besides an increase in the frequency of urination, some women experience a degree of urinary incontinence (*see* p. 341), especially when coughing, sneezing or laughing. The cause of this is usually hormonal, due to the softening of the muscles of the bladder walls and of the urethra (the tube that carries urine from the bladder to the outside), and it will usually stop after the birth.

The genitals

Hormone secretion will also affect the genital area. The labia tend to soften and become fuller, and they are often more sensitive. The increased blood flow to the pelvis may cause the veins in the labia to become distended (*see* Varicose veins, p. 344).

The clitoris, too, frequently becomes more sensitive, and tight trousers and underpants should be avoided. Some pregnant women find that, because of this increased sensitivity, they are happier with a less direct contact of the clitoris during love-making.

There is also an increased discharge from the vagina, caused by the heightened activity of the glands inside the cervix. This discharge, which is quite normal, is usually watery, whitish or pale yellow in colour, and its odour may change, although it should not be offensive.

If the discharge becomes profuse, turns thick and white or frothy and greenish and is accompanied by itching or irritation, vaginal infection may be present (*see* pp. 343-4). Because the acidity of the vaginal fluids often changes during pregnancy, you may become more susceptible to thrush.

The skeleton

The bony skeleton forms the supporting framework of your body, and is firmly held together at the joints by strong elastic ligaments. The whole structure of some 206 bones is supported, moved and returned to alignment by the muscles.

Structurally, a woman's body is ideally designed to accommodate and give birth to a child. Compared to a man's, your pelvic bones are lighter and smoother, with a wider outlet to the more rounded pelvic canal and a wider pubic arch to allow for the passage of a baby. In addition, the hormones secreted during pregnancy soften and stretch the ligaments holding the joints together; this allows the pelvis to expand and become more flexible and the body as a whole to adapt to the changing needs of your growing baby.

The spine This is the central support for the whole of your upper body, and during pregnancy, when you have to carry an extra 9 kg (20 lb) in weight, it plays a vital role by also supporting your uterus its contents.

The spine is made up of 24 bones called *vertebrae*: seven in the neck (the cervical spine), 12 in the chest (the thoracic spine) and five behind the abdomen (the lumbar spine). At its base, the vertebrae are fused to form the strong, wedge-shaped sacrum, which forms the back wall of the pelvis, and the spine ends in the tailbone, or coccyx. The weight of your upper body is transmitted through the sacrum to the hip joints and then down to the legs.

Each vertebra is linked to the next by a flat disc of fibrous tissue and cartilage. These *intervertebral discs* are spongy, enabling the spine to bend and twist, and also acting as shock absorbers to cushion the vertebrae against the jarring effects of walking or jumping. When you stand up, your body weight exerts pressure on the discs, causing a degree of compression.

Your spinal column also performs the important task of enclosing your spinal cord and protecting it from injury. Nerve branches from the cord, which make their way through openings in the vertebrae, are essential for the normal function of muscles and organs. If your spine is twisted or out of balance, pressure on the nerve branches often leads to pain and abnormal functioning of organs and muscles supplied by these nerves.

Good posture depends on the correct balance of spinal curves – forward at the neck to take the weight of the head, and backward at the chest and forward at the lumbar spine to counterbalance the weight of the chest and abdominal organs. In pregnancy, the effects of hormones allows the joints of the pelvis to expand in readiness for the birth, which causes the lumbar spine to curve forward more, thus reducing tension in your pelvic floor. This counterbalances the extra weight of the uterus. While your spinal curves will change during pregnancy, the spine's ability to counterbalance its extra load will ensure that its dynamics and functions are maintained. If your spine is off balance before pregnancy, it is likely that, without well-chosen exercise, there will be stress at the junctions of the spinal curves, causing pain in the sacrum, lower back, neck or head (*see* Back and pelvic pain, p. 327).

The pelvis In early pregnancy, your baby is protected and cradled within the bony framework of your pelvis. Later, as your growing uterus extends upwards into the abdominal cavity, your pelvis supports and holds its contents from underneath, like a bony basin.

Your pelvis is made up of four bones: the sacrum and coccyx which form the back wall and are wedged between two hip bones. Each of the latter are divided into three parts at birth – the iliac (flank or side), pelvic (groin) and ischial (buttock) bones – which become fused at puberty. The whole pelvis forms a circular girdle, shaped like a funnel, which surrounds the curved birth canal, through which your baby will pass. The entrance of the birth canal from above is known as the *pelvic inlet*, and the exit at the bottom is the *pelvic outlet*. Your pelvis is tilted forward during pregnancy so that the brim slopes downward and your baby's weight is thrown forward towards your abdominal wall, and thus pressure on the pelvic muscles is reduced.

Before giving birth, it is vital to understand the structure of your pelvic framework and how it functions, and this is described in detail on pages 136–7. You will also be greatly helped in this if you feel the various parts from the outside.

Pelvic joints and ligaments Your pelvis has four main joints which are bound together by ligaments made of tough, flexible fibrous tissue. Normally, the latter allow the joints to move only within a limited range, but this range increases during pregnancy as, through hormonal secretion, the ligaments become softened. This softening and the consequent increased flexibility of the joints plays a very important role in labour (*see* p. 136). It also may be a cause of discomfort in pregnancy (*see* Back and pelvic pain, p. 327).

Ligaments also bridge the side walls of the pelvis, thus strengthening your pelvic floor.

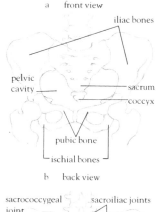

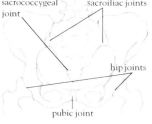

Front and back views of the female pelvis, showing the bones (a) and joints (b).

The ligaments of the pelvis.

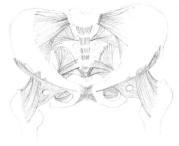

The pelvic floor muscles.

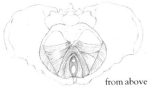

from above

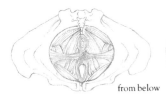

from below

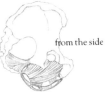

from the side

Your muscles

Your body contains mainly two types of muscles: *voluntary* muscles and *involuntary* (or *smooth*) muscles. The skeletal muscles – that is, those which are involved in the movement of our bones at the joints – are voluntary muscles because they are under our conscious control. However, the muscles that comprise all or part of the uterus, stomach, intestines and other organs are involuntary as we cannot make them do what we want – for example, we cannot consciously stimulate the uterus to contract: it contracts when stimulated by certain hormones secreted by both mother and baby (*see* p.135).

The pelvic muscles There are about 36 pairs of muscles attached to your pelvis, and in fact, most of the large and powerful muscles in your body meet there. They run up to your neck and head, down through your thighs, all round and through the abdominal wall, and enclose the pelvic outlet. Such natural positions for birth as kneeling and squatting involve almost all of your pelvic muscles.

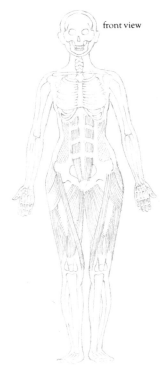

front view

The pelvic-floor muscles Your pelvic floor consists of a layer of muscle and fibrous tissue which extends across the base of the pelvis, from the lower rim of the pubic arch in front to the sacrum behind. It is a complicated structure, comprising two *levator ani* muscles which stretch from each side wall of the pelvis and meet at the midline, thus forming a hammock or sling across the pelvic outlet. They are perforated in front by the urethra, at the back by the anus and at the midpoint by the vagina.

During the second stage of labour, the levator ani muscles relax to aid the birth of the baby. As the head passes through, they are pressed against the pelvic side walls, but they return to normal soon afterwards.

Below the pelvic floor, the entrance to the vagina is surrounded by muscles which meet at a point between the vaginal opening and the anus, in an area called the perineum. These muscles help to keep the openings of the vagina, urethra and anus closed during normal activity.

The muscles of both your pelvic floor and your perineum relax when you squat. To locate them, squat and contract the pelvic floor as if you are trying to stop urinating in midstream (*see* exercise 9, p. 253).

The abdominal muscles There are several layers of muscles which encircle the abdomen, all of which protect your vital organs as well as move your abdomen during breathing and walking. During pregnancy, they expand to accommodate the enlarging uterus, and are essential in the second stage of labour in assisting the birth of the baby as you bear down.

The strap muscles, which run from the pubic bone to the breastbone on either side of your navel, are often stretched sideways during pregnancy, but they will come together again after the birth.

Your breasts

The first changes to be noticed at the beginning of pregnancy are often in the breasts, which may become fuller and feel warm, heavy, tender and sensitive to the touch almost as soon as conception occurs; they may also throb, tingle or hurt. The nipples may become larger and more sensitive, and the skin around each nipple – the *areola* – may become darker, particularly if you are already dark-skinned. Around the areolae, you may notice the appearance of little raised glands called *Montgomery's tubercles*: these secrete natural oils which keep the nipples soft and supple in readiness for breastfeeding. In addition, the increased blood supply to the breasts causes the veins in them to become more prominent; this will subside after breastfeeding or earlier. Stretch marks (described on the following page) may also develop.

By about the 20th week of pregnancy, your breasts will probably have become much larger; indeed, the increase in size – due to the increase in the number of milk-producing cells and milk ducts – can be quite dramatic. It is now important to buy a good cotton bra for adequate support, even if you do not usually wear one.

Towards the end of pregnancy, your breasts may begin to produce a thin amber or yellowish fluid called *colostrum*, which will be the first food for your baby. However, some women do not have any sign of colostrum until after the birth, so do not worry if you do not notice any. Also about this time, your nipples may become even more sensitive, in readiness for the stimulation of the baby's sucking after the birth.

Your breasts will benefit from being exposed to fresh air and moderate sunshine – taking care not to burn them. You may enjoy spending some time each day with your breasts bare in the privacy of your home, and sometimes going without a bra.

If you are planning to breastfeed your baby, your midwife or doctor will check your nipples and will also give you advice on how to prepare for breastfeeding during these months of anticipation. All this is covered fully on pages 189–205.

Breast changes are usually more dramatic with a first pregnancy than with subsequent ones.

Your skin and hair

In terms of surface area, the skin is the largest organ in your body. During pregnancy, the amount of blood flowing to it increases sixfold in the arms and slightly less in the legs. This increased flow is brought about by the dilating (widening) of the arterioles and capillaries – the tiny blood vessels which join the arteries to the veins – and is the body's way of maintaining a regular internal temperature.

The heat carried by the blood to the skin will cause your limbs to feel warm, and you may find that you are more comfortable in lower temperatures than you were before. In addition, you may also find that you are sweating more – another way that the body regulates temperature as well as eliminating waste products.

A pregnant woman's skin is usually radiant and glowing, with a healthy tone. Some of the extra fluid retained by the body during pregnancy is present in the subcutaneous tissues beneath the skin, giving it an extra fullness. Because of this, the face will often appear rounder, fuller and more glowing than before; your limbs may also become fuller.

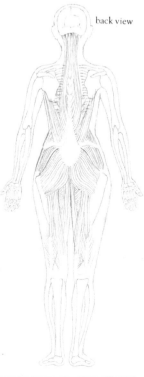

Facing page and below: The muscles which are attached to the pelvis.

back view

Occasionally, red spots appear on the face, torso, arms and palms; these are caused by the increased flow of blood through the dilated blood vessels, and will disappear after pregnancy. Pregnant women sometimes have flushed cheeks, also an effect of the increased blood flow to the skin. Women prone to acne may notice an increase during pregnancy.

Changes in skin pigmentation These are common in pregnancy and are probably brought about by increased production of the *melanocyte-stimulating hormone* (MSH). This is secreted by the pituitary gland and acts on the melanocytes – the cells in the skin which produce melanin (skin pigment).

Pigmentation changes are most commonly noticed in the darkening of the nipples and areolae of the breasts; a brown line – called the *linea nigra* – may also appear down the centre of the abdomen around the third month. Birthmarks, moles and freckles may all temporarily darken, and the latter two may increase in number and size. Occasionally the face becomes darker, giving the impression of a sun tan, particularly around the mouth. This is called *chloasma* or the 'mask of pregnancy'. These pigmentation changes tend to fade or disappear after pregnancy.

Stretch marks These often appear as reddish streaks on the breasts in early pregnancy, and are also common on the abdomen as it grows and the skin stretches in late pregnancy. They will fade and become silvery white after the birth. Stretch marks are more likely if a woman is overweight, and are more common in those with delicate skin.

It is uncertain whether there is anything you can do to avoid stretch marks except not to gain too much weight, but it is thought that stretching exercises and daily massage with oil to keep the skin supple, combined with a good diet, are helpful (*see* Part V and Chapter 7). Once stretch marks have appeared, applying vitamin E oil may help to reduce scarring.

Dry skin, rashes and itching The appearance of unexpected rashes, dryness and itching with no obvious explanation is common in pregnancy, and may be caused by allergies to certain foods or soaps. If these persist or worsen, see your doctor. (*See* Skin changes in pregnancy, p. 335.)

Your hair This usually does not change very much during pregnancy, although in a few women it darkens. Because of this, facial, arm and leg hair may become more obvious, but it will return to normal after the birth. The dryness of the scalp or the greasiness of hair varies enormously, but in general, dry scalps tend to be drier and greasy hair tends to be greasier.

During pregnancy, hair growth often slows down and the hair is finer. The latter results in more hair coming out on brushing, but this effect is reversed after the birth. After your child is born, you may find that a lot of your hair falls out, but new hair will soon grow to replace this – pregnancy never causes baldness.

The mouth, nose and eyes
The mouth The increased blood flow of pregnancy can cause the gums to swell, and they may bleed easily when you brush your teeth. It is important to pay attention to dental hygiene as such swelling may cause food to become trapped between tooth and gum, resulting in the latter becoming

inflamed. This can be minimized by a high-fibre, raw food diet as well as careful brushing. A visit to the dentist when you are pregnant is worthwhile, and all treatment will be free. If you need a filling, the local anaesthetics used by dentists are perfectly safe.

Salivating profusely is a rare and unusual phenomenon in pregnancy, and is caused by hormonal changes. It will cease after the birth of the baby.

Pregnant women often mention a change of taste in the mouth and a slightly metallic taste on the tongue. In fact, the appetite and enjoyment of certain foods can change considerably during this time, and the food cravings of pregnancy (see p. 97) are partly related to changes in the taste sensations of the tongue.

The nose and sinuses The mucous lining of the nose and sinuses is also sensitive to the effects of pregnancy. There may be an increase in the production of mucus by the nose and often swelling of the lining of the nose and sinuses. Nasal stuffiness may occur very early in a pregnancy in some women – even before the first missed period. Unfortunately, this stuffiness and nasal blockage is difficult to remedy during pregnancy, and colds and sinusitis often take longer to clear (see Colds, coughs and other respiratory infections in pregnancy, p. 301).

The eyes The lens of the eye may absorb extra fluid during pregnancy, which may slightly alter vision. This effect is not permanent, and you need not invest in a new pair of glasses. In a minority, the cornea – the transparent covering of the eyes – may also swell, and if you wear contact lenses, you may have to put them away and wear glasses for the duration of your pregnancy.

Energy and sleep

Pregnancy is a state of positive health, when your body tends towards strength and vitality. During this time, it is important to listen to the signals coming from your body and to go with them rather than against them. You will also find that physical exercise during the day will actually boost your energy and help you to sleep restfully (see Part V), and that careful attention to your eating patterns and nutrition will improve your feelings of physical well-being (see Chapter 7).

While many women feel energized throughout pregnancy, with an increased level of vitality, it is common to feel unusually drained and fatigued during the first 12 weeks or so and to need more rest during the day and more sleep at night. This tiredness is usually caused by the new demands pregnancy is making on your system, and it will be accentuated if your eating habits are disrupted by nausea or if you were not physically fit prior to conception.

During mid-pregnancy, most women find that they are full of energy, although they may still need more sleep and may require a rest during the day. However, any anxiety that you may feel about being pregnant and/or about the coming birth will reduce your energy, and it may also cost you sleepless nights.

In the last weeks, your baby will become heavier, and although your physical strength increases progressively, you will need longer periods of rest. It is, however, essential that you use your body and continue to exercise.

Getting a good night's sleep In the first 12 weeks, while your body is becoming accustomed to the hormonal changes occurring in it, your sleep may not be as refreshing as previously. You may also have to pass urine during the night.

In late pregnancy, it may be difficult to find a comfortable position for sleep: if you normally sleep on your front, the baby will be in the way; pressure on your bladder may wake you; and you may even need to prop yourself up to reduce heartburn. In addition, throughout mid- and late pregnancy, you may be kept awake as the baby continues to move.

As irritating as the inability to get to sleep may seem at the time, it may actually have a purpose: some have suggested that it is a sort of rehearsal, designed to prepare you for interrupted sleep after your baby is born. In any event, as long as you can get plenty of rest, it does not matter if you sleep somewhat less than usual. (*See also* Tiredness and insomnia, p. 338).

C H A P T E R   4

THE BABY IN THE WOMB

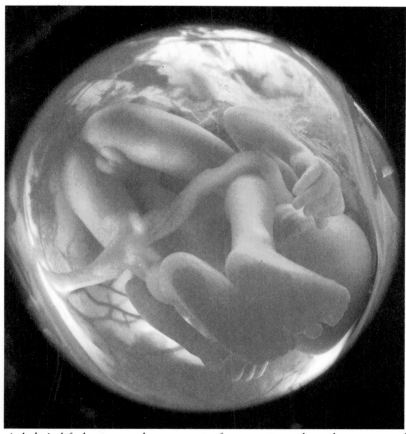

This five-month old baby girl floats inside the womb in the bag of amniotic fluid. She is fully developed but not yet fully grown.

A baby's life begins at the moment of conception when the ovum and sperm fuse to form the first cell of the embryo. During the 40 weeks of pregnancy (counted from the first day of the last menstrual period), growth is greater than at any other time in the life cycle. Even before there is any outward sign of pregnancy, vital changes are taking place in your body. During the embryonic period – that is, the first eight weeks after conception – the baby develops from a single cell into an infinitely more complex organism, in which the limbs, skeleton and all the major organs including the brain and nervous system are formed. During the remaining 30 weeks of pregnancy – the foetal period – the baby will grow and the brain and other organs of his developing body will mature in readiness for the great moment of birth. This odyssey is depicted on the next eight pages.

H O W   Y O U R   B A B Y   G R O W S · 1

The first month

Week 2 After fertilization has taken place (about two weeks after the first day of the last period), the single cell divides in two, these two divide again, and in this way the cells multiply and form a cluster known as a morula (Latin for mulberry). While this is happening, the rapidly multiplying cells are still contained within the gelatinous outer membrane of the original egg which is wafted along the Fallopian tube towards the uterus. By the time it reaches the uterus, after about four days, the morula develops a hollow centre filled with fluid and it is then called a blastocyst. This growing cell cluster floats for another two or three days in the nourishing uterine fluid.

Week 3 About seven days after conception the cell cluster loses its outer membrane and is ready for direct contact with the uterus. By now it has increased to about 150 cells which differentiate and arrange themselves into two portions: the inner cells will form the baby and the outer cells the placenta and amniotic sac.

Implantation The blastocyst lands on the spongy endometrium, whose secretions contain nutrients and oxygen, and the placental cells produce tiny

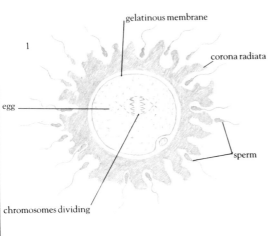

1

gelatinous membrane

corona radiata

egg

sperm

chromosomes dividing

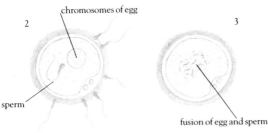

2

chromosomes of egg

sperm

3

fusion of egg and sperm

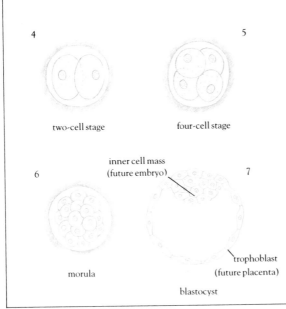

4

two-cell stage

5

four-cell stage

6

inner cell mass
(future embryo)

7

morula

trophoblast
(future placenta)

blastocyst

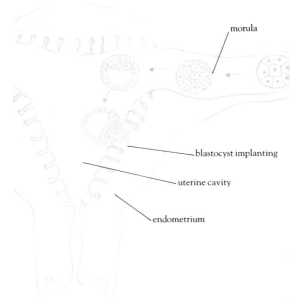

morula

blastocyst implanting

uterine cavity

endometrium

root-like projections called villi. These penetrate the endometrium and invade the uterine blood vessels to reach your bloodstream, where they draw nourishment for the developing embryo. The outer surfaces of the villi are bathed in maternal blood carrying molecules of oxygen, protein, sugars, minerals, vitamins and other substances. The villi absorb these substances like the roots of a plant, the molecules passing through their thin walls into the bloodstream of the embryo. The villi mature to form the placenta later in the pregnancy, and by means of this vital connection the foetus receives all the nourishment he needs until birth.

Week 4 The cluster of cells is firmly implanted in the uterine wall where it continues to grow rapidly; a tiny embryo now evolves, having completed the most hazardous journey of a lifetime.

How you feel Your period is now due and you may already feel different from usual. There may be premenstrual symptoms such as full or tender breasts, fullness in the lower abdomen and lower energy levels, but no period arrives. As the days pass you may suspect that you are pregnant, and you may notice changes in your appetite and dislike of or preferences for certain foods; in some women nausea and occasionally vomiting can begin at about this time. Heightened emotional sensitivity is common.

The second month
Week 5 By the end of the fifth week the embryo is 2mm (³⁄₃₂in) long and beginning to take shape. The inner cluster of cells forms a flat disc consisting of three layers. The outer layer gives rise to the skin, nervous system, ears and eyes; the middle layer will form the muscles, skeleton, heart, kidneys and genital organs; and the inner layer forms the intestinal tract and digestive system, lungs and bladder. At this stage the embryo already has the beginnings of a nervous system, the heart begins to beat and blood vessels connect it to the placenta via the umbilical cord.

Weeks 6-8 The flat inner cell mass expands rapidly and begins to bend and curl; the head and tail curve towards each other because the back is bent, and the embryo goes through phases resembling the stages of evolution. First it looks like a tadpole, then passes through a fish-like stage to become a primitive mammal and finally a tiny human being. Rudimentary eyes, ears, a mouth and limb buds appear. At eight weeks the embryo measures 13mm (½in) long, and it lies enclosed in the membranes which already contain amniotic fluid. It is now 10,000 times larger than the fertilized cell from which it originated 42 days earlier.

How you feel The extra demands on your circulation may cause breathlessness, increased kidney flow and more frequent urination. The placental hormones affect the digestive system and may lead to nausea or constipation. The demands of the pregnancy and a reduction in appetite may sap your energy, causing extreme fatigue.

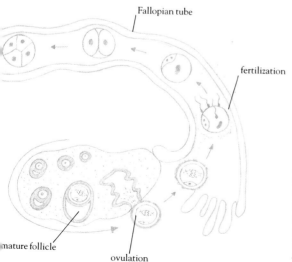

Fallopian tube

fertilization

mature follicle

ovulation

Far left: Fertilization.
1. The egg is about to be fertilized.
2. A sperm has entered the egg.
3. The male and female chromosomes are fusing.
4, 5. Early cell divisions.
6. The cell cluster multiplies and forms a morula.
7. The morula has developed a hollow centre filled with fluid, and is now a blastocyst.

Left: In the week after ovulation, the fertilized egg, growing by cell division, is wafted along the Fallopian tube and into the womb. Here it loses its outer membrane and implants in the endometrium.

HOW YOUR BABY GROWS · 2

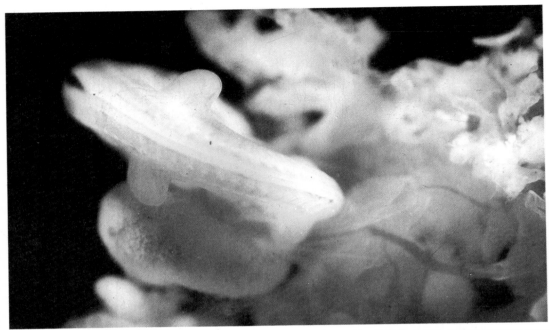

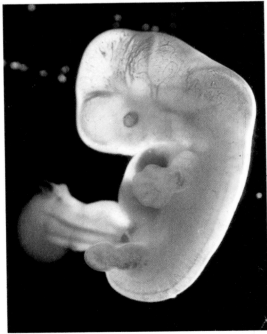

Above: In the fifth week of pregnancy the neural tube, which will become the baby's brain and spinal cord, begins to form.

Right: By the second month, the embryo has a head, trunk and 'tail'. The eyes can be clearly seen, and the hands and feet have ridges which will become fingers and toes.

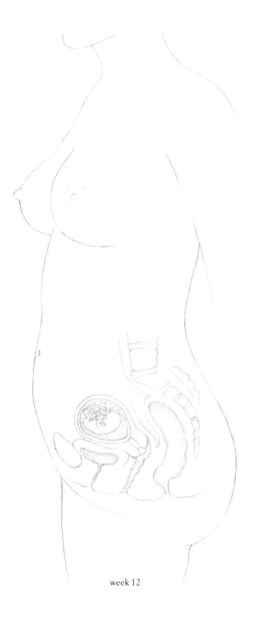

week 12

The third month

Weeks 9-10 As the second period is missed, the embryo's face is developing more distinct features, the trunk elongates and becomes straighter, and the embryonic tail shortens and disappears. By the tenth week the embryonic period has ended. The baby's human characteristics are now obvious, the fingers and toes are visible, and the kidneys produce urine. At ten weeks it is 2.5 cm (1 in) long and weighs 8 g (¼ oz).

Weeks 11-14 As the foetal period begins growth is rapid, and the placenta develops a rich network of blood vessels to support the increasing need for nourishment. The head is the largest part of the body and development is from the head downwards. Although the organs have formed, the foetus cannot survive outside your uterus until they have matured, a process which continues during the rest of the pregnancy. By the end of the third month the face has assumed a baby's profile with a large forehead, tiny snub nose and a definite chin. As the muscles and nervous system mature, movements become more active and co-ordinated. The lips move, the forehead wrinkles and the head turns: all these movements are part of the sucking reflex. Swallowing and breathing reflexes are also present. The placenta, which initially surrounded the embryo and amniotic sac completely, now occupies one area of the uterus, and the membrances of the amniotic sac cover the rest of the cavity. The baby now measures about 12 cm (4¾ in) long and weighs 110g (4 oz).

How you feel By the end of the third month the uterus has emerged from the pelvic cavity into the abdomen, and may be felt above the pelvic bone. Any nausea, vomiting or tiredness should diminish, but you may find that food preferences remain.

HOW YOUR BABY GROWS · 3

The fourth month

Weeks 15-18 The baby continues to grow rapidly
and floats in the amniotic fluid, of which there is
about 180 ml (6 fl. oz) at 16 weeks. The fingernails
develop, the eyes, ears and nose are well formed,
and the skeleton hardens and becomes more bony.
The reproductive organs continue to develop, and
the penis or vagina is easily identified. The range of
movements he can make become more intricate: he
is capable of grasping the cord, sucking his fingers
and making complex facial expressions. The
breathing reflex is well established: from now on the
baby will inhale and exhale amniotic fluid. The tiny
air sacs in the lungs are not expanded, and your baby
obtains oxygen and nutrients from your bloodstream
via the placenta. The baby also rehearses the
functions of digestion and excretion by swallowing
the amniotic fluid and passing it out through his
bladder. Taste buds are present on the tongue. By 18
weeks the baby measures about 19 cm (7½ in) long
and weighs approximately 170 g (6 oz).

How you feel During mid-pregnancy – months
four, five and six – you will probably find that the
tiredness and low energy have disappeared, and that
you have become accustomed to being pregnant. At
this time women often feel very well, their skin and
hair glow and they feel relaxed and strong as the
ligaments and muscles become more supple. This is
a good time to exercise, and to enjoy daily yoga and
deep breathing. A relaxing holiday can also be
enjoyable, as you should feel secure in the pregnancy
but not too large to be uncomfortable.

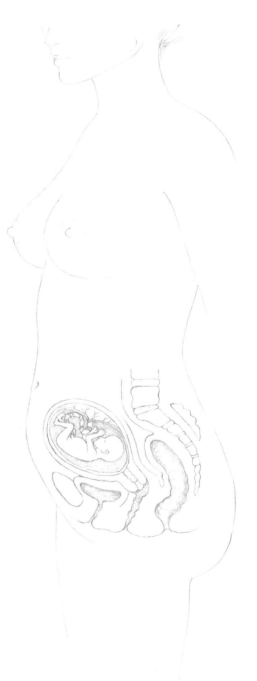

week 16

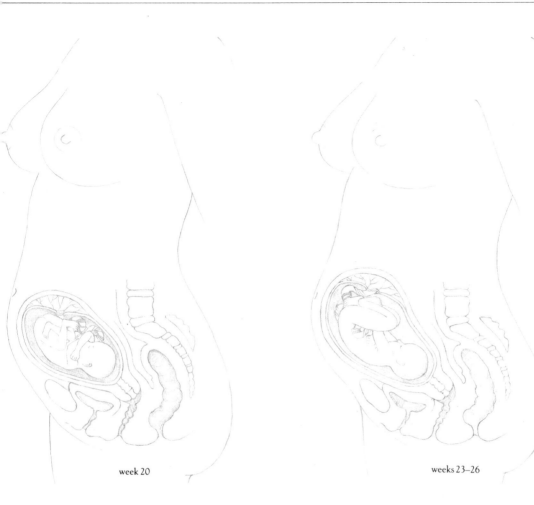

week 20

weeks 23–26

The fifth month

Weeks 19-22 Some time between the 18th and 20th week in a first pregnancy, or earlier in subsequent pregnancies, you will feel the first definite movements of your baby. The baby's skin is now covered with vernix; fine downy hair (called lanugo) covers the body; and brown fat, a source of energy in the newborn, is laid down. Hearing is acute, but the eyelids are still fused closed. The baby is about 25.5 cm (10 in) long and weighs about 340 g (12 oz).

How you feel Most women enjoy this month. Dreams may be more vivid than usual, and heightened emotional sensitivity may bring unexpected feelings to the surface. Minor discomforts of pregnancy such as back pain, cramps or varicose veins may arise.

The sixth month

Weeks 23-26 The baby's muscles and organs grow rapidly, and the cells in the cortex of the brain involved in conscious thought mature from now on. The cycle of waking and sleeping is well established, with dreaming (REM)sleep predominating. Finger- and toenails are present and reflexive movements increase. A baby born prematurely after the 26th week may survive. He is about 33 cm (13 in) long and weighs 500 g (1¼ lb).

How you feel You may feel well and full of energy and enthusiasm. You may also feel more pressure from the increasing size and weight of the uterus, and the baby may press against your bladder, causing more frequent urination. Sufficient rest and exercise and a good diet are particularly important from now on.

HOW YOUR BABY GROWS·

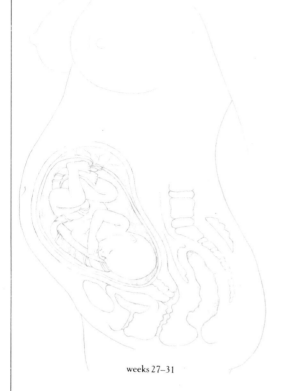

weeks 27–31

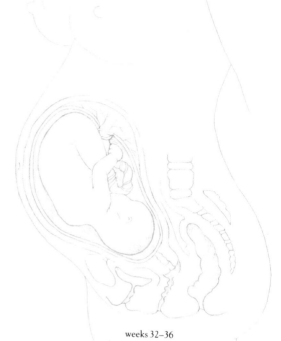

weeks 32–36

The seventh month

Weeks 27-31 The baby's eyelids open and eyelashes are present. Rhythms of moving, breathing and swallowing are well established, and the ability to orient the body in space is well developed. The amniotic sac contains up to 750 ml (26 fl. oz) of fluid, which allows the baby to move freely. At about 28 weeks the baby measures 38 cm (14 in) long and weighs about 900 g (2 lb); by week 32 he is 42 cm (16 in) long and may weigh 1800 g (4 lb).

How you feel This is the beginning of the last three months of pregnancy, and your uterus is now midway between your navel and your ribs. You will feel a variety of movements as your baby kicks and rolls from side to side. Stronger kicks may be felt under your ribs, and you may sometimes be aware of rhythmic hiccups occurring every three or four seconds. These movements may be more obvious when you are resting.

The eighth month

Weeks 32-36 The fingernails now reach the fingertips. In boys, the testicles begin to descend into the scrotum. The endocrine system is very active in preparation for birth, and the lungs secrete surfactant, a soapy fluid that keeps them open ready for breathing. Fat is deposited under the skin to provide energy and aid heat regulation after birth. Weight increases by about 200 g (7 oz) per week, and most babies now assume a head-down position. The baby responds to your moods and emotions through the hormones released by your body which pass to him via the placenta. The majority of babies born at this time survive.

How you feel The uterus almost fills the abdominal cavity, reaching to just below your ribs. Practice contractions, when the uterus hardens and then relaxes, become stronger and more noticeable. You may feel your uterus 'drop' if your baby's head engages in the pelvis, and this will make breathing easier. Pressure on your stomach from the heavy uterus may cause heartburn, especially when you lie flat. Your pelvis expands, and some discomfort in the joints at the back of the pelvis or in the pubic joint is common.

The ninth month

Weeks 37-40 The baby is now larger and roll-over movements are less frequent. The body is plump, there is progressive organization of brain activity, and consciousness is well established. Eye movements are well co-ordinated and vision improves. In the last two weeks, movements may slow down, growth rate declines to 100 g (3½ oz) a week and the placenta stops enlarging but continues to function. The baby is used to being hugged by the contracting uterus. His chest is prominent, more fat is laid down and the limbs are strong. Some 80 per cent of babies are born within ten days of day 280. The average full-term baby is about 55 cm (20 in) long and weighs 3300g (7¼ lb).

How you feel The ligaments of the pelvis reach maximum softness, allowing the pelvic and sacroiliac joints to expand. You feel your energy centring on your body and your baby as you become quieter and more meditative. You may have a strong 'nesting' instinct – a desire to prepare your home for the baby's arrival. The uterus extends up to your ribs until the head engages, and continues to contract. The cervix ripens (softens) and effaces (thins), and its mucous plug which has sealed off the uterus may be dislodged, resulting in a 'show' which may be tinged with blood. The membranes of the amniotic sac may break ('breaking of the waters') prior to the onset of labour. As birth approaches, uterine activity increases until the practice contractions merge into true labour. Your breasts may already produce colostrum.

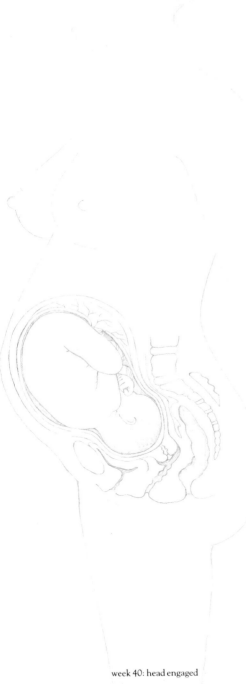

week 40: head engaged

The primal environment

In early pregnancy the placenta surrounds the embryo and blood circulates via the umbilical cord.

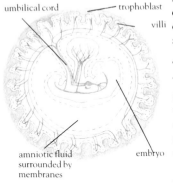

amniotic fluid surrounded by membranes

As your baby develops, the womb expands to accommodate his growing body. The baby is connected by the umbilical cord to the placenta, a remarkable organ attached to the inner lining of the uterus, which breathes, digests and excretes for the baby. The amniotic sac – sometimes called the 'membranes' – lines the interior of the womb and surrounds and contains the baby. Within it, he floats in a clear, colourless liquid known as the amniotic fluid.

The placenta and umbilical cord

The placenta is first formed by the cells of the trophoblast, which burrow into the endometrial lining of the uterus, and form little 'fingers' called *villi* which implant in the uterine wall. In early pregnancy, this placental tissue completely surrounds the baby and the amniotic sac, but eventually some of the villi disappear and the remainder become concentrated in one circular-shaped area on the wall of the uterus to form the placenta.

The core of each of the villi contains a network of very fine blood vessels which are held together by jelly-like connective tissue and enclosed within a fine membrane on which are situated placental cells. The latter pierce the walls of the blood vessels in the uterine wall, and are bathed in the pool of maternal blood that is constantly flowing past them. All nutrients and oxygen for the baby pass through or between the placental cells and those which make up the membrane, and in this way the mother's and the baby's blood are kept separate.

The primary function of the placenta is to provide the means by which oxygen, nutrients and certain protective factors can reach your baby and carbon dioxide and other waste products can be eliminated. This is accomplished in three ways:

The first is *simple diffusion*, in which substances such as oxygen travel from an area of high concentration in your blood to low concentration in your baby's.

The second is *facilitated diffusion*, which allows substances in low concentrations in your blood to pass into the baby's 'against the gradient' and vice versa. For example, if you have a low level of iron in your blood, the mineral will still pass through into the foetal circulation even though the baby's blood contains more iron than yours. This ensures that the baby will obtain all he needs even if your stores of a particular nutrient are low. Relatively high levels of waste products are passed from the baby to the mother in the same way.

The third allows large, complex proteins such as protective antibodies to be wrapped in minute bubbles by the placental cells and then transferred to the baby. This ensures that the mother's immunity to certain illnesses is passed on to her baby, and it will be effective throughout pregnancy and for some weeks after the birth.

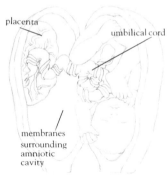

Later in pregnancy the placenta becomes a flat disc on the uterine wall.

The tiny blood vessels of the placenta eventually unite to form the two foetal arteries and the foetal vein which are contained within the umbilical cord. This connects the centre of the placenta on the side facing the baby, and the other end is connected to the baby at the navel. It acts as a 'lifeline', carrying blood from the placenta to the baby (via the foetal vein) and from the baby to the placenta (via the foetal arteries). These blood vessels are surrounded by a light bluish-green jelly which shines through the transparent membranous sheath which completely covers the cord, and the arteries spiralling around the vein give it a coiled, twisted appearance.

The placenta and the umbilical cord both grow as your baby develops. By the fourth month of pregnancy, the placenta is fully developed and a little over 7.5 cm (3 in) in diameter – approximately the same size as the baby – but by the time your baby is born, it will have grown to about 20 cm (8 in) in diameter and will weigh about 0.45 kg (1 lb). The walls of the villi become thinner and more permeable as pregnancy progresses, so that the quantity of nutrients for the baby increases and the villi's ability to eliminate waste products is enhanced. The umbilical cord gradually lengthens throughout pregnancy, until at birth it is usually long enough for the mother to hold her baby while the placenta is still embedded in the wall of her uterus – that is, about 1 m (3 ft 3 in) long.

Other functions of the placenta In addition to its involvement in nourishing your baby, your placenta produces a variety of hormones which are important in the maintenance of pregnancy and the stimulation of labour (*see* p. 32).

It used to be believed that the placenta acts as a filter, preventing toxins and other harmful substances from entering the baby's bloodstream. However, it is now known that most of the substances that a mother takes into her body will get through to the baby within an hour or two or even less. The placenta does act as a barrier in the sense that only molecules of a certain size can pass through the walls of the villi, but unfortunately this restriction does not rule out many of the gases and drugs commonly used for pain relief in labour (*see* pp. 327-8), substances such as alcohol, aspirin and nicotine or certain viruses (e.g. rubella), all of which can affect your baby.

The amniotic sac and fluid

The amniotic sac, which surrounds the baby, is made up of two separate membranes. The *chorion*, comprising a single layer of cells, is an extension of the sheath which contains the umbilical cord. Transparent with a silvery shimmer and as thin as paper, it covers the smooth side of the placenta facing the baby and lines the entire womb. Inside the chorion is a second membrane – the *amnion* – which develops from cells of the baby; it surrounds the amniotic fluid (*see below*) and the baby floating within it.

These two membranes are in contact with one another, and together are as thick as the skin of a blown-up balloon. They are strong, resilient and stretchable, and provide a wall to keep the amniotic fluid in the uterus and prevent organisms from reaching the baby.

They usually rupture at the onset of or during labour, but occasionally the baby's head may be born with the membranes intact. This is known as being born 'in a caul', which in many cultures is thought to be a sign of good luck for the baby. The membranes, together with the placenta and umbilical cord, are known as the 'afterbirth' which is expelled by your uterus after your baby is born.

During the first half of pregnancy, the clear, colourless amniotic fluid within the amniotic sac consists of water entering through the membranes and leakage through the permeable skin of the baby. Later, the major contribution is from the foetal kidneys as the baby urinates; this sterile fluid is then swallowed into the stomach, from which it passes into the baby's

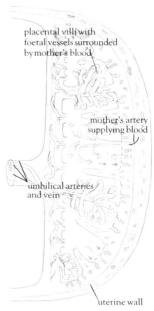

placental villi with foetal vessels surrounded by mother's blood

mother's artery supplying blood

umbilical arteries and vein

uterine wall

The placental circulation, showing the mother's arteries delivering jets of blood to surround the villi which contain the baby's blood vessels. The circulations of mother and baby are separated by a layer of cells. The mother's blood returns to her heart via the veins, and the foetal blood returns to the baby via the umbilical cord.

bloodstream to be filtered in the placenta. The amniotic fluid contains salts, minerals, sugars and proteins, all important nutrients for the baby's growth.

In the first four or five months of pregnancy, the salt content of the fluid is low, and the volume is high in proportion to the baby's size. Later, the amount of fluid increases at a slower rate than that of the baby's growth, so that, by the eighth month, he has less room to move about. At the birth, there may be between 500 and 1500 ml (17½-53 fl. oz) of the fluid in the amniotic sac, with an average of about 800 ml (1⅖ pints), and every 500 ml weighs 0.45 kg (1 lb). The pool of fluid is constantly replenished, and the entire amount is recirculated every four to six hours.

The amniotic fluid has a number of important functions:

It provides a watery environment in which the baby can exercise in freedom, free from the effects of gravity.

It maintains the baby at a constant temperature.

It provides the baby with a method of excreting waste substances in the urine.

It provides a sterile fluid for the baby to swallow and inhale in preparation for feeding and breathing after birth.

It contains nutrients for the baby's growth.

It protects the baby from blows – e.g. if you fall on your abdomen – by cushioning them and absorbing the shock. If the membranes are intact during labour, it forms a fluid wedge which protects the baby's head as the cervix dilates.

By increasing throughout pregnancy, it encourages the uterus to enlarge to accommodate the baby.

The baby's circulation

The blood circulation of mother and baby are quite separate, the baby's never leaving the placenta. Oxygen and nutrients, dissolved in the mother's blood, cross the semi-permeable membrane covering the placental cells of the villi in the uterine wall and then pass into the baby's blood contained in the foetal vein. This blood passes either through the liver or straight to the baby's heart.

Foetal circulation differs from that of an adult in that oxygen is obtained from the mother's blood via the placenta and not from the lungs. Because of this, the blood does not need to flow from the left side of the heart to the lungs to become oxygenated; rather, in the foetus it passes through an opening in one of the interior walls of the heart to travel straight to the rest of the body. At birth, this opening (known as the *foramen ovale*) closes up as the lungs expand for the first time.

In pregnancy, blood is propelled through the baby's veins and arteries by the beating of his heart, which starts by the fifth week. The foetal heart pumps at between 110 and 170 beats per minute, with an average of about 140. Its rate can vary, depending on whether the part of the nervous system which governs it – the sympathetic nervous system – is stimulated or not. For example, a healthy foetal heart will beat faster when the baby moves or kicks, and more quietly when he is asleep. The heart rate is echoed in the pulsating of the blood within the umbilical cord.

Blood is circulated through the baby's vessels at a speed of about 6.4 km (4 miles) an hour, the whole cycle taking about 30 seconds. This creates a pressure which distends the blood vessels in the cord.

The foetal circulation, showing how oxygenated blood from the placenta bypasses the lungs by flowing through the ductus and foramen ovale to the baby's body. Oxygen is not obtained via the lungs before birth.

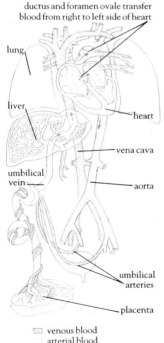

ductus and foramen ovale transfer blood from right to left side of heart

lung

liver

heart

vena cava

umbilical vein

aorta

umbilical arteries

placenta

venous blood
arterial blood
mixed arterial venous blood

The baby

With the development of psychoanalysis and the many forms of psychotherapy during this century, it has become widely understood that, as adults, we may be deeply affected by our early experiences in infancy, during birth and even in the womb.

In the early 1970s, the French obstetrician Frederick Leboyer reminded us that the newborn child is an exquisitely sensitive creature whose primal needs were being neglected in hospital delivery rooms. A few years earlier, two paediatricians, Marshall Klaus and John Kenell, had focused on the first hours and days after birth, and found that the instinctive mother-child communication after birth – which they called 'bonding' – was being disturbed by unnecessary intervention and routine medical procedures. They pointed out what most mothers already knew: that a mother and her newborn baby have a vital need to be together, uninterrupted, at this time, and these early bonds help to establish a smooth relationship in the future.

It is now known that, from the early months of life in the womb, the unborn child is an aware, remembering, feeling and reacting being, and that communication between the mother and her unborn child is well established long before birth. The bonding that occurs after childbirth has its roots in this early communication, which occurs on a multitude of levels and begins soon after conception, becoming more intricate as the baby develops.

The skin and touch

As well as the brain, the outer layer of the embryo – the *ectoderm* – gives rise to the skin, which is formed by the sixth week of pregnancy. Thus we experience our first sensations through the skin before we can see or hear. During pregnancy, we float in the amniotic fluid, unaware of our body weight or the force of gravity. In the early weeks of development, sensations and feelings are focused on the skin: the warmth of the amniotic fluid; the smooth amniotic membranes lining the uterine cavity; and the pulsating cord which can be grasped in play. We suck our fingers and toes, and are also aware of vibrations in the fluid arising from external noises.

It is through the skin that, as unborn babies, we become aware of the relationship between our own bodies and our surroundings, and this gives us our earliest sense of self. During early pregnancy, the embryo is tiny compared with the volume of amniotic fluid, and is free to float, somersault and move his limbs and spine. Later in pregnancy, although the amount of fluid is increased, the baby grows rapidly and cannot move as freely.

During the last weeks of pregnancy, the baby's body fills the entire uterus, and the skin is close to the uterine wall as the volume of amniotic fluid decreases. At this stage, the baby can feel your hands when you stroke or massage your belly, and is also massaged by the contractions which become increasingly frequent and powerful as your uterus prepares for birth. Movement is restricted to the arms and legs.

After birth, the cooler temperature of the air on the baby's skin stimulates the breathing reflex. When babies are born underwater, they do not breathe until lifted to the surface, oxygen being provided by the placenta and cord. Immediately after birth, contact with your warm skin and the gentle touch and massage of your hands will instinctively soothe and comfort your new child.

Hearing and body sense

In the womb, the foetus can hear by the 12th week, and during pregnancy, this sense becomes very well developed. The baby lives in a dark world filled with sounds transmitted through fluid. Intestinal rumblings of food passing through your digestive tract are clearly audible, as is the rhythm of your breathing; and there is the constant rhythmic beat of your heart, as well as the sound of blood whooshing into the uterine muscle and placental pool with each contraction of your heart.

Your heartbeat alters when you exercise, become angry or excited, are calm and meditative and when you sleep. These rhythms surround the baby in the womb every minute of the day, playing an important part in the communication between you. When recordings of a maternal heartbeat are played to newborns, this often calms and quietens them and helps them to sleep. You will also find this to be true after the birth when you hold your baby to your breast so that he will again be able to hear the familiar sound of your heart.

Your baby can also hear your voice clearly in the womb and may respond to its tones when you are calm or angry and when you sing or laugh. After the birth, your voice, as you talk to your child, will be a familiar sound which links the outside environment with the sounds he has heard in the womb. Sound is also transmitted through your abdominal wall, and your baby may know and recognize the voices of your partner and others.

The rhythm of the maternal heartbeat forms the primal rhythmic beat from which our musical sense develops. Unborn babies react to music: many are calmed by gentle music – e.g. that of Mozart and Vivaldi – and often kick vigorously when they hear loud rock music. Singing to your baby and playing an instrument while you are pregnant are delightful ways to communicate with your unborn child.

The ears, as well as containing the organs of hearing, also contain the structures which control balance and orientation in space. Even though your baby develops in the relatively 'weightless' environment of the amniotic sac, he will be aware of moving and turning somersaults, and will be affected by your movements. In most pregnancies, babies lie head down for months and thus are quite used to being upside down. Later, you will notice how your baby will be quite comfortable and relaxed when held in this position.

Movement

Babies begin to move by the eighth week of pregnancy, when they are about 2.5 cm (1 in) long. The newly formed muscles of the limbs and trunk begin to be used as movement increases, and during the rest of pregnancy they become stronger and more powerful and coordination improves. Swallowing and tongue movements are present at 12 weeks, and complex lip movements, sucking and facial expressions such as frowning and grimacing begin by 14 weeks. The first movements you are aware of – called the 'quickening' – can be felt at any time between 16 and 24 weeks.

By mid-pregnancy, your baby floats peacefully, kicks vigorously, turns somersaults, hiccups, urinates, swallows and inhales amniotic fluid, gets excited at sudden noises, calms down when you talk quietly and is rocked to sleep as you walk about. In the second half of pregnancy, when the baby has less space in which to move, you may be able to tell if your baby is asleep or awake: when awake, he may either move quietly or vigorously.

Babies may express their likes and dislikes by kicking – for example, vigorous kicking may be stimulated by loud noises as well as by any feelings of anger or excitement their mothers may communicate. They may also kick strongly when exercising and when they feel good, as frequently happens when you are at rest and relaxing after a day of physical activity. Other movements that can be felt at this point will vary. Mothers are commonly aware of 'roll over' movements as their babies turn from one side to the other, the sensation of their bottoms rising upward as they extend their spines and, sometimes, a fit of hiccups which may last a few minutes.

As you get closer to term, the movements that indicate that your child is rolling over will decrease because space is limited, and his limbs will tend to move in the same general area, often causing discomfort under your ribs. Although some babies move more than others, an active baby is usually a healthy one, and you should only be concerned if the pattern of movements changes noticeably and suddenly, particularly if movements decrease in intensity or frequency. After 38 weeks, the activity of some, but not all, babies will lessen.

Movements can also continue during labour. Babies may sometimes rock or otherwise move their heads during the first stage to assist their progress through the pelvis. During the birth itself, they may participate by kicking to help their bodies descend through the birth canal.

Breathing, digestion and excretion

In the womb, your baby obtains oxygen and eliminates carbon dioxide through your bloodstream via the placenta. He will take the first breath of air into his lungs seconds after birth.

During the months in the womb, he practises in readiness for this event. From the 12th week, he inhales amniotic fluid into his lungs and thus uses and exercises the breathing reflex. The lungs themselves do not expand and there is no oxygen transfer at this time. Your baby also swallows amniotic fluid, which is also absorbed. Waste products are carried to the placenta, and he gets rid of the rest of the liquid by urinating into the amniotic fluid.

The sucking reflex, so vital to the survival of newborn babies, develops during pregnancy. By the time they are born, all the muscles involved in sucking are very strong, and you may be surprised at the force with which your baby begins to suck just moments after birth.

During pregnancy, a baby's bowels become filled with a greenish-black liquid called *meconium*, derived from bile produced by the liver and cells shed by the bowel. Defecation will not usually begin until some hours after birth. Occasionally, however, babies do defecate in the uterus, in which case the amniotic fluid will become stained a greenish brown (*see* p. 323).

Taste

Taste buds are present on the tongue by the 12th week of pregnancy, and the baby will be able to taste the amniotic fluid. Although it is unlikely that taste preferences are set by the taste of the amniotic fluid, research has shown that unborn babies react to certain tastes and prefer sweet ones. Certainly, as soon as your baby is born, he will enjoy the taste of your first milk, and it seems logical that the taste buds mature in readiness for feeding. Within hours of birth, your baby will be able to identify the taste and smell of your milk and distinguish it from that of other women.

Your baby's weight

Your baby's weight increases throughout pregnancy, although there is a wide variation. The following are the average weights a baby will achieve from the middle to the end of pregnancy:

Week	Weight
26	500 g (1 lb 2 oz)
28	900 g (2 lb)
30	1350 g (3 lb)
32	1800 g (4 lb)
34	2270 g (5 lb)
36	2720 g (6 lb)
38	3175 g (7 lb)
40	3300 g (7 lb 4 oz)
42	3400 g (7 lb 8 oz)

Sight

Although not yet fully developed, the eyes are formed by the seventh week after conception, and by the tenth week, the optic nerves which connect the eyes to the brain are present. Eyelids are formed by the 12th week but are fused, only opening at week 28.

Because the eyelids are fused and the uterus is deep within the abdomen, your baby, although aware of light by 16 weeks, essentially lives in a dark world. However, if you expose your pregnant belly to the sun after the 28th week, light filtering through the abdominal wall may be seen by the baby as a reddish haze.

At birth, your baby will have coordinated movements of both eyes – that is, the binocular vision which makes us see things in three dimensions rather than as flat pictures. He will prefer complex to simple patterns, curves to straight lines, and irregular to regular shapes, all of which adds up to a preference for the rounded contours of your head and the features of your face. He will see light and colour for the first time, and will be able to focus at 22–30 cm (9–12 in), the ideal distance to see your face as you hold him in your arms.

Weight gain and growth

A baby's final birth weight may vary for a number of reasons. It can be low if the baby is premature or is one of a pair of twins, or if the mother is undernourished, suffers from certain diseases, smokes, drinks excessively or uses drugs such as heroin (see Low birth weight, p. 321). On the other hand, it may be high if the mother is diabetic (see p. 307). However, the most common determining factor is the mother's own size, regardless of that of the father.

In general, the tallest and heaviest mothers have babies which, at birth, are heavier than those of shorter and slighter women. The race of the mother also has an influence – for example, Oriental babies are usually smaller at birth than Caucasian babies.

Memory

Nerve circuits in the cerebral cortex – the part of the brain we use for conscious thought and remembering – develop throughout pregnancy, and by the 32nd week, they are already as advanced as those of a newborn. Unborn babies will not 'remember' in the same way as adults do, but they are acutely sensitive, highly impressionable and responsive, and it seems logical that as they are capable of many complex functions, they should also have a developing memory base.

Under hypnosis or during regressive therapy, some people are able to recall birth and even pre-birth experiences, and it seems that we all unconsciously remember experiences in the womb, and these early memories play an important part in the foundation of the self. Schools of psychotherapy have emerged to help adults contact primitive emotions originating from their own birth and infancy, and dramatic therapeutic changes can occur with the release of such emotions.

Sleeping, waking and dreaming

During the second half of pregnancy, your baby will have periods of wakefulness, when he moves around, and periods of quiet and sleep, and the pattern of waking and sleeping established then often continues after birth. For example, towards the end of pregnancy, as your growing uterus presses on your bladder, you will probably find yourself getting up two or three times a night to urinate, and after birth, your baby may tend to wake up during the night at about the same times.

There are two types of sleep, depending on brain-wave activity: rapid eye movement (REM), during which we as adults dream, and non-rapid eye movement, or deep sleep. Brain wave tests on sleeping unborn babies have shown that up to 80 per cent of their sleep comprises REM sleep. (By contrast, in old age this drops to 15 per cent.) Although it is impossible to prove that the babies are actually dreaming during this REM sleep, it does indicate that they are mentally active while asleep.

Communication

It is often noticeable how even the very youngest children seem to be affected by their mothers' emotional state: if the mother is calm and relaxed, the baby will tend to be at ease and peaceful, and when she is tense or anxious, the child may be fretful, too.

During pregnancy, mothers and babies are so closely linked that, in many ways, they form one biological unit, and their reciprocity is psychological as well as physical. The emotional 'radar' of babies is already greatly developed before birth, and they respond not only to the more obvious emotions such as love and hate but are capable of much finer emotional distinctions. Even in the womb, babies need to feel wanted and loved in order to thrive best, and your baby's awareness of the variations in your moods will help to prepare him for the rich emotional texture of life.

There is a physical basis to this sharing of emotions. In the mother, changing moods will trigger off the release of different hormones and other substances (see p. 33) into the bloodstream, and these will cross the placenta to affect the baby. For example, if the mother is anxious, she will produce more adrenalin, but if she is calm or happy, the manufacture of endorphins may predominate. Thus babies are also biochemically in harmony with their mothers; and the biorhythms, sleeping patterns, eating habits and physical state of the mother all affect her baby. A certain amount of stress and anxiety is part of normal life, and experiencing these is an important part of your child's development. Only when negative feelings or depression are extreme is there the possibility of a harmful effect on the baby, and in this case, help needs to be sought.

It should always be borne in mind, however, that babies are very much separate beings. The degree to which they are affected by what they experience will differ according to the inherent nature and resilience of each individual child. Indeed, many thrive despite circumstances which would appear to be far from ideal.

In ancient China, pregnant women were encouraged to enhance their babies' development by trying to ensure that they spent time each day communicating with their babies in the womb, as well as maintaining a lifestyle most conducive to their children's emotional well-being. This practice, known as *tai-kyo*, was based on the principle that the mother's health and happiness can affect her baby both physically and emotionally. When we see newborn babies, moments after birth, it is easy to believe that the ability to respond emotionally must have begun to develop while they were in the womb, and that the psychological ties between mothers and babies are a continuum of their relationship during pregnancy.

C H A P T E R   5

THE EMOTIONAL ASPECTS OF PREGNANCY

Discovering that you are to become a parent – particularly for the first time – is the beginning of a new era in your life. The birth of a baby signals the birth of a family, a time of change and transformation. As this adventure unfolds, you may well find that becoming a parent is a fundamental challenge which not only introduces a new life but also a wide variety of new emotions and experiences.

Pregnancy is an eventful time. As the birth approaches, you will have to accept the inevitable and long-term responsibilities of being a fully fledged adult and parent. Such an abrupt transformation is achieved with ease by some people but with greater difficulty by others.

Many problems can be avoided if you have planned to have a baby and there is little conflict with other aspects of your life. However, whether the pregnancy is intended or not, you will inevitably undergo many changes, both physical and emotional, and there are also bound to be alterations in your relationships, occupation and lifestyle.

Although the experiences that lie ahead are relatively unknown and unpredictable, there is a lot you can do by preparing well to make your transition to parenthood as successful as possible. The nine months of pregnancy will provide you with a marvellous opportunity to become more open and aware, more deeply in touch with yourself and with your partner.

The pages that follow highlight some of the more common emotional aspects of impending parenthood, and are intended as a guide to encourage you to explore and find your own way through the joys and difficulties, the ups and downs of the daily challenges that are all part of becoming a parent.

Becoming a mother

Entering motherhood involves a dramatic and all-encompassing change for most women. For many, having a child satisfies a deep and instinctive biological need which is the natural outcome of the process of maturation from childhood through adolescence to adulthood. The transition from 'woman' to 'mother' can be smooth and proceed quite effortlessly as your baby grows inside you, but most find that pregnancy and, indeed, parenthood involve considerable challenges emotionally.

Sometimes it may be difficult to accept the new role, and it often requires courage and considerable adjustment to bridge the gap between carefree young adult and mature, responsible parent. If you have a career, you will find that, for a time at least, you will shed your previous role and assume the new responsibilities, status and expectations associated with becoming a mother. After the birth, your life will be dominated by your baby's need for constant care, and your former priorities and values will be called into question in the light of this new experience.

Part of the excitement of having a baby is going through this transformation, with its difficulties, conflicts and anxieties balanced by the positive energy arising from the joy of creation and mothering.

Personal change

As pregnancy advances, you may discover that unexpected emotions arise as your self-awareness deepens, along with inexplicable rapid mood changes and feelings that may seem irrational and contradictory. Some women find that, while they are pregnant, deep-seated memories may surface, consciously or in dreams, which relate to past relationships or experiences in childhood or even further back — as far as their own infancy or birth.

Our past experiences are part of us and need to be well understood or resolved as we mature, but often this all-important aspect of pregnancy is neglected or overlooked. Allowing your feelings to surface and coming to terms with your past are vital parts of your evolution into motherhood. Some of these memories may be pleasant, while others may involve painful or more difficult feelings. Although the re-experiencing of these emotions may be painful at the time, they are positive events which will free you to grow and accept motherhood with grace and equanimity.

Usually this process unfolds naturally without your needing to think about it, and most women may only notice that they are unusually moody or emotional during pregnancy. If, however, you feel overwhelmed, confused or under a great deal of stress, it may be helpful to seek professional counselling and guidance so that any difficulties can be resolved during pregnancy and, in this way, prevent problems such as post-natal depression after the birth.

Finding out that you are pregnant can come as quite a shock, even if you have planned to have a baby and more so if you have not. At first, some women feel a sense of anxiety and doubt about whether they will be able to measure up emotionally and physically to this new event in their lives.

What is important is to be honest with yourself and open with your partner about your feelings, and to expect that, while you are adjusting to the reality of being pregnant, your emotions are bound to be turbulent and your feelings, hopes and fears very mixed. Accepting, understanding and allowing for this is the way to begin to come to terms with the reality of becoming a parent.

Freedom and independence

Along with the joys and rewards of having a baby, motherhood is likely to impose many new demands upon you. There is a considerable loss of freedom, and sometimes a total change of lifestyle may be involved. Even if you have planned to have a baby, you may feel trapped as you realize that, for the next few years, your time can no longer be your own. You will need to adjust your activities and rhythms to your baby's needs and be available to her at any time of the day or night, or make sure that someone else is.

Caring for a baby is a 24-hour job, and it is helpful to have realistic expectations about this, and to explore ways of making the most of this time. Usually the path of least resistance is the most successful! A young baby can be a great teacher, and by consciously deciding (if your circumstances allow) to give your all during the years of early infancy, it is possible to derive great satisfaction and joy from the experience, and to help lay a secure and healthy foundation for your child's developing personality. If you plan to return to work, it is imperative that you arrange for another person with similar ideas to your own to care for your baby while you are away (see Working mothers, p. 346).

Although many working women look forward to staying home to prepare for the birth and parenthood, if you have an interesting career or a job which you enjoy, you may find it difficult to leave as the birth approaches. For some, the loss of contact with colleagues at work and leaving an existence outside the home can be upsetting. You may also find losing your own income and the financial independence it brings hard to adjust to, as well as spending most of your time at home waiting for your child to be born without the challenge and the responsibilities of either a job or motherhood to absorb you.

A sensible way to approach motherhood is to try to accept your new reality as a challenge rather than a curse. Now is a good time to explore new friendships and to seek out other pregnant women or mothers of young children with whom you can share experiences. Involve yourself deeply in the pleasures and joys of being pregnant and having a baby. Although at first you may not realize it, those early years can be deeply satisfying and will very soon be over.

Your changing body

Many women enjoy the physical changes of pregnancy when they occur smoothly and naturally, and feel healthy and relaxed with a wonderful sense of earthy fullness, strength and vigour. Your new rounded and sensuous body may seem more beautiful than ever; your skin, hair and face may appear to glow as you sense your baby growing inside you; and you may display your changing shape with a feeling of pride by wearing maternity clothes long before it is necessary.

However, for some women it is difficult to feel positive about these changes, particularly if they are accompanied by nausea, stretch marks, indigestion, tiredness or any of the other discomforts brought about by the hormonal changes in the body. Occasionally women experience pregnancy mainly as a state of obesity, or they may refer to their new shape as that of a normal person with a lump attached, and attempt to hide it for as long as they possibly can.

There can also be a fundamental conflict in the way in which a woman perceives her body before, during and after pregnancy. Before pregnancy, the body is often thought of as primarily an object of sexual attraction, whereas with pregnancy and childbirth, it becomes a functional carrier and subsequent feeder of a child, with its sexual aspects taking second place. For some, these two views are hard to reconcile.

It is useful to remember that the female body is ideally designed to bear and give birth to children. By developing a positive attitude towards it and trusting its natural ability to change and adapt to the needs of your baby, many of these problems can be overcome. Although your body will undergo a major transformation as it accommodates your growing child and prepares for birth and breastfeeding, miraculously these changes are only temporary and your body will return to 'normal' in its own time.

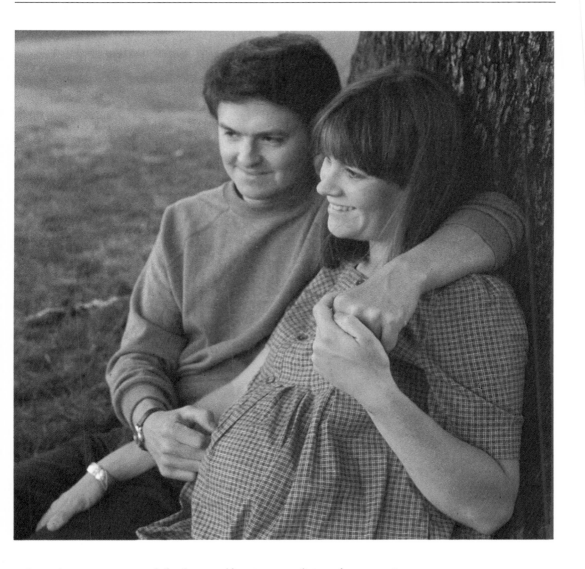

It is also important to defend yourself against conditioned expectations of the ideal female physique and to enjoy your body during pregnancy. True beauty depends far less on ideal images than on your own inner feelings about your physical self, and pregnancy provides a marvellous opportunity to deepen your consciousness of your body's range of sensory experience. In this way, you will feel good from the 'inside out', and this inner glow will be reflected by your external appearance. Spending some time without clothes, preferably in the sunshine if the climate and season allow, and dancing, walking, swimming, exercising or a massage are all ways to feel good during pregnancy.

By accepting the physical changes you go through as appropriate to your new role as a mother, as well as eating and exercising well before and after the birth, you will discover a sense of radiant health and contentment more deeply beautiful than any conventional image.

Maternal instinct

In traditional societies, women are exposed to childbirth and mothering throughout their lives, and their maternal instinct is encouraged and nurtured during childhood and adolescence. Older girls may attend the births of their brothers, sisters and cousins and take an active role in the home, including caring for babies. However, in many Western societies, where the nuclear family is prevalent and some women embark on parenthood alone, it is rare for a new mother to have witnessed a birth, and often she will never have held, bathed, clothed or fed an infant.

The ability to care for and nurture a child is partly instinctive and partly a learned experience. Sometimes, this learning must be done for the first time through trial and error, and it may take some time before you feel confident and relaxed about mothering your baby.

Although some degree of ambivalence is normal, it is rare for a mother to have no maternal feelings for her child; this only occurs when there is an emotional disturbance. Motherly feelings usually flower with the birth of the baby, even if it takes you a little time to realize it. For most women, the maternal instinct is powerful and arises quite spontaneously as a consequence of the continuum of events that occur during pregnancy and birth. However, for some, maternal feelings are not strong, and some relate better to their children later on or in adolescence.

To give maternal feelings the best chance to develop, it is helpful if the physiological processes of pregnancy and childbirth progress naturally and the transition into feeding and mothering takes place undisturbed. The ability to mother will come with practice, and you can trust your baby to teach you most of what you need to know. There are no ideal standards to which you should aspire: all mothers are different, and circumstances vary.

Many women choose to devote themselves to motherhood full-time, while others may need or want to work as well and manage to do both successfully by sharing the task with a suitable helper. What is most important is to understand the primal needs that are common to all young babies and to do your best to satisfy these so that your child feels loved, understood and secure.

It is natural to be somewhat apprehensive about your ability to love and mother your baby. It will help to bear in mind that nobody is right all the time, and that we all make mistakes and learn by them. As long as you do your best and are open to new ideas, you are bound to be the perfect mother for your baby.

Relating to your unborn child

Around the 18th week of pregnancy, you may begin to feel the first movements of your baby inside you: these very light, fluttering sensations are described as the 'quickening' of the baby in the womb. Throughout the next few months, your awareness of the child inside you will increase physically and psychologically, and by the time your baby is born, the bonding process will already have begun.

The simple ways in which you alter your life and plan for your baby are part of this process – for example, giving up work and changing your lifestyle, moving or altering your home, shopping for your new son or daughter. Bonding before birth also occurs on a deeply subconscious level, not only between babies and their mothers, but also between them and their fathers and brothers and sisters.

During the months of pregnancy, your unborn child will have already become familiar with your body rhythms and your moods and with the sound of your voice (*see* pages 58-61). The last three months are especially important in establishing these links, as by this time your baby has developed great sensitivity towards you both emotionally and physically. One of the best ways to help this natural process is to spend time with young babies.

Babies in the womb enjoy and respond to chanting, singing and the sounds of musical instruments, and will also benefit from the rhythmic movements of your body when you exercise or dance. Meditation and deep breathing in which you focus your attention inward will help you to connect with your baby (*see* Part V).

In late pregnancy, women often stroke and massage their bellies. You will be interested to feel how your baby lies in your abdomen and learn to tell the different parts of her body — your doctor or midwife should be able to help you to do this. Your child will be aware of this contact, and your partner and other members of your family may also enjoy communicating with your unborn baby in this manner. Swimming or bathing in warm water is also a good way to connect with your baby, by immersing your own body in water, you not only relax yourself but, like your baby, you too are in a warm fluid environment.

Most women have, at some time in their pregnancies, a fear about whether their baby will be normal. It is quite common to doubt whether you are actually 'good enough' to produce a perfect infant, and immediately after delivery, many women express first surprise and then delight that they have done so. Since the vast majority of babies are perfectly normal, to dwell on this issue is unnecessary.

You may also have a strong desire or expectation about the sex of the baby. While a mother's intuition is generally right, it sometimes does happen that she is surprised or disappointed by her child's gender. Although the best approach is to be ready to accept the role of destiny in this matter, it is often impossible to alter a strong preference that you and your partner may have. However, it is important to realize that your baby may be affected by your expectations and is likely to be aware of your pleasure or disappointment at birth.

Whatever the circumstances in which you find yourself, try to give some time each day to your baby, long before it is born. By giving your attention to your unborn child and doing things you both enjoy, you will allow the natural and instinctive connection between you to flower of its own accord.

Dreaming

Although not everyone remembers them, most pregnant women have vivid, varied and interesting dreams. They often become even more so during the last three months of pregnancy when, as a woman is less mobile, she naturally becomes more psychically oriented. The dreams often feature the unborn baby, frequently in the rather strange and sometimes unusual form of an animal or perhaps with some sort of defect, and while they may sometimes be disturbing or frightening, they are often pleasant and colourful. This is a natural phenomenon and is a way in which we work out our fears, expectations, desires and anxieties while we sleep.

Remembering dreams is one way of bringing feelings into consciousness

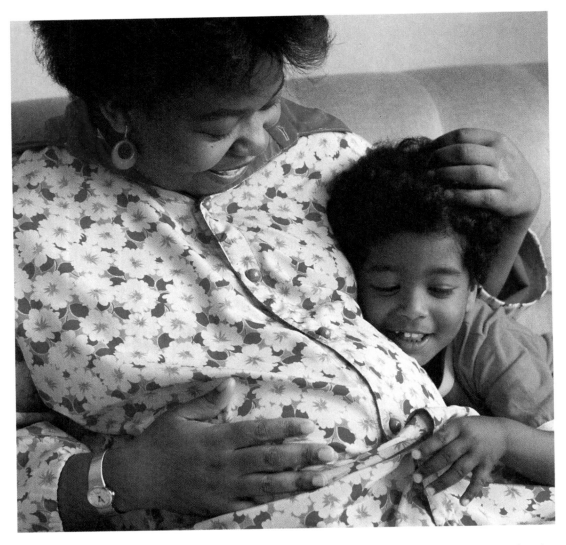

so that you can deal with them. Try discussing your dreams with other pregnant women, your partner or your birth attendants: you will discover that even frightening or macabre dreams are not unusual and have no harmful effects, either on you or the baby.

There is also some conjecture that pregnant women communicate with their babies through dreaming and vice versa.

Your relationship with your partner

If you are married or live with a partner, you may well feel some apprehension about how having a baby is likely to affect the man in your life. Perhaps the decision to have a child was mutual or perhaps the pregnancy has come as a surprise to him or to both of you. Either way, he is going to need to come to terms with the reality of impending parenthood just as you are. He may take longer to realize he is to become a father as he will not have the advantage of having the baby already growing inside his body. Socially, too, men's feelings and emotions about pregnancy are often ignored or made fun of, even though, for them, this may also be a time of great emotional turbulence and psychological change. For some, the prospect of the new responsibilities and commitments of fatherhood can be quite terrifying.

Occasionally, these feelings may be so extreme that they cause the man to abandon his pregnant partner, then feel so guilty about it that he cannot return. This sort of extreme situation can sometimes be avoided by considering your partner's feelings from an early stage and making a special effort to understand and share with him.

Many men, before the birth of their first child, have very little experience or knowledge of childbearing, and may at first feel reluctant to involve themselves too deeply in what traditionally have been women's affairs. It is important that your partner should not feel that he is being pressured into becoming involved and that he retains the option of remaining at a distance if this is where he would really be more comfortable. Of course, if your partner chooses to take an active part in your pregnancy, the birth and baby care, he can be a great help and support to you, and is likely to have a close bond with your child.

Even if your partner is delighted that you are pregnant, you are bound to be apprehensive about how he will react to your physical changes. Will he still find you attractive? Will he love you as much? Will he still want you sexually having watched you give birth? Some women may worry that their partners may turn away from them and be attracted to other women. Although this does sometimes happen, most men mature with their partners during pregnancy, and find the soft maternal contours and bloom of pregnancy both beautiful and exciting, arousing new feelings of protectiveness and tenderness.

You may also be concerned about the loss of freedom that is the inevitable consequence when a baby has entered your life. Certainly you will both need to find a way to accept this third person into your relationship and to balance your baby's needs with your time together as a couple. This can be a very difficult adjustment to make, requiring great forbearance on your partner's part as your attention is likely to be increasingly absorbed by the baby.

Your relationship with your partner can be one of the most important factors in a successful pregnancy and birth. How you feel about each other will also affect your baby and is the basis of happy family life. It is important that you are open with one another and share your feelings, both positive and negative, and that you spend time together doing something you both enjoy. If there is any serious conflict that you cannot sort out yourselves, it can be greatly beneficial to seek professional guidance.

Pregnant again

If you are about to embark on a second or subsequent pregnancy, you have all the advantages of your previous experience to make the territory more familiar. You will have gone through the initiation into parenthood that is so intense the first time around and will probably approach the pregnancy with more confidence. That is bound to make things easier in some ways, although every pregnancy offers new challenges. If you have had a difficult experience with a previous birth, you may need to resolve any residual feelings about it in order to approach this experience afresh, and perhaps make different decisions in the choice of the place of birth, your attendants and ways of preparing during pregnancy.

Adjusting to another pregnancy

Whether you have planned another child or not, you will need to come to terms with the reality that another baby is on the way, very much as you did the first time. If you wanted another baby and the timing is right, it may all be plain sailing. However, perhaps you have conceived again unexpectedly; or your other child or children may still be very young, demanding a lot of your time and attention. It may seem almost impossible to make space for another baby. It is also quite common to wonder whether you will have the sheer capacity to love and care for another child and to give her as much attention as your other child or children seem to need.

Besides your own reaction to another pregnancy, you may find that others are less enthusiastic than they were about your first pregnancy. Your partner, too, may have mixed feelings or a negative reaction to the news; he may feel trapped or frightened at the increased responsibility, both emotional and financial. Although, in the end, he will probably be delighted with the new baby, he may first need to come to terms with conflicting emotions, as indeed you may have to yourself. Do not forget to talk things through to try and understand each other's feelings.

New challenges

Once again you are going to need to adjust to the changes in your body. In physiological terms, you will find that your abdomen tends to enlarge somewhat sooner in a second or subsequent pregnancy than it did the first time round. More importantly, this time you may find the physical adjustment to another pregnancy rather difficult.

If you already have one or more young and energetic children to look after, you will probably have less time to yourself to rest and exercise, to concentrate on and dream about the new baby, and you may feel tired much of the time. Perhaps you have a lively toddler jumping into bed with you or waking you up at night. It is easy to slip into a pattern of looking after everyone else and neglecting your own needs so that you feel drained and exhausted.

One way to help is to make sure that you look after yourself properly and do not neglect your own health and appearance. Ensure that you eat well and get enough sleep even if you need to plan in advance to do so. If you are lucky and your other child or children have a nap during the day, make the most of this time to rest yourself, leaving chores for another occasion. It will certainly help you to replenish your energy if you make a point of doing some essential stretching exercises every day (see Part V). You will find that you can include these in your daily activity with your child(ren) so that everyone benefits. Do not neglect such pleasures as being massaged or massaging your partner, and try to organize your schedule so that there is a special time for you to concentrate on this pregnancy.

Many women feel guilty about not being able to devote as much time and attention to their second and subsequent babies as they did to their firstborn – either during pregnancy or after the birth. Then, you had only to adjust to your baby's needs and rhythms, but this time the newborn has to become part of an established family, and you may feel that you have to compromise on her needs. Nevertheless, you will gradually find a time for everything, and a new order and harmony will slowly evolve. The answer lies in sorting out your priorities. If you give time and attention first of all to what is most important, then somehow all the other things seem to get done, and you are more likely to feel calm and relaxed.

Becoming a father

The decision to take on the responsibility of fathering a child is probably one of the most important that you are likely to make in your life, and whatever your age or whether you are married or not, having a baby is bound to affect your life in a great number of ways. In particular, the level of commitment between you and your partner will deepen and create an inextricable link between you for many years to come.

Entering parenthood can be a very optimistic time in your life, offering new social, emotional and financial challenges. There are likely to be a variety of problems and difficulties to smooth out and obstacles to overcome, but the joy that comes of having your first child can be one of life's most rewarding experiences.

Fathering a child will involve your emotions at a very deep level. When you hear the news that your partner is pregnant, you may feel an amazing surge of pleasure, confidence and pride in yourself, both as a father and as a man, and you may look forward to the prospect of taking on the new responsibilities of fatherhood.

In the early months of pregnancy, the physical reality of the growing child will be far more immediate to your partner as rapid and dynamic changes take place within her body. It may take you a while to absorb the news that you are to become a father. When you have, the reality of the pregnancy, whether planned or not, can come as something of a shock as you begin to reflect upon how this is going to affect your life.

You may be proud and delighted, although apprehensive about the new challenges. On the other hand, many men find the transition into fatherhood quite difficult, and it is not unusual for a man to suffer from depression or to feel isolated and left out, particularly if his feelings are not understood, either by himself or by family and friends. In such a situation, a man may become preoccupied with his work or other outside interests and retreat emotionally into himself – thus creating a rift of understanding between him and his partner, as well as from his own feelings.

Occasionally this emotional alienation may be so acute that some men find it impossible to cope and may need to seek help. This may be given by your family doctor or, alternatively, family and/or friends may have useful advice to offer. In certain circumstances, a professional counsellor or therapist may be able to help you through a crisis.

So perhaps the first step towards fatherhood is to accept this as a time of change, when you are likely to have conflicting and intense emotions to deal with as you come to terms with what is bound to be a major step in your life. By openly sharing your thoughts and feelings with your partner, you will encourage her to do the same, and thus a new special closeness and friendship between you can evolve.

Male attitudes towards impending fatherhood

Throughout the world, men differ in the degree of their involvement and participation in the events of pregnancy, birth and infancy, but in recent years, the accepted sexual stereotypes and expected roles regarding parenthood have become much more flexible. Although some feel more comfortable as observers on the sidelines than as active participants, many men now enjoy some degree of direct involvement.

This may include being interested in ante-natal care, and being present during labour to provide important emotional support. Others want to take a more active role in pregnancy and birth and share the experiences involved in having a baby, including attending ante-natal classes and being present during labour and the birth. Some fathers will try to take time off work after the birth to help out with household chores.

Some men are perhaps even more interested in parenting than their partners. They may have strong ideas and preferences about the way in which their children should be born, and will participate in all preparation and decision-making during pregnancy and the birth.

Men often need to find a new balance between their lives at work and at home if they are to have the time they need to be with their families. Often there is a choice to be made between career prospects and deciding to make family relationships a priority. Having a baby can, therefore, stimulate change in your lifestyle, giving you an opportunity to re-evaluate your choices and possibilities and to question your basic values.

New responsibilities

The financial implications of parenthood are usually underestimated. Certainly, having a baby is going to involve new expenses and perhaps a need to increase your income. There are likely to be new constraints such as the loss of your partner's earnings and the cost of providing suitable housing for your family and other necessities.

Often women find the challenges of pregnancy so enveloping that their partners have to take on the primary responsibility concerning finances. This can occasionally become overwhelming, especially if you need to work overtime, move or decorate your home or acquire extra capital while at the same time providing emotional support for your partner. These new demands may lead to feelings of tension, anxiety and even depression in some men, and it can be a great help if you can find a way to ease the situation and view it in perspective.

Your feelings about the baby

Even though, like most fathers, you may be proud and delighted that your partner is pregnant, you will probably ask yourself how the presence of this new being in your family is going to affect your life. Certainly, it is realistic to expect that for some years at least your movements and decisions will have to be adapted to the needs of your child. It will be more difficult to be carefree and spontaneous, and for some people, this realization results in considerable conflict.

There is also the emotional challenge of fatherhood. How, in fact, will you be able to respond and relate to your child? You may already be quite familiar with babies, or this may be your very first encounter with one. Perhaps you have never held a baby, let alone changed a nappy or dressed or bathed one. In addition, you may or may not be satisfied with the way

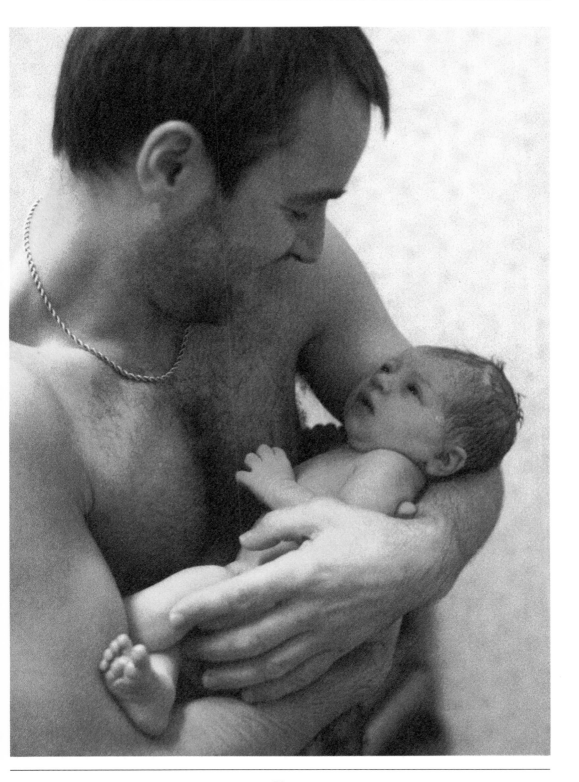

that you were treated by your own parents, and now is an appropriate time to reflect upon this and to give some thought as to how you would like to parent your own children.

Your relationship with your baby begins long before birth, when she is still in the womb. She will be able to hear your voice and feel your touch long before she is born, and will recognize and be soothed by your presence after birth (*see* Chapter 14).

During the second half of pregnancy, as the baby grows larger, you will be able to feel with your hands her movements within your partner's abdomen. Towards the end, these movements will become more obvious, and it may be possible to recognize parts of the baby's body as she changes position in the womb. In these later months, you may find it interesting and helpful to accompany your partner to her ante-natal checkups. There you might ask the midwife to show you how to feel the baby lying in the uterus and also to let you listen to her heart beating. You can do this very simply by pressing your ear against your partner's lower abdomen or by using an ear trumpet or stethoscope.

An excellent way to find out what a real baby is like is to spend time with one. If you are able to have some contact with the babies of friends or relatives and to observe another father, this can help to give you a realistic sense of what it will be like once your child is born.

Jealousy

Your relationship with your partner is bound to change during pregnancy because there is now another person to include in your lives. You may feel somewhat neglected, or that you are losing your partner's attention and affection as she becomes increasingly absorbed in the child growing within her, and these feelings may become even more acute once the baby is born.

If you are the type of man who prefers to be involved in things, you may feel excluded because childbirth and caring for a baby is, inevitably, chiefly the mother's concern, at least until the baby is some weeks old. Your partner's mother may well have an increasingly dominant role in the discussions and decisions about the baby's needs, and this may be difficult for you.

In addition, people usually pay all their attention to the mother, the person who carries, gives birth and nurtures the baby, and tend to neglect the father's needs. It is both common and normal for a man who is basically delighted to become a father to feel some jealousy of the baby and to be somewhat envious of his partner's procreative powers. If, however, you experience intense or persistent feelings of anger or jealousy, it is best to find some way of discussing these either with your partner or with friends, family or a counsellor.

Living with pregnancy

Aside from your own personal feelings and reactions to impending fatherhood, living with a pregnant woman is no mean challenge. She is bound to be more emotional and moody than normal, and she may develop strange food fads and cravings or be more demanding emotionally, needing to be nurtured. She may be more self-centred and may experience unusual fluctuations in her energy and capacity to fulfil her role as your companion, not to mention her preoccupation with everything concerning pregnancy, birth and mothering.

As a result of all of this, she will need a great deal of understanding and loving support, and this may be trying and demanding for you. Generally, the first three months, as the pregnancy is being established, and the last three, when the birth draws nearer, are the most turbulent emotionally.

As pregnancy advances, your partner's body will become softer, fuller and more motherly, and this temporary voluptuousness can be a source of comfort and delight. Many men find the maternal contours of their partner's body very attractive and thus treasure this time, although it is true (though rare) that some actively dislike the way their partners' bodies change during pregnancy, a feeling that may be difficult to come to terms with. However, once the maternal period is over, your partner's body will return to normal, provided she eats and exercises well. Understanding the changes happening in her body will help you to understand her changing moods and her need to allow her feelings to surface and flow at this time (see Chapter 4).

Although your partner provides the essential primal environment that your child needs during pregnancy, your presence and support are also most important to the well-being of both your baby and your partner. During the birth itself, your help can make all the difference, and you can also provide your partner with support and encouragement in the early months of motherhood and breastfeeding. Your baby can be doubly blessed by having two parents central to her growth and development.

One of the most important adjustments that prospective fathers have to make is to the changes and fluctuations which pregnancy can introduce into their sexual lives. Once pregnancy has been established, your attraction for one another and sexual needs and desires may be altered, and you may need to explore new ways of expressing your love and affection.

Living with a pregnant woman can be an extremely rich and certainly a very challenging experience which is bound to increase the depth and dimension of your partnership. You have the chance to discover new and unexpected resources within yourself, to increase your self-awareness and to become closer to the person with whom you are about to share the ups and downs of parenthood.

Couvade

This term was coined by an anthropologist to describe the physical symptoms that some men experience when their partners become pregnant and go into labour. In certain tribes, it is considered normal for men to experience physically a false labour, and lesser degrees of the couvade are very frequently observed in Western men during pregnancy.

They often gain weight and experience abdominal symptoms which may include indigestion, nausea, vomiting or diarrhoea, or suffer abdominal cramps or minor injuries which are frequently a sympathetic reaction to their partners' impending labour. Usually these are quite mild, and provided there is no underlying cause for the symptoms, they are much easier to deal with if you are aware of the phenomenon.

Men who experience the couvade are often the ones most deeply affected by the events surrounding birth. Perhaps these men identify very closely with their partners: they can sometimes become distressed when their partners are in pain during labour or if they need any form of intervention. If this is the case, it is important that such men should feel free to withdraw and leave the room and not feel pressured to participate.

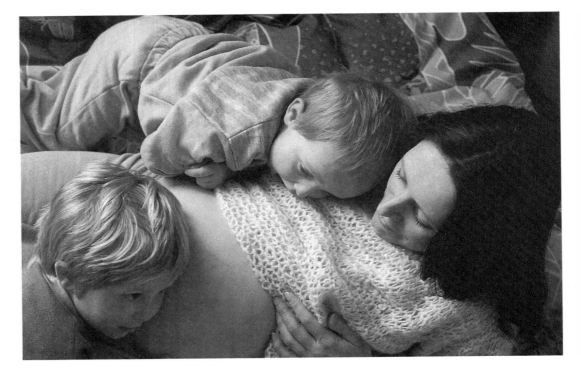

The rest of the family

With the coming of a new baby into the family, other family members, particularly children, need to make an emotional adjustment, and there are a number of ways that parents can help them. Expand their world so that, when you are busy with the new baby, they will have other interests to occupy them. Help them to establish other relationships – perhaps with other children of the same age, with a loving grandparent or a friend or helper who would enjoy spending some time with your children on a regular basis.

Older children

This is an appropriate time for older children to become closer to their fathers and to spend longer periods of time with them. If he does not do so already, the father could perhaps take over some daily routines so that the mother can have some time to concentrate on the coming baby. Taking on these new responsibilities can be a delight, and the relationship between a father and a firstborn child can become much closer at this time.

Another way to help the firstborn to accept a new baby is to include them in the interesting events of pregnancy. If they accompany you to some of your ante-natal checkups, the midwife can help them to listen to the baby's heartbeat. They should also be encouraged to feel the baby's movements and to 'talk' to the baby through your abdomen.

If you plan to change your children's sleeping arrangements, it may be a good idea to do so long before the new baby comes.

When choosing where to have your baby (*see* Chapter 8), you might

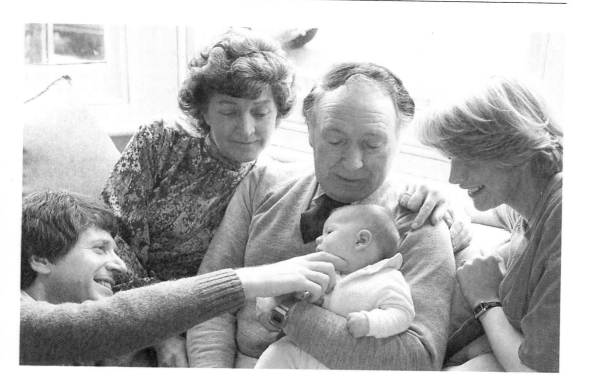

consider a home birth if circumstances allow, as this has many advantages for your other children. You will not need to go away; life can continue more or less as normal; and they can be included in everything, possibly even seeing their brother or sister being born. They will be able to have contact with the new baby right from birth, and will be able to hold and explore the baby at leisure. If a home birth is not possible, you could try to find a birth centre or hospital which will allow siblings to be present during the birth itself or shortly thereafter.

Apart from their separation from you, the greatest anxiety of your older children will probably be that they will be displaced in your affections by another. If you can somehow reassure them that this is not the case, they should manage to include the baby in their world without difficulty. It is important for you to understand the emotional adjustments they have to make but, at the same time, not make too much fuss about it as these things do have a way of coming into balance of their own accord. The fascination with a brand-new companion that siblings usually develop should ultimately be stronger than their feelings of having been made to take second place. (*See also* p. 234.)

Your parents

It is an exciting, meaningful and important experience to become a grandparent, particularly for the first time. You may find that having a baby brings you closer to your parents and/or parents-in-law, and if this is the case, you will probably enjoy sharing the experience of bringing a new life into the family and make the most of their help, company and love.

However, becoming a grandparent also requires a psychological adjustment. For some, this is not easy: they have to get used to the idea of you as the parent and hand over the primary responsibility to you. It is not uncommon for a couple having a first baby to experience conflict with parents or parents-in-law, especially if the latter try to take too dominant a role and interfere with too much advice and help, no matter how well-meaning they might be.

If this is the case, you may need to make quite firm decisions about where and how you are prepared to share your baby. Try not to feel overwhelmed by the wishes and expectations of parents or parents-in-law: you are the parents from now on and the ones who will make the decisions and be responsible for your child.

In many ways, it should be from the older generation of women that the skills of birth and motherhood are handed down to a first-time mother, and this is often the case. However, we live in times when there is often a 'generation gap' and this process sometimes does not occur. A pregnant woman may find that her mother, aunts or mother-in-law may not be able to be very helpful because the ways in which they gave birth or looked after their babies do not coincide with the expectant mother's way of thinking.

Men, too, may find that, if they decide to take an active part in the birth of their children and share in the jobs involved in bringing them up, they may meet with surprise and, possibly, disapproval from their own fathers, who very likely were excluded when their children were born and actively discouraged from sharing in such tasks as changing nappies. It is important, however, that both new parents do what they believe to be correct in relation to the birth and upbringing of their children, even if this is at odds with 'normality' as perceived by their family or friends and they are put under a great deal of pressure to conform.

That said, your parents can play an important role when your baby is small, providing you with a rich source of support, reassurance and help. Their willing participation in your life – whether it be emotional, practical or both – will allow you the opportunity to have some time for yourself, and can relieve the cumulative effect of constant responsibility.

It is also important to remember that there is a very special bond between children and their grandparents which gives great pleasure to both generations. Even if lifestyles and ideas change, this fundamental relationship is a deep one, giving grandparents a sense of continuity and children a sense of their ancestry and heritage.

Having a baby alone

Some women face the challenges of pregnancy, birth and parenthood alone. Taking responsibility for a new baby and coping with the ups and downs of pregnancy and birth without the love and support – both emotional and financial – of a partner is not easy, but many women do manage very well on their own and for some it is the preferred choice.

There are a number of reasons why a woman may find herself alone at this time. Perhaps the pregnancy was unplanned, unexpected and the result of a fling, and somehow it was too late or you did not want a termination. Perhaps your relationship with the baby's father ended during pregnancy, or you found yourself rejected and abandoned by a man for whom the challenge of fatherhood was too difficult or undesirable. Perhaps the father of the baby is unable to participate due to illness, or even death. Or perhaps you have decided to have a baby alone rather than miss out on parenthood altogether.

Whatever your situation, as any lone mother will tell you, you need all the help you can get. For a start, it is a good idea to contact one of the organizations which have been set up to help parents coping alone (see p. 347). They will be able to offer practical advice to help you overcome any financial, emotional or other problems you may experience, and will know the social security benefits to which you are entitled, and through them, you will be able to meet others in a similar position.

It will also be very useful to join an ante-natal preparation class, preferably one which begins in early pregnancy (see p. 87). If you let the teacher know that you are alone, she will be able to offer you special help and support. If you do not like the idea of being in a class with couples, you can go to one for women only.

Think ahead to the birth, and try to choose a place to have your baby where you will feel relaxed and comfortable. You might also consider asking someone to be with you for emotional help and support during labour and the birth. This person could be a women friend, relative, ante-natal teacher or a male friend who is not the father of the baby but who would like to offer you his support when you have your baby. Such a companion could also accompany you to preparation classes. If you do not know anyone who could fulfil this role, the hospital, your doctor or your ante-natal teacher may know of someone who would like to help, whom you could meet in advance. If you ask, some hospitals, even if this is not their usual policy, will also try to help by introducing you to one or two midwives who may attend you in labour.

On your own

You may have the support of your family, but very often – particularly if your parents are very conventional – they may be unwilling or unable to accept the fact that you are having a baby alone. This can be very hurtful and distressing. In addition, if most of your friends are married or living with a partner or, perhaps more especially, if they are single and have no children, it may be difficult for them to understand you.

Loneliness and having to manage alone are probably the most difficult problems that you will have to face. In fact, many of the problems ahead of you will be the same as those faced by a woman with a partner, but may be intensified without the presence of someone to offer you love and support and take over when you cannot cope. Put pride to one side and accept help that is offered, and consider in advance where and how you are going to live, so that you can make life as easy as possible.

Think beforehand about maintaining other interests as well as how you are going to manage to be a mother and still have a bit of time and freedom to yourself. For some while, your life will certainly revolve around the needs of your baby, and you are bound to find that your ability to go as you please is restricted. Although you can take a baby with you to most places, some things will be difficult or even impossible to manage. In the long run, it will help if you surrender to the inevitable from the beginning: accept that your life will be greatly circumscribed by the very fact that you have a baby, but take heart that, little by little, as your child grows and becomes more independent, you will regain an increasing amount of your freedom.

If the father of your baby has unexpectedly refused to take responsibility, you will need to come to terms with your feelings. You are bound to feel rejected, abandoned, angry and resentful, but for your own sake and that of your baby, try to reconcile yourself to the situation and, if possible, find emotional equilibrium.

Do everything you can to ensure that your baby will have everything he or she needs to remain contented and satisfied. Make your relationship with your son or daughter your top priority. The closer the bond between you and the smoother the transition during late pregnancy and contact immediately after birth, the easier it will be to cope with the early months of motherhood.

Financial considerations

Facing parenthood alone, you will probably have lost the luxury of choosing between working and staying at home. If you must work, you will also have to provide alternative childcare for your future son or daughter. If you can, try to sort this out before your baby is born; in some areas, nursery places, childminders and nannies are hard to come by. As a first step, check with the social services department of your local council. You should also make sure that you keep your employer informed of what is going on, and that you carefully follow every procedure for getting maternity benefit and allowance and for ensuring your right to return to work.

Having to depend on someone else to care for your child during most of her waking hours can be a very worrying and, sometimes, depressing prospect; it is also usually quite expensive. You may have feelings of inadequacy or that you have somehow failed your child or are not a 'proper' mother. However, if you choose your carer carefully, making sure it is someone that you *like* and can talk to as well as someone who has the right kind of facilities, you may find the arrangement not only enables you to work without worrying about your child, but also is a source of support. The presence of other children will help your child learn to become a sociable person, willing to share and take part in the rough and tumble games of childhood.

If, on the other hand, you stay at home (either by choice or circumstance), you may find it very difficult to manage financially. In effect, you must become a star performer in the art of cheap living. This can be very upsetting when all you want is the best for your child, but again, priorities are important here: your son or daughter is the most important thing in your life, and her happiness does not really depend on a continual supply of new clothes or the latest toys. Rather, it depends on you and your relationship. It is all too easy to let money worries blight your pregnancy and the first years of your child's life, and you must be firm with yourself to ensure that this does not happen.

Although it certainly helps to have two people available to parent a child, so long as your son or daughter has your love and feels wanted by you, he or she has every chance of becoming a healthy and happy child despite the difficulties you may encounter.

Emotional aspects

The emotional aspects of labour and birth, and of the establishment of a new family, which are just as important for a single parent, are described in Chapters 9, 12 and 17.

C H A P T E R   6

PREPARING FOR PARENTHOOD

After confirmation of your pregnancy, you will need to prepare for parenthood by ensuring your physical and emotional well-being throughout pregnancy. Ante-natal care is a part of this, and you can opt for care at a hospital-based clinic, shared care between a hospital and your family doctor or complete care by your GP and a community midwife.

Ante-natal care

Hospital-based ante-natal clinics offer new and sophisticated screening techniques to assess well-being and ensure safety of both mother and baby, but they can have two major disadvantages: a conveyor-belt atmosphere; and a clinical approach geared towards detecting abnormalities although the majority of pregnant women and their babies are perfectly healthy. Hospital-based care usually focuses on birth as an endpoint in itself, and the importance of preparing for and coping with the first months after the birth and the social, psychological and emotional needs of the parents may be neglected.

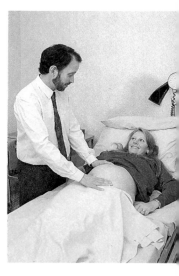

Checking the growth and position of the baby is an essential part of ante-natal check-ups.

Many women feel dissatisfied with hospital-based clinics, finding them too impersonal, and often involving them in a long wait before they are seen by staff who are working under tremendous pressure and are unable to give them sufficient or individual attention. Most hospitals are aware of the sorts of problems women experience, and many attempt to find ways to make visits to them more pleasant. However, this is still one of the unsolved problems of modern ante-natal care.

One of the great advantages of a home birth is that the woman receives both ante- and postnatal care from the same people, who will also attend the birth. In hospital, ante-natal care is usually separate from the labour ward. One solution to this – and to the problem of crowded hospital clinics – is the system of *shared care*, whereby routine checks are carried out by the family doctor and also occasionally by the hospital. Usually the GP will be more involved in early pregnancy, and as the due date draws closer, the hospital-based checks become more frequent.

Your first ante-natal visit

Your first ante-natal visit to your doctor, midwife or hospital clinic after pregnancy has been confirmed is an important occasion. It is an opportunity to meet some of the people who will be involved in your care during pregnancy. They will gain an overall view of your general health and pregnancy and will be able to advise you about the months to come. At this visit, you may wish to discuss the sort of birth you would like and your preferences as to the environment for birth (*see* Chapter 8).

The visit will continue with a thorough physical checkup, including a detailed exploration of the medical histories of both you and your partner, and that of both your families. This will provide an opportunity for discovering any obvious diseases or health problems, as well as ensuring that you are perfectly fit. You will also be given nutritional advice, genetic counselling (if appropriate), general information and reassurance. You may already have covered some or all of these things if you have had a pre-conceptual consultation before becoming pregnant.

The following are some of the topics that are usually investigated during both pre-conceptual and the first ante-natal checks:

Age Very young women may need extra help in preparing for motherhood. In women over 35, the risk of genetic abnormality is slightly higher, so they may be offered an amniocentesis test (*see* p. 86).

Reproductive and genital organs A full history of your menstrual function will be taken, to help estimate your expected 'due date', and an internal examination may be done to check your uterus and ovaries. A cervical smear test may also be performed. The urine is also tested (*see* below).

Digestive tract Nausea, vomiting, constipation and, sometimes, diarrhoea can all occur during pregnancy. Attention to nutrition beforehand can help to prevent these problems.

Respiratory system Women with chronic respiratory congestion, asthma or bronchitis may need special attention. Avoiding smoking and using certain homoeopathic remedies and physiotherapy, as well as good nutrition and exercise, are helpful.

Spine and pelvis Back pain and headaches are common problems, mostly arising from a postural imbalance of the spine. They may be aggravated by pregnancy (*see* Back and pelvic pain, Headache, p. 327).

Past illnesses and/or operations It is important to assess whether these will have any bearing on pregnancy or labour.

Social and family history The age, education and marital status of both partners, as well as your attitudes towards pregnancy and childbirth, will be discussed. Your hopes and fears as well as your own experiences during infancy and childhood are all relevant as you contemplate parenthood. In addition, it is important to discover if any of the following have occurred among members of your families: multiple births, diabetes, high blood pressure, heart disease, congenital abnormalities.

Diabetes If you have a family history of diabetes or if your urine contains sugar, you may be given a glucose tolerance test (*see* p. 85) to exclude diabetes (*see* Diabetes, p. 307).

Previous obstetric history A detailed obstetric history is vitally important in every pregnancy, and should include details of previous abortions and/or miscarriages, any difficulties with fertility and any previous problems during pregnancy, labour and childbirth.

Congenital abnormalities These are rare, and the incidence is particularly low in well-nourished women. However, women over the age of 35 (and possibly those whose partners are well into middle age) and couples with family histories of genetic defects need special genetic counselling (*see* pp. 87, 302) about the risk of abnormalities. Vitamin and mineral supplements before conception may reduce the incidence of spina bifida (*see* Neural tube defects, p. 324).

It is important to avoid having X-rays taken when you are attempting to conceive and when you are pregnant (*see* p. 333). However, as long as you are adequately protected, essential dental X-rays are generally safe.

Lifestyle If you are in the habit of smoking, taking medications, drinking alcohol or using drugs, you should consider their effects during pregnancy.

Nutrition One of the most important functions of pre-conceptual or ante-natal counselling is careful attention to your diet and eating habits; your nutrition during infancy and childhood may also have some bearing on the pregnancy. Now you have the opportunity to correct deficiencies or imbalances, and to learn how to improve your diet. (*See* Chapter 7.)

Your emotional state If you have any emotional or psychological difficulties – for example, if you suffer from depression or anxiety – or if you are having problems with relationships, you may benefit from counselling or psychotherapy before, during and/or after the pregnancy. Post-natal depression can sometimes be prevented in this way, and you may also be able to resolve any fears about pregnancy and parenthood.

Subsequent anti-natal visits

At every ante-natal visit, your blood pressure, weight and urine will be checked and recorded. Your attendants will examine your abdomen to check the growth of your baby and its position, the amount of amniotic fluid surrounding it, the size of the uterus and, at the end of pregnancy, whether the head has engaged (i.e. entered your pelvis). Your baby's heartbeat will also be checked in the later months, and near your due date you may be given an internal examination to assess your pelvic capacity and to ascertain whether your cervix has softened and thinned (effaced) prior to the onset of labour; however, such an examination is not always necessary. If there is an indication that your baby's growth is either reduced or excessive, other tests may be needed.

Most women want to find out whether their babies are well, how large they are, when labour is about to start and whether it is likely to be easy or difficult. However, while it is usually possible to assess the well-being of your baby, the onset or outcome of labour can never be predicted with certainty.

During the first 28 weeks of pregnancy, you will probably be advised to visit the ante-natal clinic once a month. Thereafter, the frequency of the visits increases until, during the last month, you will be asked to attend once a week. This means that you will have between seven and ten ante-natal appointments during pregnancy, although if problems arise you may wish to see your doctor more often.

An important part of each visit should be time spent in the discussion of any queries or problems that you may have.

Routine ante-natal tests

During pregnancy, a number of tests are carried out routinely, some only once and others at each visit.

Urine analysis At every ante-natal visit, you will be asked to bring a sample of your urine for testing. This should be a 'mid-stream' sample – that is, one collected midway through emptying your bladder – which will avoid the presence of vaginal secretions which can produce a false positive protein result. It is not necessary to collect this first thing in the morning.

As well as being tested for protein, which may be due to either urinary infection or occasionally (if associated with high blood pressure) pre-eclampsia (*see* p. 315), it is also tested for sugar, which may indicate diabetes. Sugar may occasionally be present in the urine of a non-diabetic woman because of the increased blood flow through the kidneys during pregnancy. Diabetes is proven by taking a glucose tolerance test (*see bottom of opposite page*).

Urine taken at your first visit is often sent to be cultured to test for infection. Bacteria and other organisms may be present without symptoms during pregnancy, and prompt treatment will prevent a flare-up of any infection later on.

Weight The primary reason for being weighed at each visit is to make you aware of the rate of your weight gain so that you can prevent an excess which may be difficult to shed after the birth. A low gain in the last few months may indicate slow growth of the baby and the need for special observation. If the baby is growing normally, slight weight loss in the mother at the end of pregnancy is not a problem. (*See*. pp. 321, 345.)

Blood pressure Your blood pressure will be measured each time you visit your doctor and also at frequent intervals during labour. The upper limit of normal blood pressure is 140/90 mm of mercury. High blood pressure (also called hypertension) can be a complication of pregnancy; if it is combined with fluid retention and/or protein in the urine, it is called pre-eclampsia and may need treatment (*see* p. 315).

Blood tests

Haemoglobin This is the red pigment in red blood cells that transports oxygen, and reduced levels indicate anaemia (*see* p. 292). A level of less than 10 grammes per 100 millilitres is abnormal. Haemoglobin is usually measured in early pregnancy and again during the last ten weeks.

Blood group Your blood group will be ascertained so that, in the rare case of an emergency arising, you can have a blood transfusion.

Rhesus (Rh) factor This is a biochemical molecule found in the red blood cells, and establishing its presence or absence is also part of blood grouping. (*See* Rhesus disease, p. 334.)

Rubella (German measles) A blood test will be performed to check whether you have ever had this. Since the symptoms of rubella are often so mild (and can be mistaken for those of other illnesses and vice versa), only a blood test can tell you if you have definitely had it. (*See* Rubella in pregnancy, p. 334.)

Syphilis A blood test for syphilis is also performed on pregnant women and, if present, the disease can be treated with antibiotics. (*See* p. 343.)

Special tests

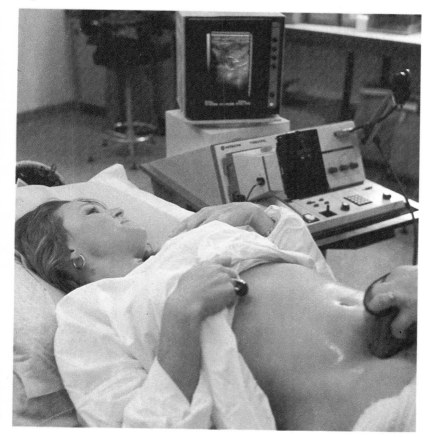

During an ultrasound scan, the image of the baby in the womb seen on the screen can offer valuable information about its well-being.

Ultrasound

This is a method of observing the baby in the womb by directing high-frequency sound waves through the mother's abdominal wall and into the amniotic fluid. Like radar, the sound waves bounce back to be picked up by a sensor on the abdominal wall and converted into electrical signals. These produce an image on a television screen which can be seen simultaneously by the mother and by the ultrasound operator.

To date, this sophisticated new technology appears safe for mother and child, although its long-term safety will not be known for a few decades. It is not necessary to screen all pregnancies routinely with ultrasound; however, in Britain the majority of pregnant women are offered a scan at 16 weeks to assess foetal well-being. (*See* pp. 340-1).

Blood tests

Glucose tolerance test This is performed if there is a likelihood of diabetes (*see* p. 307) – e.g. a family history or sugar in the urine. Blood samples are taken before and 2½ hours after drinking water containing a large amount of sugar (glucose) to assess the body's ability to clear glucose from the blood. If the blood glucose levels remain high, diabetes is present.

Alpha-foetoprotein (AFP) This is a protein which circulates in the baby's blood before birth, and small amounts escape from the foetal circulation into the mother's during pregnancy. AFP is measured between the 16th and 18th weeks of pregnancy because elevated levels may indicate an abnormal development of the brain or spinal cord – i.e. anencephaly (malformation of the skull) or spina bifida (malformation of the spinal column). If a higher than normal level is present, an ultrasound scan is essential to exclude causes such as twins, threatened miscarriage, inaccurate dating of pregnancy or maldevelopment of the baby's abdominal wall or intestinal tract. (*See* Neural tube defects, p. 324.) This test is done by taking a sample of maternal blood.

Hepatitis There are two types of this liver disease, both caused by viruses. Women who are carriers of hepatitis may pass on the infection to medical staff at the time of delivery. Screening for hepatitis is therefore becoming increasingly common.

Toxoplasmosis and cytomegalovirus Both of these infections may affect foetal development. Cytomegalovirus (*see* p. 306) probably affects more babies than rubella, but toxoplasmosis (*see* pp. 338-9) is common only in communities where undercooked meat is eaten. Vaccines are not available for either infection, and routine screening is not usually undertaken.

Sickle-cell disease and thalassaemia All women in high-risk groups are screened for these disorders of haemoglobin function (*see* p. 334).

AIDS The virus responsible for acquired immune deficiency syndrome can affect an unborn baby. The incidence of AIDS (*see* p. 290) is bound to increase over the next decade, and may make routine screening necessary.

Amniocentesis

In this test, a sample of amniotic fluid is withdrawn from the uterus by the insertion of a hollow needle through the mother's abdominal wall. The cells in the fluid are cultured and analysed to exclude a variety of congenital abnormalities. Amniocentesis is mainly performed to detect Down's syndrome (*see* Chromosomal abnormalities, p. 300), but also if there is a family history of certain congenital disorders (*see* pp. 300-1). The test is done at about the 16th week of pregnancy. Because there is a one per cent chance that the test itself may cause a miscarriage, it is only carried out if there is a significant risk of an abnormality. (*See* p. 291.)

Chorion biopsy

Cells from the placenta are obtained in about the ninth week of pregnancy by the insertion of a small needle through the cervix. Developed in the 1980s and used as an alternative to amniocentesis, this test gives results at an earlier stage, but its safety is still under evaluation. (*See* p. 291.)

The baby's well-being in late pregnancy

If you have had problems during pregnancy, you may require special tests in the later months to ascertain your baby's well-being.

If your baby is suspected of being 'small for dates' (*see* Low birth weight babies, p. 321), your obstetrician may suggest an ultrasound scan to help assess the baby's growth rate. If it is found that your child is small given the length of the pregnancy, you may be asked to record the pattern of the baby's movements on a 'kick chart', and the foetal heart rate may be monitored and recorded. Another ultrasound scan may be used to measure blood flow to the uterus, placenta and baby.

Genetic counselling

In every pregnancy, there is a small risk of the baby being born with a congenital abnormality. However, the vast majority of problems occur as one-off phenomena, and it is unlikely that even a significant minority of congenital defects will be diagnosed in the months before birth.

Nevertheless, if by virtue of your age, ethnic background or family history, your baby has a significant risk of an abnormality, genetic counselling may be needed, either before you become pregnant or after you have conceived. This is usually begun by the family doctor and continued by the midwife or obstetrician, and in some circumstances, a specialist genetic counsellor may also be involved. You may need advice about conception, whether ante-natal tests are available, what risks are involved and what your options are. (*See* pp. 301-2.)

Education during pregnancy

Entering motherhood or fatherhood is a stage in the life cycle known as a 'rite of passage' and is as significant as the transition from childhood to adolescence and from adolescence to adulthood, and it is immensely helpful to meet other people at the same stage in their lives, to share experiences and gain knowledge together. At ante-natal classes you can meet other pregnant women who live locally, and couples classes will provide men with a similar opportunity.

These are sometimes called 'parentcraft' classes, a name which is perhaps misleading as it implies concentration on the practical rather than the emotional aspects of birth and parenthood. Ante-natal classes involve exploring the options available to you in giving birth and caring for your baby, increasing self-awareness and understanding and helping you to have the best possible experience of pregnancy, labour, childbirth and early infancy. They usually cover the basic physiology of labour and birth, and include practice for labour with breathing, relaxation, massage and positions for labour and birth. They are also valuable sources of information about all aspects of birth and parenthood, medical practices and other topics.

Classes are offered at a variety of places. If you are having your baby in hospital, the classes offered there may, among other things, provide you with an opportunity to discuss the policies and practices of the hospital, and may be very helpful, even if you attend classes elsewhere as well. In addition, classes are held by ante-natal clinics and local health centres, and there are also several organizations which run them (*see* p. 347).

The quality of classes varies widely, as does the approach, ranging from the more didactic, academic way of teaching with lectures and discussion to classes run on lines of group participation. Both these factors can depend on the teacher, so it is wise to investigate what is available in your area by talking to other women who have attended them as well as to the teacher before making your final choice of which ante-natal class to attend.

Some classes run for a period of six to eight weeks with meetings every week. It is advisable to attend such a course in the last three months of your pregnancy.

Other classes are ongoing throughout pregnancy and may include activities such as yoga-based exercise, meditation and massage. These tend to make the most of the marvellous opportunity for change and healing in pregnancy, rather than concentrating on the last few months, and promote your health during pregnancy, ensuring that you approach the birth physically fit. Yoga-based exercise is particularly effective in helping women to discover their instinctive potential for giving birth, and to develop ease with the upright and supported postures natural to labour and birth. If such a group is not available in your area, you might consider starting your own, working from the self-help guide in Part V.

It is essential that ante-natal classes should also include advice about feeding and caring for babies in the days and weeks after birth. You may not realize how important it is to prepare during pregnancy for the postnatal period, but adequate knowledge and previous practical experience will prove to be very helpful during the first weeks of your baby's life. Take any opportunity you can to attend events where parents and their babies will be present, so that you can become familiar with infants and what is involved in early parenthood. Baby massage and baby gymnastics groups are becoming more popular, and there pregnant women and their partners have a chance to hold and massage young babies and observe how other mothers and fathers handle and care for their children.

In addition, you may learn from your own parents, other members of your family and friends, and your midwife, family doctor and obstetrician.

An ante-natal class offering yoga-based exercise.

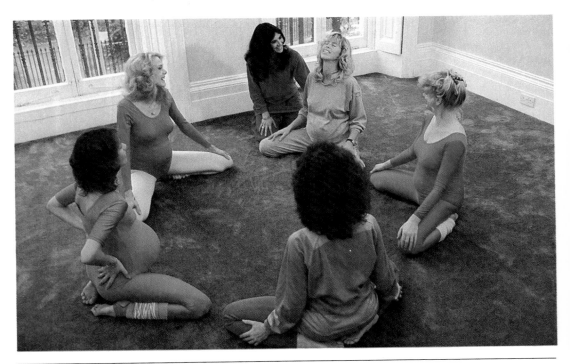

Your lifestyle during pregnancy

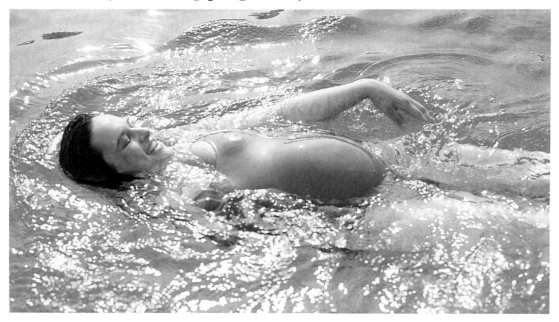

Rest and sleep

Ideally, every pregnant woman should be able to sleep as much as she needs to. The amount varies enormously – from five to ten hours – but on average, most people require about eight hours. It is also a good idea to put your feet up for a while every afternoon, and this may be particularly needed during the first and last three months. Sometimes, due to the pressures of work or of other children, this is difficult to achieve, but you should try to rest whenever the opportunity presents itself.

Your body will soon tell you if you need more sleep than you are getting. Ideally, it is best to follow the messages it is sending you, sleeping a lot when you feel like it or relaxing in other ways when you do not. (*See also* pp. 43-44, 338.)

Fitness, exercise and nutrition

You will find that physical fitness is a tremendous asset during pregnancy, in labour and during the postnatal months. If you were in the habit of exercising before pregnancy, you can continue, but you may have to alter the amount and type of exercise you do. Exercise usually improves your vitality and feeling of well-being, but you should obey your body and not overdo it. (*See* Part V.) A balanced diet with regular, nutritious meals will help you to feel your best. (*See* Chapter 7.)

Going out

Many pregnant women are tired at night, and do not enjoy going out as much as they did before. It is best to listen to what your body tells you. Crowded, hot and smoke-filled places may make you feel sick, faint or uncomfortable. If you feel faint, go out into the fresh air.

Swimming is excellent exercise in pregnancy.

Looking good and feeling good

How you look can certainly influence how you feel and vice versa. Taking special care of your appearance during pregnancy will boost your confidence, as well as give pleasure to you and those around you. This is a perfect time to pamper yourself, to be comfortable and to have fun with your appearance, experimenting with new ideas and even adding a touch of humour to your pregnant form.

Clothes Maternity clothes are widely available but can be expensive, especially if you do not plan another pregnancy and they cannot be adapted to non-pregnant life. You could investigate second-hand shops which specialize in maternity clothes (and also usually babies' and children's clothes). It is possible to find unusual clothing combinations that express your individuality, so that you do not have to accept the first smock or pair of maternity dungarees that comes your way. Tracksuits are very comfortable and ideal for exercising.

Increased sweating is common in pregnancy, and clothes made of natural fibres – i.e. cotton, wool, silk, linen – are advisable as these will allow your skin to breathe and you will be more comfortable. The same holds true for underwear: well-fitting cotton bras (with plenty of support) and cotton underpants. Avoid tight clothes, especially if they constrict the abdomen.

Wear sensible, flat-heeled shoes. Make sure that your feet can breathe, going barefoot indoors and outdoors in warm weather, and wearing open sandals if possible.

Skin, hair and nails Your skin mirrors your health, so the most important way to improve your skin is through rest, exercise and a good diet. However, it too needs individual attention. Use a good cleanser and moisturizer daily, preferably ones without a chemical base.

It is a good idea to take a relaxing bath every night. Use oil instead of soap: put a few drops of coconut, almond or olive oil or lanolin in the bath. A few drops of essential oil – e.g. basil, cedar, camphor, cypress or flower-fragrances – can be soothing or revitalizing. You can also use oil to massage your whole body after your bath, concentrating especially on your breasts and belly.

Take extra care of your hair, getting a good haircut and using conditioning treatments so that you make the most of the shine and glow of pregnancy. Treat split-ends and dandruff, and be sure to wear a hat in hot sunshine. You should probably avoid changing your hair colour while you are pregnant, so that chemicals are not absorbed through your scalp.

If your nails have become brittle, as very occasionally happens in pregnancy, apply oil to them every night.

Making love during pregnancy

Being pregnant is bound to affect your feelings about sexuality and those of your partner. Carrying a baby and giving birth are major events in your sexual life: during pregnancy, your love-making is bearing fruit, and giving birth can be a profound and deeply orgasmic experience. You may feel an increased interest in sex throughout pregnancy and enjoy the freedom from concern about contraception. On the other hand, you or your partner may be less interested in sexual intercourse and more inclined to express your tenderness and affection in other ways.

The first trimester Once the pregnancy is confirmed, many find that there is an increase in sexual desire and a new sense of relaxation – ironically enough, because there is no concern about falling pregnant!

It is also true that, in the first trimester, you may find the physiological and hormonal changes you are experiencing quite difficult. You may be tired and suffering from nausea, and therefore not particularly interested in making love. Instead, you may want to be held or given a massage.

Either you or your partner may have certain anxieties about making love at this time. A common fear is of losing the baby, but there is no need to be concerned about this – sexual intercourse normally has no effect on whether or not a woman miscarries (*see* Miscarriage, pp. 323-4.).

Sometimes making love can cause slight spotting because the blood vessels around the cervix are more plentiful during pregnancy, and some of them may rupture. If this happens, you should abstain from intercourse until after you have consulted your doctor so that he or she can rule out any other cause for the bleeding. It may be wise to try out some different positions and perhaps avoid deep penetration. Also, if you have miscarried often before, you may be advised to avoid intercourse for the first 12 weeks.

Another possible worry may be that making love will cause an infection, or that deep penetration and pressure on the cervix and uterus will somehow harm the tiny developing baby. This is impossible as the growing baby is protected by the membranes of the amniotic sac and by the amniotic fluid. Also, the cervix is tightly closed and sealed by a protective plug of mucus until labour starts. In fact, the baby is well above the vagina and cannot be injured while you make love.

These anxieties are very common and can cause conflict and frustration. It is important to communicate and to be open with one another because, if one partner is worried and makes love just to please the other, this will merely lead to tension. True love-making means staying in touch, emotionally as well as physically.

The second trimester This is generally the most comfortable time for love-making, as the initial adjustment to pregnancy has been made. Many of the physical discomforts of the first three months tend to disappear at this stage, and the fear of miscarriage is lessened. Although your abdomen begins to bulge in these months, it is not yet large enough to present any obstacle to love-making. You will also become more aware of your baby moving inside you at this time. For most women, it is the most relaxed part of pregnancy, and many find that they make love with greater abandon than ever before; it is not uncommon for a woman to have her first real orgasm. Orgasm causes the uterus to contract, and during pregnancy, the post-orgasmic phase (when the uterus relaxes) tends to be slower, so that the uterus tightens and remains contracted for some time before altering. This is natural and very common, but often a woman experiencing this for the first time may be startled or worried that something may be amiss. Neither of the two old folktales about orgasm – that it either deprives the baby of oxygen or brings on premature labour – is true.

You may find that new positions that you have never tried before will be enjoyable and more comfortable, and this is a good time to experiment with different ways of expressing your love and affection. Oral and manual sex, as well as masturbation, are enjoyed by many during pregnancy, and there is no danger to the baby in these practices.

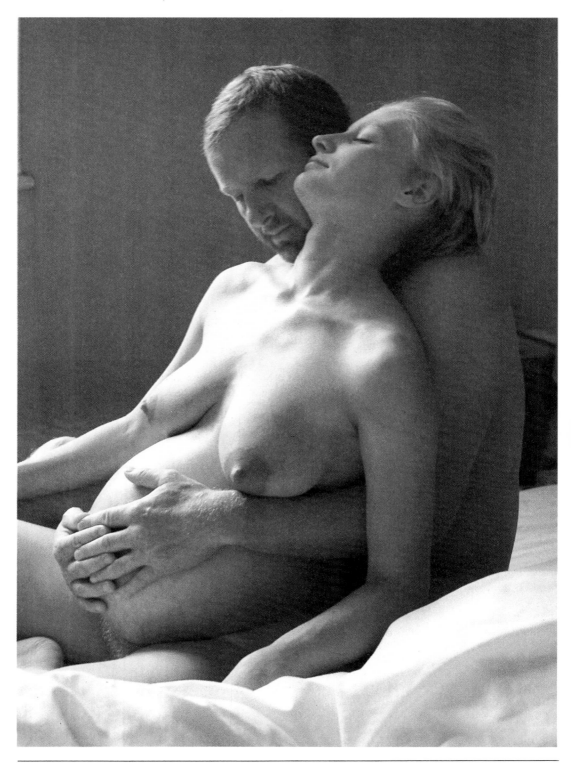

It is helpful to know that the tissues of the vagina often become fuller and more abundant during pregnancy, and that the secretions and lubricating fluids also increase, so that the normal taste and feel of your genital area may be quite different.

Moving and preparing your home

Despite the fact that it is preferable to avoid moving house during pregnancy, it is surprising how many couples do so. You may well find yourself moving to a larger flat or house or even to a different area. Or perhaps you will decide to make alterations to the home you are in.

A change of home can be an exhausting and disturbing as well as an exciting event. You can make it less traumatic by having a relaxed attitude. Put your pregnancy before anything else, and let other people help.

Your baby will not mind at all if your house is chaotic; so long as you are near him and you are calm, that is all that is needed. It is not necessary to have a bedroom for the baby organized and decorated. For the first few months it is preferable to have your baby in your own room.

Travel and driving

Undertaking short trips generally presents no problems, and many enjoy a holiday or change of environment during pregnancy. Longer trips can be fatiguing, particularly jet travel, and it is important to ensure that you get adequate rest before, during and after the journey, especially if there is a change in time zone. When travelling by air, make sure that you drink plenty of fluids to avoid dehydration.

The ideal time to travel in pregnancy is between the 16th and the 28th weeks. In early pregnancy, when the baby is going through the vital embryonic period and your energy may be low, travel is generally not advisable, and in the weeks approaching birth, it is best to stay close to home. However, sometimes travel is necessary during these times and should not be harmful if you are well cared for.

If you are travelling by air, check with the airline before you do so as they have different regulations concerning pregnant women. Some demand a medical certificate from your doctor, which states that it is all right for you to travel; most will not carry women more than 36 weeks pregnant.

It is quite safe to continue to drive a car during pregnancy. Many women are anxious that their baby may be harmed in an accident, but since the baby is protected by the amniotic sac and the strong walls of the uterus, this rarely happens. If driving is uncomfortable during the last few weeks, or concentration lessens, it may be advisable to stop driving until after the birth.

The third trimester In the last three months, as the time of the birth approaches, your belly will become much larger and you are bound to feel somewhat heavier and less comfortable. You may also be sleeping restlessly and thus may feel quite tired and need to rest more. Many couples feel unnecessarily anxious that their baby will be disturbed either physically or emotionally if they make love.

Your interest in sex may decrease and so may that of your partner, but if the opposite is the case, there is no need to abstain. Some women feel more sexual than ever when approaching childbirth, and it is possible to make

Hazards at work

If you enjoy your work, there is no reason to stop unless you are employed in an environment that can be harmful to your baby – for example, if you work:

- with paint or lead or mercury compounds.
- in a big industrial complex.
- in a place which produces chemical waste.
- in a hospital operating theatre or anywhere else where anaesthetics are frequently used.
- with visual display units (VDUs), as found with computers and word processors.
- with X-rays.

If any of these are the case, you should be adequately screened (if possible) or given alternative work away from areas of danger.

love right up to the last minute, provided the waters have not broken. Whatever your inclinations, your need for sharing and affection will almost certainly be increased. Your partner, too, will need to feel that your love and attention is not only directed towards the baby; he needs to know and feel that some of it is his.

Sex in pregnancy can be a shared intimacy that will nurture you during your adjustment to parenthood. Most important of all, expressing your emotions, however you do it, and being open with one another about your difficulties, likes and dislikes will help you to keep in touch and enjoy the deepening and maturing of your relationship.

Many men find their pregnant partners immensely desirable, and like to make love frequently and passionately. However, some do experience problems in adapting their sexual needs to the fact that their partners are pregnant. The change in the pattern of love-making is an important aspect of adjusting to the advent of a new baby and the demands the child will make on the parents' relationships.

There is often a deep fear, which men frequently do not express, of injuring the baby or their partner, who may seem very fragile to them. Some also worry that the baby, who is able to hear and feel, is like an intrusive onlooker, and that making love in late pregnancy is no longer a private event between two people.

It is important to remember that touching and physical contact is very important during pregnancy and childbirth. If full sexual intercourse is not desired, other ways of making love, or massage, may be very satisfying.

Working during pregnancy

Many women feel very fit during pregnancy, and working until labour begins poses no problem.

If you find that work is tiring or even exhausting, it may be advisable to leave or try to improve the facilities or routines at work so that you are able to rest. For instance, in a flexitime system, it may be possible for women to arrange working times to suit their pregnancies. In any case, it is common to stop work sometime during the last three months, especially if continuing makes you feel drained and exhausted. However, if financial or other circumstances make leaving your employment impossible, try your best to put your feet up during the day, and do not overstretch yourself unnecessarily.

Many working women are legally entitled to return to their previous jobs after having a baby; most others (but usually not the self-employed) are also entitled to statutory maternity pay, provided the correct National Insurance contributions have been paid. This benefit is payable from 11 weeks before your due date – i.e. at the end of the 29th week – and continues for up to eighteen weeks altogether (unless your trade union has negotiated a better deal). The conditions under which you can receive this pay and other allowances, and for keeping your right to return to work, are quite complicated, so you should read carefully the relevant pamphlets from the Department of Health and Social Security (for maternity pay) and the Department of Employment (for returning to work) and ask your trade union representative.

Some women need or want to return to work soon after the birth, and thus must make adequate plans for someone else to care for the baby during working hours (see p. 346).

C H A P T E R 7

NUTRITION

The quality of our food and the way we eat it plays a vital role in the maintenance of our health and well-being. During pregnancy, nutrition becomes even more important, as your body now has to provide you *and* your baby with essential nutrients, drawn from your daily diet and from your body stores. Making sure that you are eating well is one of the most important ways to ensure that you will be at your best for pregnancy, childbirth and motherhood.

Over the past century, with the development of industry and mass production, food has become increasingly processed and refined – in fact, over two-thirds of the foods now eaten were developed after 1945. Animals are factory-farmed and often fed or injected with antibiotics and hormones; cereal grains are stripped of their nutritious husks while being refined into flour; vegetables are often frozen or canned months before reaching the table, and even fresh vegetables and fruit are sprayed with pesticides and herbicides. The largest growth area has been the massive rise in the consumption of sugar, food additives and 'junk' foods. These products add to our calorie intake and increase the size of our food bills while reducing the nutritional quality of our diet. Poor nutrition plays a major role in the cause of many common illnesses and diseases. To overcome this, our diets should include more fibre-filled raw foods, cereals, vegetables and grains, and fewer highly processed and fatty foods and additives.

Selecting ingredients to achieve a well-balanced diet can be confusing. The following is intended as a guide to help you understand the nutritional value of different foods, and to ensure that the way your food is prepared and cooked preserves its valuable nutrients.

Nourishing your baby

While you are pregnant, your baby receives from your bloodstream via the placenta all the nourishment needed for her development. Amino acids (for building proteins), saccharides (for sugars), fatty acids, minerals and vitamins as well as complex molecules such as antibodies – all cross the placenta into your baby's bloodstream. Even when a woman is nutritionally deficient, her body will try to ensure that the baby receives the nutrients required for normal development. For example, if the mother is anaemic, she will become even more so as the placenta extracts from her blood as much iron as is required to build up the baby's store of this vital mineral.

Nevertheless, it is obviously preferable to be at your physical best and avoid dietary deficiencies by making sure that your diet is well balanced so that your bloodstream contains all the nutrients you and your baby need. Adequate nutrition is available to most women in Western society.

Your needs during pregnancy

Nutritional requirements are individual, varying from woman to woman. They depend not only on climate and occupation but also on lifestyle, basic metabolism, the amount of exercise a person undertakes and so on – there is no perfect formula. Nutritional needs increase during pregnancy, due to the extra energy needed to circulate the blood through the body to the placenta to nourish the baby as her organs and skeleton develop. The blood supply needed for the growth and functioning of the placenta is equivalent to that required by an extra vital organ.

Weight and weight gain

In pregnancy, the overall quality of the diet is more important than weight gain. A woman who is overweight is less likely to be malnourished than someone who is underweight, although excessive weight can be difficult to lose after the birth (see p. 345). In addition, women differ in their tendency to put on weight during pregnancy: some gain a lot in the beginning and find that their weight levels off later on, while others gain more at the end. This is discussed in full in Chapter 3, page 34.

If you were overweight before pregnancy, attention to your diet is essential to ensure that you are eating well but avoiding foods that will increase this tendency. Similarly, women who are underweight before pregnancy need to be particularly careful to concentrate on the quality of their daily diets to make up the weight and nourishment.

If your weight before pregnancy was normal, it is more important to eat a well-balanced diet than to watch the scales. While every woman should gain some weight during pregnancy, you do not need to 'eat for two'. In fact, you only need approximately 500 extra calories a day, and this can be found in a very small amount of food – for example, 100 g (3½ oz) of nuts or 200 g (7 oz) of muesli. Instead, you can safely follow your appetite to satisfy your nutritional needs, as long as you make sure that your diet is well balanced and contains all the nutrients you need.

Your needs at different times

While optimum nutrition should be maintained before and throughout pregnancy, the demands on your body and those on your baby's will change during this time.

Pre-conception Experts believe that this is the most important time nutritionally. Attention to diet in the weeks and months leading up to conception will ensure that your bloodstream contains adequate quantities of the minerals, vitamins and other nutrients needed during the important embryonic phase in the early weeks of pregnancy.

First trimester During the first three months of pregnancy, your baby's organs are developing, and this is a period when it is best to avoid extremes. It is unwise to change your diet drastically from, say, one that includes meat to a wholly vegetarian one: it will take your body months to adjust to the alteration. Rather, try to eat unrefined and unprocessed foods.

This is also a time when nausea may make it difficult for you to eat whatever you want, but the baby will be able to use the nutritional reserves your body has stored until a fully balanced diet can be achieved. Try eating small snacks including complex carbohydrates and proteins, while eliminating stimulants, particularly refined sugar, from the diet (*see* Essential foods, *below*).

Second trimester The fourth to sixth months of pregnancy are generally the most comfortable. This is when your nutritional state is often at its peak, as you enjoy your pregnancy and look forward to the birth. You will probably have a hearty appetite, and care should be taken to eat well while avoiding excess. Nutrition is important now as your baby will be growing rapidly.

Third trimester Good nutrition remains essential as you approach childbirth and motherhood. Take particular care to avoid foods that cause indigestion or constipation. Balancing your diet will help to reduce excessive weight gain, will help you to sleep and will provide you with the strength and energy you need for labour and breastfeeding.

Appetite

Generally, your appetite will increase, reflecting the increased nutritional needs of pregnancy. If the appetite is reduced in early pregnancy because of nausea, or if in the last three months it is physically difficult to eat very much at one sitting, try eating small amounts more frequently. This can mean eating several times a day: early morning, mid-morning, lunch, mid-afternoon and dinner. It is also important to eat slowly and chew your food thoroughly, thereby prolonging the meal, avoiding overeating and preventing indigestion.

Sometimes a lack of appetite may be caused by dietary deficiency, especially a shortage of B vitamins and/or zinc. By eating foods rich in these (*see below*) for a few days, even if you do not feel like it, you will probably find that your appetite soon returns.

Food fads and cravings

Women may sometimes find that certain foods – especially coffee and fried or rich foods – are intolerable during pregnancy. On the other hand, some develop cravings for particular foods – often sweet ones, but also unlikely combinations of foods – or (rarely now that most people are well nourished) for substances not intended to be eaten, such as coal, soil and toothpaste. This last is a condition called *pica*. It may be due to some nutritional deficiency, often of iron or other minerals such as calcium, zinc or cobalt.

Cravings for or intolerance of certain foods may be caused by changes in the balance of hormones in the body which occur during pregnancy and which, in turn, affect the taste buds. As long as the liking or disliking of certain foodstuffs is kept within reason, it is not harmful. However, excessive eating of soft fruit, puddings and cakes, refined foods, chocolate and other sweets, fizzy drinks, fruit juices and ice cream will cause excess weight gain.

If you develop a craving to eat between meals, snacks could take the form of slow-burning carbohydrates, such as nuts, raisins and other dried fruit, and raw vegetables and fruit – e.g. carrots, celery and apples. Keeping a small supply of these with you is useful. If your diet is well-rounded and nourishing, you will find that food fads will be reduced.

Essential vitamins and minerals

Vitamins

	Effect on the body	Best food sources
A	Raises resistance to infections; feeling of well-being; promotes tooth & skin health; keeps mucous membranes moist & aids healing; helps regulate the thyroid gland.	Parsley, kale, spinach, greens, chard, broccoli leaves & flowers, turnip greens, carrots, apricots, red peppers, sweet potatoes, dried peaches, lettuce, egg yolk, whole milk cheese, fish-liver oils, Chinese cabbage, butter, liver.
B_1 (thiamin)	Calms & soothes nervous system; aids digestion & metabolic function of body cells.	Wheatgerm, dried beans, peanuts, dried chickpeas, buckwheat, hazelnuts, wheat bran, oat bran, green leafy vegetables, egg yolk, fish roe, Jerusalem artichokes, fresh pineapple, roast pork, kidney, liver.
B_2 (riboflavin)	Essential for breakdown & assimilation of carbohydrates; oxygenation of cells & maintenance of healthy tissue; anti-stress & anti-itching.	Brewer's yeast powder, egg yolk, cottage cheese, green leafy vegetables, poultry, mushrooms, milk, liver.
B_3 (nicotinic acid, niacin)	Dilates blood vessels; reduces levels of cholesterol; helpful for circulatory problems; regulates blood sugar.	Green leafy vegetables, fish oils, peanuts, mushrooms, brewer's yeast powder, liver, beef.
B_5 (pantothenic acid)	Helps cortisone release; increases energy.	Calves' liver, beans, chickpeas, soya beans, brown rice, bulgar wheat, nuts, molasses, egg yolks, avocado pears.
B_6 (pyridoxine)	Anti-pollutant; essential for absorption & conversion of proteins; reduces fluid retention; anti-stress; needed for hormone formation; combats nausea.	Soya beans, brewer's yeast powder, green leafy vegetables, seaweeds, oat & wheat bran, sunflower seeds, black treacle, salmon, liver, beef.
B_{12} (cyano-cobalamine)	Plays vital role in synthesis of nucleic acid; vital for cell formation; important in production of red blood cells.	Brewer's yeast & yeast extracts, dairy produce, fish, organ meats, seaweeds, wheatgerm, oysters, beef, pork.
Folic acid	Aids in iron use & maintaining blood volume; body requires double the normal amount during pregnancy.	Dark leafy greens, brewer's yeast, root vegetables, whole grains, oysters, salmon, whole milk, dates, mushrooms, orange juice, liver.
C (ascorbic acid)	Increases resistance to infection; natural antibiotic; tones capillary walls; prevents formation of ulcers; anti-pollutant; needed for healthy teeth, gums & connective tissue; important in absorption of iron.	All citrus fruits & juices, onions, garlic, red & green peppers, parsley, blackcurrants, horseradish, green leafy vegetables, rosehips, oregano, paprika, strawberries, watermelon, potatoes. Absorption enhanced by bioflavonoids found in grapes & citrus fruits.

D	Necessary for absorption of calcium phosphate; essential for health & growth of bones, functioning of nervous system & teeth formation; especially needed during breastfeeding.	Sunlight, fish liver oils, butter, milk, egg yolk, chicken & beef liver.
E	Controls formation of fibrin (the blood-clotting agent); keeps blood flowing smoothly; helps tissue oxygenation.	Wheatgerm, butter, eggs, lettuce, peanuts, whole grains, milk, spinach, black treacle, soya beans, sunflower, pumpkin & sesame seeds, avocados.
F	Essential fatty acids. Reduce cholesterol; prevent heart disease.	Polyunsaturated, cold-pressed oils, nuts, sesame seeds.
K	Important for blood flow; helps to clot blood; especially needed during last trimester of pregnancy for baby's clotting system; made by bacteria in bowel & can be reduced by antibiotics.	*Precursors:* alfalfa sprouts, brewer's yeast, dark green leafy vegetables, soya beans, sunflower oil, seaweeds, egg yolk, black treacle, cauliflower.

Minerals

Iron	Carries oxygen in blood throughout body; stimulates vital processes of cells; most important mineral in pregnancy; one-third is absorbed by baby to form blood & store in liver.	Cherry juice, seaweeds, brewer's yeast powder, brown meats, liver, green leafy vegetables, whole grains, pulses, sprouted seeds & grains, sunflower seeds, dried fruits, watermelon, egg yolk, nuts, mushrooms, beetroot.
Calcium	Essential for structure of bones & teeth of mother & baby, & normal functioning of nerves and muscles; natural tranquilliser.	Whole milk, milk products, dark green leafy vegetables, shellfish, salmon, black treacle, prunes, almonds, egg yolk, nuts, seeds, sprouted seeds & grains, seaweeds, sesame seeds, oranges, papayas, watermelon, bone meal, carrots.
Phosphorus	Works in conjunction with calcium & vitamin D; essential to healthy bones & teeth; helps maintain alkalinity of blood; necessary for gland function.	Wheat bran, wheatgerm, dairy products, whole grains, pulses, egg yolk, peanuts, white meat, nuts, tuna, all seaweeds.
Potassium	Activates many enzymes; essential for muscle contraction; keeps sodium in balance in body.	Bananas, avocado pears, dates, elderberries, papayas, stewed prunes, pulses, dried apricots, sunflower seeds, whole grains, vegetables, kelp.
Magnesium	Helps in absorption of proteins & utilization of fats, carbohydrates & enzymes; keeps calcium in balance; tranquilliser & anti-depressant.	All sprouted seeds & grains, green leafy vegetables, wheatgerm, seaweeds, seafood, black treacle, nuts, avocado pears, dates, dried apricots, bone meal.
Zinc	Needed for healthy growth & brain & nerve formation; works in conjunction with other minerals; involved in enzyme production; speeds healing; anti-nausea. Essential in breastfeeding.	Bananas, wheat germ & bran, whole grains, meat, fish, seeds, seaweeds, nuts, pulses, all sprouted grains & seeds, dairy products, oysters.

Essential foods

All foods consist of proteins, carbohydrates, fats, vitamins and minerals in varying proportions. Your digestive system breaks down complex foods into their constituents for absorption through the intestine into the bloodstream, after which they are used or stored by the body.

Protein

The most important increased need in pregnancy is for protein which, in the form of long chains of amino acids, supplies the 'building blocks' for the growth and repair of cells in your body and your baby's, as well as energy. A woman normally needs approximately 46 g (about 1½ oz) of protein daily, but in pregnancy this can rise to 75–100 g (2½–3½ oz) per day, an increase of between 63 and 117 per cent, depending on the individual.

Your protein intake should be spread throughout the day, incorporating foods which satisfy your palate while providing other essential nutrients for your body. Protein concentration is highest in meat, fish, cheese, eggs (an especially well-balanced source in pregnancy), most nuts, dried peas, beans and lentils, and in grains such as rice, wheat, oats, barley and maize.

Of the 20 different types of amino acid, the body manufactures all but eight, which must be found in food. Some protein foods are used more efficiently by the body than others. Vegetable proteins generally contain what are known as 'limiting amino acids', and in order to provide the full amount of essential amino acids, they must be combined in complementary groups. This is easy to do if you make sure that pulses (e.g. peas, beans, lentils) are always eaten in combination with grains. For example, the protein in peanut butter is more accessible if it is eaten with bread, and beans should be combined with rice, and lentils with rice or wholewheat pasta. On the other hand, soya beans and products made from them contain the most complete vegetable protein, equal to that of cheese. Animal proteins are more digestible eaten without carbohydrates.

Carbohydrates (sugars)

All carbohydrate foods are broken down in the intestine into sugars which are used in the body for energy. However, the way in which they act within your digestive system and in your bloodstream can differ dramatically. They can be divided into two sorts: refined and unrefined.

Refined carbohydrates are those which have been processed in some way from the raw plant material. They include brown and white sugar, molasses, treacle, maple syrup and glucose. While they are absorbed by the bloodstream quickly and so provide energy at a faster rate than unrefined carbohydrates, this is not usually needed if the diet is a balanced one.

Blackstrap molasses, *real* maple syrup and honeycomb (preferably not from bees fed with sugar) contain a variety of nutrients including calcium, iron and potassium as well as traces of B vitamins. Refined white and brown sugar have virtually no nutritional value – which is why they are called 'empty calories' – and eating too much can upset blood sugar balance and use up B vitamins. All refined sugars can cause tooth decay.

Unrefined carbohydrates are found in a wide variety of foods, particularly wholewheat flour and bread, brown rice, wholegrain cereals, dried pulses (lentils, beans, etc.) and unpeeled potatoes. These foods are also valuable sources of vitamins and minerals.

In addition, unrefined carbohydrate foods contain varying amounts of indigestible cellulose and other substances which form the cell walls of the plants from which they come, and this *dietary fibre* is vital for proper digestion and bowel movements. It virtually eliminates constipation if eaten in sufficient quantities, and ensures that the energy contained in the food is delivered to the body slowly and steadily.

Refined white flour and white rice do contain about the same amount of protein and carbohydrate (of the refined type) as their wholemeal and brown counterparts, but they are absorbed very quickly, and lack the important vitamins and minerals found in the discarded husks (although manufacturers have by law to add iron and two B vitamins to white bread). Some bakers make bread brown by adding brown sugar, so be careful always to buy bread that is marked as 'wholemeal' or 'wholewheat'.

Fats

Fats consist of chains of fatty acids which are essential for the normal functioning of the body, particularly the nervous system. However, weight for weight, they provide more energy (i.e. calories) than any other food.

By metabolizing carbohydrates and protein, the liver is capable of producing some of the fatty acids that the body requires. However, fats must remain an important part of our diets as they carry the fat-soluble vitamins A and D, as well as other essential fatty acids. Fats can be broadly divided into two categories: saturated and polyunsaturated. *Saturated* fats have been found to raise levels of cholesterol in the blood and have thus been implicated in heart disease and other degenerative illnesses. They tend to be solid at room temperature and usually come from animals – e.g. butter and other dairy products, the fat on and in meat, lard and dripping.

Polyunsaturated fats, on the other hand, somewhat lower the amount of cholesterol in the blood. They tend to be liquid at room temperature, and are most frequently found in plant foods, although fish oils generally contain large amounts. In addition, all nuts and the husks of wholegrain cereals contain small quantities of polyunsaturated fats, sufficient for the body's well-being. The best types of oils to use are sesame, sunflower, corn and walnut, all of which are primarily polyunsaturated, and olive oil, which is mono-unsaturated and thus does not affect the blood cholesterol.

Cold-pressed oils are preferable because the fat is released when the plant is compressed and heat, which can cause polyunsaturated fats to decline, is not involved in the process. Frying foods at high temperatures can cause the release of toxic 'free fatty acids', as well as adding calories – for example, fried potatoes contain five times the number of calories as the same weight of jacket potatoes.

Although our diets will contain both saturated and unsaturated fats, the latter should comprise most of our intake of this essential food.

Vitamins and minerals

Essential constituents of the body, vitamins and minerals are needed for the normal function of the blood, tissues and all the cells. In conjunction with other nutrients and enzymes, they work within each system of the body as well as in each cell to ensure that our metabolism performs at its best. None of the minerals and only insufficient amounts of vitamins can be manufactured by the body, and so they must be taken in with our food or in the form of supplements.

Delicate mechanisms within the body ensure that, for the most part, we maintain optimal levels of each. However, consumption of excessive amounts of any one may overload the body and cause harm – e.g. an excess of sodium (as found in table salt) can contribute to high blood pressure (hypertension), and too much aluminium and copper (both dangerous) can be obtained by cooking in pots and pans made from them. By contrast, too little of a mineral or vitamin will deplete the body's stores and may lead to one of a number of deficiency diseases, such as anaemia from too little iron, scurvy from low amounts of vitamin C and rickets from lack of vitamin D.

Poor dietary habits will reduce the amounts of vitamins and minerals available to be used on a daily basis. Some types can be stored in the body for months, but others have to be replenished daily or weekly. The way in which you prepare your food can be significant; high temperatures will destroy vitamins such as vitamin C, and boiling vegetables and meat can result in vitamins and minerals leaching out into the water. Steaming, pressure-cooking and stir-frying avoids this, and it is also essential to eat some raw vegetables and fruit.

The nutritional value of cereals such as wheat, rice and barley and fruit and vegetables can be affected by processing. Minerals are present in highest concentration in the outer husks of the grains and in the skin of fruit and most vegetables, and will be lost if the outer layer is removed.

In addition, farming methods can reduce the amount of nutrients, particularly minerals and trace elements, available in food. For example, deficiency in zinc – which is now thought to be essential for the growth of the baby and the health of the mother – has become relatively common because phosphate fertilizers decrease zinc absorption by plants.

It is now possible to analyse the mineral content of the blood and hair to determine whether there is a dietary deficiency.

It is best to obtain vitamins and minerals from a variety of foods and not to rely on only a limited number of sources. By doing this, you will obtain a natural balance of these nutrients, and will overcome the enormous seasonal variation in mineral and vitamin content in different foods. The table will give you some creative ideas for adding vitamins and minerals to your diet. In some instances, vitamin and mineral supplements may be needed before or during pregnancy.

Sources of essential nutrients

Protein, carbohydrates, fats, vitamins and minerals can be found in varying quantities in virtually all foods. The following will give you some idea of the foods that are ideal for a balanced diet.

Meat, fish, poultry and eggs These have high concentrations of protein, vitamins and minerals, although red meat contains a high proportion of saturated fat. Fish, on the other hand, is low in this. The amount of fat – and thus calories – will increase if any of these are fried.

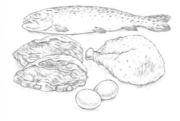

Animals reared for meat are often given hormones to increase their yield and antibiotics to avoid the infections that can be rampant in factory-farming. Although difficult to obtain as well as expensive, free-range meat is free of these. It is a good idea to eat less meat, and to make sure that it is of a very good quality when you do. It is not necessary to eat meat every day if your diet contains other types of protein foods.

Eggs are an excellent source of nutrients during pregnancy, containing a balance of protein and fat as well as vitamins A, B complex, D and E, iron and other minerals. Eggs laid by battery hens contain only about half the vitamin B_{12} and less folic acid than that in free-range and 'deep litter' eggs.

Cereals and grains Most of the world's population relies on cereals and grains for the bulk of its protein, calorie and mineral intake, and these can form the basis of an excellent diet.

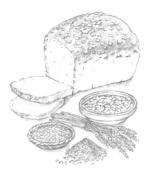

All cereals and grains consist of an outer protective husk and an inner core which mainly comprises carbohydrate. When refined, as in white flour and white rice, the outer husk is removed, thus depleting the diet of essential vitamins, minerals and fibre.

Unrefined cereals may provide important nutrients, calories and fibre, but they should not form the *whole* diet. This is because, in addition to their valuable constituents, they also contain phytic acid which may reduce the absorption of calcium, iron, magnesium and zinc, and they also lack some important vitamins. The diet should be balanced with the inclusion of vegetables, fruit, pulses and/or animal foods, and ideally, cereals and grains should be eaten at meals in combination with pulses as this will ensure that the protein in both is more efficiently metabolized (*see above*). A diet containing as much as one-third cereals and grains will be a healthy one, provided they are unrefined.

Pulses 'Pulses' are all the different types of dried beans, peas and lentils that play such a large part in vegetarian diets, supplying vitamins (particularly the B group), minerals and protein. Only soya beans (and beancurd and paste – also known as *tofu* and *miso* – made from them) contain all the essential amino acids needed for a balanced diet. However, if you eat the other pulses with whole grains and cereals – e.g. rice, wheat, barley, millet – at the same meal, your total protein needs will be met.

Dried pulses, when cooked, do not regain all the water that was in them originally and so, weight for weight, they contain more calories and more protein than fresh pulses. Some beans are difficult to digest and cause 'wind'. To avoid this, allow the beans to sprout and then eat raw or cooked (particularly stir-fried); this also increases their vitamin content. Dried red kidney beans should always be boiled for at least ten minutes to eliminate a poison they contain.

Nuts and seeds These are valuable sources of protein, especially in a vegetarian diet. Walnuts and sesame and sunflower seeds are particularly useful as they contain a high percentage of polyunsaturated fat. As well as having high concentrations of minerals, nuts and seeds also contain calcium, and can prove useful sources of this if you are allergic to dairy products. However, although all kinds of nuts and seeds are very nutritious, eaten in excess they can be fattening and indigestible.

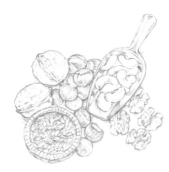

They can be eaten raw as a snack, and peanut butter and sesame seed spread can make nourishing sandwiches. Nuts and seeds can also be used in main dishes, in the form of nut roasts or added to salads. Lightly roasting them without oil over direct heat in a frying pan may make them easier to digest. Salted nuts should be avoided.

Vegetables A diet containing a large quantity of vegetables means that you will be consuming a great deal of dietary fibre. As a result, you will feel less hungry than if you were eating concentrated calories and proteins such as occur in dairy products and meat, in addition to all the other benefits that fibre can bring.

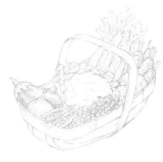

A glance at the chart on pages 98–9 will quickly show you that green leafy vegetables, potatoes and carrots have high levels of essential vitamins and minerals. The highest concentrations of these are frequently found in their outer skin and so, whenever possible, peeling should be avoided. Instead, only the outer leaves should be removed or they should be scrubbed clean.

To preserve their vitamins and minerals, vegetables should be lightly steamed, pressure-cooked or stir-fried using only a little oil; boiling should be avoided. Any cooking water left over can be used in soups and stews so that you can get the benefit of any minerals that have leached out.

Potatoes can be a useful part of your diet. They are now known to be a vital slow-burning carbohydrate, especially if they are baked in their jackets or steamed in their skins. Avoid frying potatoes or eating crisps as the oil used will add a massive calorific value while reducing the nutrients. Ageing and green potatoes should be discarded.

Seaweeds Also called sea vegetables, their nutritional value has been known in the Orient for centuries, and their use is becoming more common in the West. They are exceptionally rich in minerals and trace elements, and they contain high concentrations of iron and other minerals essential for pregnancy, including iodine, needed by the thyroid gland.

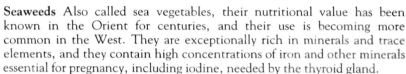

Available from health food shops and Oriental groceries, they can be cooked and eaten on their own, added to stews or to other vegetables, washed and soaked and incorporated into a salad, or roasted and crushed and sprinkled on top of food. Most seaweeds are of Japanese origin, with names such as *noi, kombu, arame* and *hijiki*; in addition there are the red seaweeds popular in Ireland – carragheen (also called Irish moss), dulse and laver, which is also eaten in Wales.

Fruit Fresh fruit consists mainly of water (80-90 per cent), but also contains sugar, vitamins (particularly vitamin C) and some minerals. Most tend to be acid, particularly citrus fruits, and although moderate amounts are beneficial in pregnancy, eating too much can result in hyperacidity. In addition, the sugar content is very high, especially in soft fruits such as grapes, plums, peaches and melons, and this may be a major source of excessive calories and weight gain. Eating two pieces of fruit daily is probably sufficient.

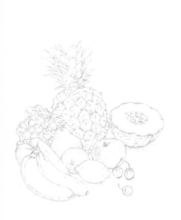

In season, it is best to choose fruits grown locally as the vitamin content declines the longer the fruit is stored. Vitamins and minerals are contained in the skin of apples and pears, so peeling these is not recommended.

Dried fruits contain far more sugar than fresh varieties and, therefore, should only be eaten in small quantities. However, they are a rich source of potassium, and dried apricots contain useful amounts of iron, as well as copper which balances with zinc in the body.

Fresh citrus fruit juices are a very reliable source of vitamin C; other types tend to lose their vitamin C content during processing (although this may be put back in). Fruit juice made from concentrates may be hard to digest, can cause heartburn, is high in calories and may erode tooth enamel because of its high acidity. If you drink it, dilute it with water first. Fruit 'drinks' and squashes have very few nutrients and usually contain relatively vast quantities of added sugar; you should avoid them altogether.

Dairy products These provide calcium, protein and fats in a convenient form, and are consumed by many pregnant women. However, their importance as a source of calcium, protein and vitamins is often overestimated, even though many women feel that they ought to have significant quantities of milk, yogurt, cheese and other dairy products in their diets. Some people are sensitive or allergic to milk products, including butter (*see* Allergies and hypersensitivity, pp. 290-1). Moreover, they have low bulk (and may cause constipation), and they are high in calories and in saturated fats.

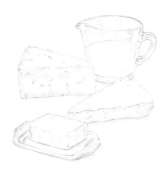

It is certainly not necessary to drink a pint of milk a day during or after pregnancy. You can obtain all the nutrients contained in dairy products by eating other types of foods containing these – such as nuts, seeds, pulses, lentils and vegetables. In many Oriental cuisines, dairy products play a very limited role, and some nutritionists believe that they are not needed at all.

The best advice, then, is to eat dairy products in moderation if at all. Live low-fat yogurt is useful to provide *Lactobacillus* which protects against thrush (*see* p. 343). Hard cheeses such as Cheddar and Cheshire are perhaps preferable as they have a higher protein content than soft ones such as cottage cheese, cream cheese and Brie, but you should avoid cheeses that are excessively salty.

Vegetarian diets

Over half the world's population are vegetarians, and this type of diet, if well planned, can provide a complete balance of nutrients. It is essential to ensure that the protein, vitamin and mineral content is adequate, and that vegetable protein is eaten in combinations of pulses and grains.

During pregnancy, extra nutrients can be added by means of such protein-rich foods as tofu (soya beancurd), beans, lentils and wholegrain cereals (e.g. rice, wheat, barley, millet), and seaweeds, nuts and seeds which contain valuable minerals. Particular attention should also be focused on the vegetables, fruits and pulses that contain the most iron, folic acid and calcium. Refined foods and cooking by frying or boiling should be avoided. It is usually possible to achieve an ample intake of all the nutrients you need from food, but if not, supplements may be needed, particularly iron, zinc and some vitamins.

The above assumes that you will be eating some cheese, eggs and/or milk. However, if you are a vegan and you eat no animal foods whatsoever, you may find that you are deficient in vitamin B_{12}, which is present only in animal foods, apart from yeast extracts such as Marmite and Barmene (which should be included in your diet). Vegans should take supplements of vitamin B_{12} during pregnancy.

Occasionally women find meat unpalatable when they are pregnant and so become vegetarians for the first time. While it is preferable not to change your diet drastically during pregnancy, if meat is intolerable, ensure that you have an adequate intake of protein, fats, minerals and vitamins. On the other hand, if you became a vegetarian as an adult after a non-vegetarian childhood, you may find that, now that you are pregnant, you desire to eat meat again. In this case, it is wise to follow your body's signals; it is always possible to give up meat again after birth.

Things to avoid

During pregnancy, your baby depends on you for nourishment, and any substance you take in – be it nourishing or harmful – will cross the placenta and enter your baby's bloodstream too.

Nature tends to be very efficient, and your liver and kidneys do the work of removing harmful toxins from your blood. While your growing baby will be unaffected by the majority of these substances, any unnecessary drugs or inappropriate foods or drinks should be avoided, especially in the first eight weeks of pregnancy when the baby is most vulnerable. In cases where medication is essential for your well-being, the risks to the baby will be balanced with your needs and your medication should be carefully monitored by your doctor.

The following substances may be harmful to your baby:

Drugs The risks of tranquillizers and other prescribed or over-the-counter drugs, alcohol, cigarettes and illegal drugs are discussed in detail on pages 290, 308-9 and 335.

You may be given iron tablets (usually combined with folic acid) by your doctor when your pregnancy is confirmed; however, not everyone needs supplements of iron or any other mineral or vitamin, and some women prefer to eat foods rich in such nutrients. Any other medicine should only be taken in consultation with your doctor.

If you suffer from disorders for which there is no safe or effective orthodox treatment, you could try homoeopathic remedies that are considered to be safer for use in pregnancy (*see* pp. 315-6). You will need the advice of a qualified homoeopath before taking any of these, as the correct remedies are always chosen on an individual basis. You should also inform your doctor of any remedies you may be taking.

Coffee and tea The amount of coffee and tea you drink is best reduced during pregnancy as they both contain varying amounts of caffeine, a stimulant drug that is addictive and can over-activate the nervous system. It may cause the heartbeat to become faster, and could have a similar effect on your baby as caffeine can cross the placenta. When taken in excess, caffeine causes the stomach to secrete more acid, can raise blood pressure levels and encourages the adrenal system to overwork. If tea is drunk at meals, it will reduce the absorption of iron.

If you decide to reduce your intake of coffee or tea or give it up entirely, you may experience a few days of withdrawal symptoms such as headache, muscle pain, irritability and cramps as your system clears itself. It will help to drink plenty of mineral water or other fluids at this time. Your energy level and vitality will soon increase.

There is a wide range of delicious and comforting herbal teas and cereal-based coffee substitutes. Camomile, raspberry leaf and rosehip teas are useful in pregnancy. Decaffeinated coffee is not preferable to the untreated variety due to the chemicals used to remove the stimulant.

The best drink of all is water. Try bottled spring water, drinking it in between rather than during meals.

Processed foods and food additives Highly flavoured and easily prepared, refined and processed foods are widely available. However, they are more expensive and less nutritious than natural foods, and do not promote health.

Processed foods frequently contain an excess of saturated fat and highly refined sugars to provide flavour and improve shelf life. Nitrites (and nitrates which can be converted into nitrites in the digestive system), often added as preservatives, especially in cheese and cured and pickled meats, can combine with the oxygen-carrying haemoglobin in the blood so that the latter becomes less effective. Babies are particularly susceptible to this.

Food flavourings and colourings are usually chemically based and, with preservatives and other additives, are frequent ingredients in processed foods. Colourings, preservatives and other additives (but not flavourings) are listed by 'E' numbers and their use is controlled. However, some quite common ones cause allergic reactions in certain individuals – e.g. the orange colouring *tartrazine*, known by its number 'E102' – and adverse symptoms have occurred with others.

It is best to eat a minimum of preserved and processed foods and those which have had many chemicals added to them. Always check labels when you shop.

Salt An appropriate amount of salt is essential for the body to maintain fluid balance, and a woman's requirement for salt – or, rather, the mineral *sodium* that it contains – will increase during pregnancy because of the rise in blood volume. However, only moderate amounts should be eaten as an excess of salt may be harmful – for example, it has been implicated in high blood pressure (hypertension), and it can be responsible for excessive thirst, which can lead to drinking a great deal of fluid and thus to possible fluid retention.

Most people eat far more salt than they need, often adding it to food during cooking or at the table before they eat it, or eating salty crisps and nuts, and thus acquiring a taste for it. Most foods already contain salt, and provided your diet contains adequate amounts of good-quality vegetables and fruit eaten in their natural state, this should be sufficient for your needs. When cooking or preparing food, unrefined sea salt, which contains other trace elements, or a good soya sauce are better to use than refined salt.

It is advisable to avoid salty flavour enhancers such as *monosodium glutamate* (MSG), sometimes called 'Chinese taste powder'. This sodium salt is a familiar additive in processed foods and, as its alternative name suggests, is a common constituent of Chinese food. It can cause dehydration, headaches and sweating.

If you suffer from high blood pressure or pre-eclampsia (see p. 315), eliminating salt from the diet is not advisable: this will simply reduce blood volume and may worsen the situation. Rather, you should continue with a moderate salt intake.

Sugar and sweeteners These refined carbohydrates (see above) can cause many problems. Besides the damage they can do to teeth, an intake of too much sugar can affect normal blood sugar levels. A vicious circle may develop, which starts when your blood sugar and energy levels fall and you crave something sweet to give yourself that much-needed lift. A bar of chocolate, a sweetened drink and you are 'up' again, but the lift is only temporary and fairly soon you are again feeling low and lethargic and in need of something else to make you feel energetic – and so it goes on. If you are pregnant, your baby will also experience this cycle of ups and downs.

You can maintain a constant stream of energy by eating enough slow-burning unrefined carbohydrates – for example, jacket potatoes, wholemeal bread and unsalted nuts. If you have a sweet tooth, eat more fruit, being careful to watch calories to avoid excessive weight gain. In particular, dried fruits may provide the answer to an urge for something sweet. Select those that have not been dipped into glucose or treated with sulphur. You could either eat them as they come, or soak a selection – apples, peaches, raisins, sultanas, apricots, pears – in water for a few hours until they are soft.

For cooking and baking, dispense with white sugar and instead use honey, malt extract, blackstrap molasses, black treacle, maple syrup or a good-quality dark brown sugar. (If you use a liquid sweetener, be sure to increase the dry ingredients in your recipe slightly.) Although these are also refined carbohydrates, they do have the advantage of containing at least some other nutrients, although often in minute amounts. It is far better to sweeten your recipes with dried and fresh fruits, freshly squeezed orange juice or apple juice concentrate.

Cooking and eating

Food should be cooked carefully, and cooking methods such as steaming, grilling, stir-frying and pressure-cooking are preferable to frying or roasting (both of which will require a lot of fat) and boiling. Try to cook food only lightly to preserve the majority of the nutrients it contains.

Balance your meals by making sure that you receive an adequate amount of protein, with at least one protein-rich food daily (*see* p. 100). By selecting fresh foods available seasonally, you will help to ensure that the nutrients in your diet are varied and sufficient for your needs. You will benefit from planning your meals carefully, keeping the colours, textures and flavours in mind. This need not take a long time and the result will be worth it: a beautifully presented meal is an aid to digestion.

Try to make every meal an enjoyable occasion, by preparing a pleasant setting and eating in a slow and leisurely way, whether alone or in the company of others. Chew each mouthful well so that the first stage of digestion can take place in your mouth. In this way, you will absorb all the nutrients in your food more fully, and you will also feel satisfied without having overeaten.

CHAPTER 8

THE ENVIRONMENT FOR BIRTH

Once pregnancy is confirmed, you will begin to think about where to have your baby and the sort of labour and delivery you would like. In choosing where and with whom to have your ante-natal care as well as deciding on the place of birth and your birth attendants, you will be making some of your first major decisions as parents.

If this is your first baby, you may be learning about pregnancy and childbirth for the first time and it may take you a while to acquire knowledge and information and to explore alternatives before making your final choice. Of course, this choice is not irrevocable: women often change their minds as pregnancy advances and their ideas and preferences become clearer. The first step is to ask your family doctor about local choices, and to talk to friends in your area. It can also be helpful to contact local birth centres, associations or information services.

Once you have ascertained what is available, it is important to investigate the possibilities personally rather than relying on hearsay. It is particularly worth while to take the trouble to visit hospitals you may be considering and to ask any questions you may have regarding policy and general approach, so that you can get a 'feel' of the atmosphere before committing yourself. You will be going through a deeply personal experience when giving birth, and it is most important to find the best possible environment to suit your needs, one which will allow you security, safety and privacy for this important event.

To find the right place to have your baby, trust your instincts and base your choice on what really feels best. For some women, the right choice is to have their babies at home; for others, it may be a hospital which encourages natural active childbirth while offering good medical back-up if intervention is needed; and for some, it means a hospital offering the latest in high technology. You may live in an area where the choice is very limited; then it may be up to you to persuade your attendants to cooperate with your ideas.

Birth in hospital

Consultant units The most popular hospitals are often very busy, so the earlier you begin your enquiries, the greater your chance of being booked into the consultant unit at a hospital of your choice. You can go and see the hospital yourself or ask your GP for a letter of referral. Every hospital has a catchment area, and if you are outside this or the hospital is heavily booked for your estimated date of delivery, you may have trouble being accepted. However, sometimes persistence or a letter to the consultant explaining why you would like to have your baby there may be effective.

In an uncomplicated hospital birth, a midwife will attend you in labour. If assistance is needed, there is always a resident doctor on hand to help, and the consultant in charge will be contacted if further advice is required. In addition to a consultant unit, there may be other options in your locality (*see* below).

GP units In some areas, there are separate small hospitals staffed by midwives and local general practitioners who are trained in obstetrics (sometimes referred to as GPOs). Alternatively, some hospitals have GP units within them, so that your own GP and community midwives can supervise your ante-natal care, deliver your baby and follow you up after the birth with all the facilities of the hospital at hand in case of need. This system allows for continuity of care, and many women feel very reassured to be attended by people they already know.

The domino scheme 'Domino' stands for 'DOMiciliary IN and Out'. In this case, the community midwife and GP undertake the ante-natal care. When labour starts, the midwife comes to your home and takes you into hospital to deliver your baby; your GP and hospital staff are only involved if needed. If all goes well, you can go home within a few hours and the same midwife will take care of you and and your baby after the birth. This scheme works very satisfactorily for some women, combining continuity of care with the safety of hospital facilities and the advantages of the home.

Your birth attendants

Midwives The primary attendants at birth, midwives have had special training and experience in looking after women and their babies during pregnancy, birth and the postnatal period. They work in hospitals and in GP or ante-natal clinics as well as in the community. Some midwives work independently, and their services can be obtained to deliver babies at home (*see* pp. 119-20).

A senior midwife is known as a 'sister' or nursing officer, and she is usually in charge of junior and student midwives, some of whom will become involved in your labour and delivery. The most senior midwife is called the senior nursing officer, previously known as 'matron'.

A woman in labour needs the help of a midwife who will be able to empathize with her, provide her with reassurance and inspiration and encourage her to let herself go without disturbing or distracting her. Being a midwife – the word means 'one who is with the mother' – is an intuitive art, and the presence of a skilled one is essential to the birth. An experienced midwife will understand your needs and help you to feel relaxed and secure, will be aware of your need for privacy and will also know when you need guidance, firmness or help. She will check your well-being throughout labour and also that of your baby.

Ideally, every pregnant woman should meet the midwife (and doctor) who will be attending her so that there is an opportunity to get to know each other and discuss important issues, but in a busy hospital this is not always possible. It is helpful to visit the labour ward and meet the midwife in charge – particularly if you are hoping for an active birth. She will then be aware of your needs, and may be able to help on the day by scheduling a midwife who has had experience of active birth or one whose ideas are compatible with yours.

Hospital doctors For many women, the additional presence of a doctor or obstetrician is important and reassuring.

Every woman is booked into hospital under the care of a consultant during her period of pregnancy and childbirth. However, a junior doctor (a house officer or registrar) may attend to you at your ante-natal clinic and in the labour suite, and may be involved in your baby's birth if there are any minor difficulties. For more serious problems or if decisions regarding the conduct of labour are needed, the consultant may be involved.

When birth is active, however, the doctor's main function is to provide a feeling of security by his or her availablility. Sometimes the doctor may help to support the mother physically or take on the role of midwife and primary helper.

The general practitioner This may be your family doctor if he or she is qualified in obstetrics, or another GP who is. You are entitled to change your doctor for the length of your pregnancy and the birth, and then go back to your family doctor afterwards. Your doctor may elect to share some of your ante-natal care with the hospital and may also be involved with the birth and after-care.

Other supporters It may be helpful if your partner or another person of your choice can give you support during labour – either in hospital or at home. This person should be someone who is likely to be a positive presence in the labour suite; he or she will also need to be free from anxiety and have the ability to tune in to your needs in a supportive but non-intrusive way.

Very often, the ideal person is the baby's father – many couples enjoy sharing the intimacy of labour and the birth of their child. However, sometimes the helper is a close friend or relative, ideally a woman who has had a positive experience of childbirth herself. Sometimes there may be more than one helper; this can be useful in a long labour, as they can take turns being with you. It is important, however, not to have too many people present as this may distract or inhibit you and prolong the labour.

One vital aspect of the helper's role is to shield the mother from outside distractions or disturbance. He or she also often protects her from feeling that she is being watched or expected to behave in a certain way or perform in a specified amount of time. It is best if both helpers and attendants avoid giving instructions; rather, they should respond tactfully, helping the woman in labour to trust her own instincts and intuition.

The birth setting

Until very recently, most women giving birth in hospital have done so in the recumbent position – that is, semi-reclining or flat on their backs – on an obstetric bed. The main consideration in the design of delivery rooms was the medical safety of mother and child: childbirth was seen mainly as a medical event and the woman in labour as a 'patient'. For this reason, most conventional delivery rooms look more like operating theatres than the kind of setting that might encourage a woman to give birth spontaneously without inhibition. Today, there is a greater awareness of women's needs during labour, and the emotional and sexual aspects of birth are better understood. Many maternity units are being adapted to reflect these changes.

Who's who in the maternity unit
The midwives' team
Senior nursing officer (matron)
Nursing officers (sisters)
Staff midwives
Student midwives
The doctor's team
Consultant obstetrician
Senior registrar
Registrar
House officer (houseman)
Medical students

What to take with you into hospital

You will feel more at home and comfortable in labour if you take a few simple items with you to supplement what is provided by the hospital. It is a good idea to pack two bags in readiness – one containing the things you will require during labour, and the other, items you will need after the birth. During labour, you may need:

● Your own nightgown or a large cotton shirt or pyjama jacket.

● A tape recorder and a good selection of music you might enjoy.

● A large bean bag or one or two large floor cushions for leaning on, if these are not already supplied by the hospital.

● Fruit juice (such as apple or red grape juice), honey, glucose tablets to keep your blood sugar level up.

● Food for your partner or other supporter(s).

● A water spray and sponge.

● Homoeopathic remedies that may be helpful in labour, provided the staff have no objection (see pp. 315-6).

● Some pure vegetable oil or talcum powder for massage.

● A simple hand-held fan.

● A pair of warm socks. The hospital will tell you what you will need after the birth.

When going through the intense and intimate experience of giving birth, you will need to feel safe and secure, to have a sense of privacy, peace and calm and to have the right people with you. You should be able to feel free to adopt any position that feels comfortable, to let youself go, to empty your bowels, to shout or cry, to express your feelings, to move or be held. You will need to be able to concentrate – to listen to your own body with the minimum of external distractions.

In many hospitals, labour wards are being redesigned to produce birth rooms that are as comfortable and homely as possible. Sometimes circumstances make it impossible to change the physical setting radically, but the vital element is really just a change in attitude. With this, and a few simple improvisations, even the most basic delivery room can become an appropriate setting for an active birth.

If you are having your baby in hospital, it is helpful if the environment is already familiar to you. For this reason, it is important to visit the labour ward and delivery rooms beforehand, and to participate in ante-natal activities (see p. 87).

What is needed Preferably, an obstetric bed or any other furniture that confines a woman to one position should be pushed to one side or removed. This is also true of expensive borning-beds and other costly, complicated equipment: even though the position the mother adopts is more upright, her freedom of movement is still greatly restricted. In their place, a simple foam mattress covered with washable material can be placed on the floor, together with cushions and a large bean bag (see below for a list of useful equipment). A low wooden platform, about the size of a double bed, covered with a comfortable, firm mattress and plenty of cushions would be ideal, but a bean bag or some large floor cushions can be used on the conventional delivery bed just as well.

If you are giving birth in a hospital where it is preferred that you remain in bed, it is possible to use the surface of the bed and the backrest in a variety of ways suitable for active birth. A low stool, a low wooden 'birthing' chair or an ordinary straight-back chair may also be useful and are to be found in most conventional labour wards. With these few simple props, you will find it easy to change positions and move your body spontaneously. The baby's heartbeat can be checked with an electronic hand-held heart monitor, no matter what position you have assumed; if this is not available, an ordinary stethoscope will suffice.

The room should be well heated, with extra heat available to ensure that it is very warm when the baby is born. An overhead heater on wheels is useful for this. To create the right atmosphere during labour, it is helpful if there are curtains which can be drawn or dimmers on the lights, as you may feel more relaxed in semi-darkness.

Many women find it helpful to be in water when they are in labour. It is important that there is easy access to an ordinary bath or shower or, ideally, a small pool, jacuzzi or double bath in which you can immerse your whole body in any position – immersion in water is one of the most efficient ways to relax and to relieve the pain of labour. If none of these is available, a sponge rinsed out in cold water or a water spray will be refreshing.

Your own nightgown, a man's shirt or your partner's pyjama jacket will feel more personal and comfortable than a hospital gown. They can also be

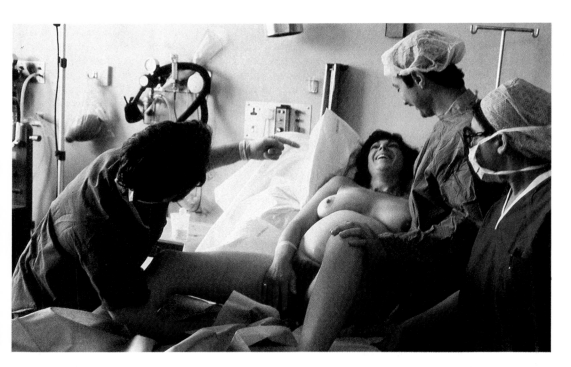

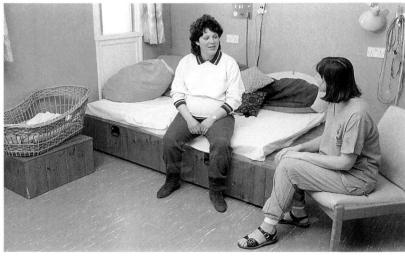

Above: A delivery suite in a consultant unit.
Left: A birth room in a maternity unit.

easily removed if you prefer to be naked or to allow skin-to-skin contact with your baby. Alternatively, a hospital gown can be worn back to front, so that it opens in front.

Water, honey and fruit juices, and perhaps some herbal teas and an electric kettle with which to make them, are necessary to prevent dehydration and to keep up blood sugar levels. Finally, if you bring a cassette player or stereo, together with a set of headphones, you will be able to listen to quiet, calming music – an effective aid to relaxation.

Helpful hospital equipment for women who would like an active birth

Helpful hospital equipment for women who would like an active birth

- A bath, shower, pool or jacuzzi, to be freely available to the mother in labour.
- Two large beanbags – preferably with removable linen covers.
- A small, low stool or birth stool for squatting on.
- A simple upright chair.
- Plenty of pillows.
- An inexpensive and valuable addition to the usual labour ward is a small mattress about half the size of a normal one on a hospital bed and about 5 cm (2 in) thick, covered in thick, washable, anti-static material. This can be placed on the floor anywhere to receive the newborn baby. Additional mats can be provided for the midwife and supporters.
- A clean sheet and a sterile towel to be placed on top of the mat when the baby is born. This will absorb the amniotic fluid and provide a soft surface for the baby.
- An electronic hand-held heart monitor.
- An overhead heater on wheels for keeping the mother and baby warm.
- Fruit juices (not citrus) and simple facilities for making fresh tea.

'Rooming in' and feeding

In order that you can get to know your baby and for breastfeeding to get off to a good start, it is important that you and your child are not separated either during the day or at night and that hospital routines do not interfere with the establishment of the first communication between you. Find out whether the hospital encourages 'rooming in' – that is, babies allowed to stay with their mothers at all times, day and night. You will want to get to know your baby at your own pace without having to comply with rigid routines.

If you are intending to breastfeed (*see* Chapter 15), it is best if the first contact between you and your child is not disturbed, and that the people who will be caring for you after the birth share the same attitudes.

It is also important to discover whether mothers are free to feed their babies whenever necessary, or if there are routine feeding times. In some hospitals, babies are taken to a nursery at night and given supplementary feeds while their mothers sleep. This practice can disturb the establishment of breastfeeding, as the breasts need the stimulation of the baby's sucking in order to produce the right supply of milk. The baby would be deprived of the warmth and security of his mother's familiar body as well as her responses to his cries.

Although the post-natal care in some hospitals is particularly good, if there is no alternative to a busy ward where you are not happy with the approach, it is well worth considering this in advance and perhaps arranging for an early, 48-hour discharge; then you can be cared for at home by a community midwife. You are likely to be much more relaxed and comfortable in your own home, provided you have plenty of help and can devote yourself completely to your baby.

It may also be helpful to establish contact before the birth with a good breastfeeding counsellor (*see* p. 197), so that if you run into difficulties, you can obtain advice at short notice.

Asking questions

During your ante-natal visits and in preparation classes, many topics are bound to arise for discussion, and you may have specific questions that you would like to ask your birth attendants. If they are not able to help, you can make an appointment with the senior midwife or with a member of the medical staff to discuss these issues. It is a good idea to write down your questions beforehand and take your partner with you if possible. Your preferences should be written in your notes so that this information is readily available when you are in labour.

Some hospitals welcome the idea of you compiling a 'birth plan' which states clearly and simply your wishes and preferences for the birth and after, and which can be attached to your notes. You will not want to discuss these things once you are in labour, and a midwife coming on duty will benefit from reading your birth plan.

How long to stay in hospital

With a first baby, mothers are expected to stay in hospital for anything up to ten days after the birth. Some women benefit from this, while others prefer to go home as soon as possible. It is normally easier to extend a short-stay booking than it is to arrange to be discharged early, as the community midwives need to be available to care for you at home.

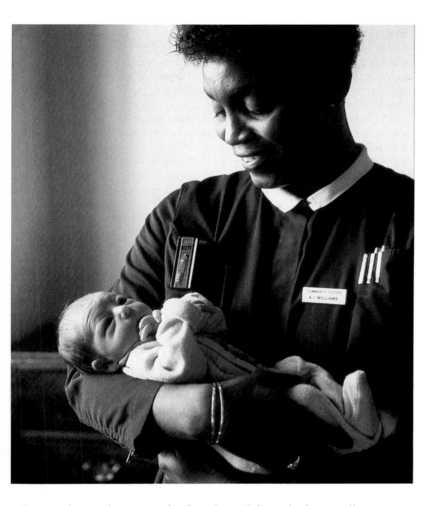

In some hospitals, you can book a 6- or 48-hour discharge, allowing you to leave soon after the birth provided it was straightforward and there are no complications. Then the community midwife is obliged by law to visit you at home every day until the baby is ten days old. These visits, during which she will check the well-being of both of you and advise you about feeding and caring for your baby, can be very enjoyable and helpful.

Birth at home

Giving birth at home has many advantages, and for some women and their families this is the right choice.

At home, the birth can take place within the environment you have created yourself, as one of the highlights of your family life. The successful outcome of any birth depends on the skill of the attendants and the way that the mother feels. To be at your best and most relaxed during labour and while giving birth, you may need to remain in the surroundings you are used to, where you are assured of privacy, peace and comfort.

Practical reasons for a hospital birth

You may prefer to have your baby in hospital if:

* your domestic situation and/or home environment are not suitable for a home birth.
* you would like to have the full back-up facilities offered by a hospital.
* the supportive atmosphere in hospital will make you feel more at ease.
* it is important for you to have contact with other new mothers during the first few days after the birth.

Making a choice

Before deciding on a home birth, you will need to reflect carefully on the advantages and disadvantages of your own specific circumstances. In addition, if you opt for either a home or hospital birth, it is important that your partner should feel comfortable with your choice and that there is no conflict between you about this.

There are no absolute rules when choosing the place for the birth of your baby. There are always factors which may complicate birth, and although it is usually assumed that hospital is safer than home, there are statistics to show that this is not necessarily true. While the overall fall in the neonatal death rate has been attributed to the high level of hospital births, the improvement in general health standards and ante-natal care are also major factors. This is clear in countries such as Holland where home birth is common, and hospital births are generally for women whose labours are likely to be complicated. The mortality rate in Holland for both mothers and babies is one of the lowest in the world.

Although birth at home should only be considered for women having uncomplicated labours following normal healthy pregnancies, occasionally a 'high risk' mother may be more suited to individual and specialized care at home. There is no conclusive evidence to prove that it is safer for 'low risk' women to give birth in hospital rather than at home, provided the care given at the time is of an adequate standard, nor that it is necessarily safer to have a first baby in hospital.

Choosing a home birth

Although some hospitals endeavour to provide women with a home-like atmosphere and respect their need for privacy and calm, many women choose to have a home birth because they feel that a hospital is not the right environment for birth and are not satisfied that their individual requirements will be understood as well as they might be at home. For these women, giving birth is primarily a normal biological function, an expression of health and vitality and very much a family, rather than a medical, event. It can also be an intensely private and personal experience, and a home birth may be especially important if the mother feels a need to be alone.

Freedom and autonomy are important issues. In her own home, a woman can choose any position that is comfortable for her, and can listen to music, make as much noise as she likes, eat or drink, spend time in the bath – in fact, she is free to do as she pleases. She does not need to worry about disturbing or being disturbed by other women and their families, or breaking hospital rules, and can therefore be more relaxed.

In any busy hospital, there are bound to be routines not to everyone's taste, and in some, a woman wanting natural childbirth may need to work hard to get what she wants. A home birth is sometimes chosen as a way of avoiding active management of labour by medical staff as well as the routine and sometimes injudicious use of intervention, particularly if this has been the experience in a previous labour. Even if the hospital is willing to assist a woman to have as natural, active and drug-free a labour as possible, staff may lack the necessary confidence and experience to do so.

With a home birth, you will not have to travel, nor be obliged to move from one room for admission to another for labour and then to a final one for the birth, all of which can slow or disturb the progress of labour.

At home, continuity of care by a familiar midwife and supporter of your choice is also usual. Some women particularly enjoy being cared for by their family doctor and community midwife during pregnancy, childbirth and in the days that follow. In addition, all these people will be guests on your territory – often an important attitudinal factor.

A home birth unites rather than divides the family. Since it occurs as a normal part of family life, other children need not be excluded, nor will they have to cope with separation from their mother. This can be important for a toddler, who will be losing his place as the baby of the family and will need to be reassured and given plenty of love and attention in order to learn to accept the new baby. For the father, being separated from his partner and new baby after the intensity of the birth can cause feelings of isolation and depression.

In a home birth, your partner will be able to share fully in the experience on his own familiar territory. Communication between you will retain its continuity, and will be as warm and spontaneous as you are usually accustomed to in the intimacy of your own home. Close, physical contact between partners and the uninhibited release of emotion will enhance the flow of hormones to help the smooth progress of labour.

Welcoming your baby into the world at home can help to ensure that his very first experiences after birth are exactly as you would like them to be, something you could discuss with your attendants in detail beforehand. You can arrange soft lighting and make sure that your baby is handled as gently as possible to take into account his exceptional sensitivity at this time. You can also bathe your baby or have a bath together, and make the most of the sacred atmosphere that can surround the birth of a child.

After the birth, the home environment will offer the most conducive conditions for an undisturbed first contact and bonding with your new baby. It is easy to ensure that there is no separation of mother and baby, and he can be kept beside you in bed where you can attend to his needs immediately; this may be particularly important to a woman whose baby was taken away to a nursery or special-care unit after a previous labour.

In the days following the birth, you can be sure of the privacy that you and your family will need to get to know the new baby at leisure. You will be fully responsible for your child from the start, caring for him yourself. You will be able to look at, talk to, handle and hold him as much as you like, and can rest and sleep undisturbed when your baby does, so that you can slip more easily into a rhythm together. The relaxed atmosphere at home can also provide the ideal conditions for starting to breastfeed.

At home, your baby will also be protected from the infections that can flare up in hospital nurseries. His resistance will be highest to the familiar bacteria of your home, to which he will also obtain a natural immunity from the antibodies in your milk if you decide to breastfeed.

Important considerations Home births are not, however, right for everyone, and the following factors should be considered when assessing your suitability:

● *Number of previous pregnancies* Although each pregnancy is individual and should be assessed as such, a woman having her first baby is usually considered to be slightly more at risk than a woman having her second after a previously successful birth. The risk also increases statistically for women having fifth babies and more. However, there is no evidence that having a baby at home in the presence of skilled attendants will increase the risk.

● *Height* Particularly if she was inadequately nourished in childhood, a woman under 1.5 m (5 ft) tall may sometimes find that her pelvis is too small for her baby to get through. However, genetically small-boned women tend to have matching small babies and thus usually experience no difficulty. If the baby's head engages in the pelvis shortly before labour starts, a home birth can be considered.

● *Social circumstances* Poverty and poor ante-natal care (which often go together) may make a home birth more risky.

● *General health* If you suffer from any of the following, you may be advised not to have a home birth: diabetes, heart, kidney or circulatory disease, pulmonary tuberculosis, epilepsy, sexually transmitted disease such as gonorrhoea or active genital herpes. A home birth should not be contemplated if you are a heavy smoker or drinker or habitually use drugs such as heroin or barbiturates.

● *Health in pregnancy* You should not have a home birth if you are anaemic (*see* p. 292), or have placental insufficiency (*see* Low birth weight and prematurity, p. 321) or consistently high blood pressure as well as protein in your urine (i.e. possible pre-eclampsia, *see* p. 315).

● *Previous difficult labour* Some difficulties are likely to recur – e.g. a retained placenta or post-partum haemorrhage – and some are not. The possibility of something going wrong a second time should be discussed with your birth attendants and the risks considered.

● *Premature labour* If a previous child was premature and/or weighed less than 2.5 kg (5½ lb), this could recur and it would be best to plan to give birth in hospital so that, if your baby's lungs are immature and he has difficulty in breathing, he can be specially cared for. Women who have had repeated miscarriages are more at risk of giving birth prematurely. If, however, the pregnancy progresses to full term and the baby is a good size, a home birth can be contemplated. A hospital birth is also best if your labour starts when your pregnancy has lasted for 36 weeks or less, even if you have planned a home birth.

● *Post-maturity* If pregnancy continues for more than 14 days after the due date, the usual advice is that birth should take place in hospital. This is debatable, however, and each case should be assessed on its merits since the pregnancy can last as long as 44 weeks without problems arising.

● *Low-lying placenta* If the placenta is actually covering the cervix in late pregnancy, this is a contra-indication for a home birth.

● *Breech position* If a baby is in the breech position (*see* pp. 139, 296-7) after 36 weeks, a hospital birth is generally recommended. However, the baby may turn spontaneously at any time. If this is your second or a subsequent baby and your pelvic size is large, or if you have a confident and experienced doctor and midwife, a home birth may still be possible if unusual.

● *Multiple pregnancy* Although the birth of twins is often easier because the babies tend to be smaller, there is an increased risk that labour may be complicated. Because of this, it can be difficult to arrange for a multiple birth at home, and these are generally carried out in hospital.

● *Rhesus factor* If your blood is Rh negative (*see* p. 334) and this is your first child or if you have had an anti-D injection after a previous birth or pregnancy, there is no reason why you should not have a home birth unless blood tests show the presence of antibodies.

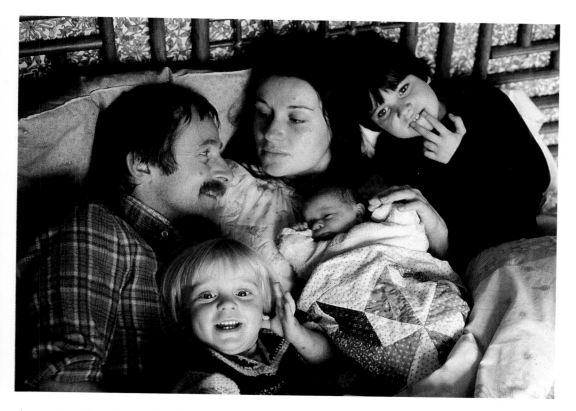

Arranging for a home birth

The first step is to be absolutely sure in yourself that you want a home birth. It is important that both you and your partner, if you have one, feel strongly that a home birth is the right choice.

Once you are sure, talk to your family doctor and find out his or her general attitude towards home birth. If your doctor believes that all babies should be born in hospital, you can try to find another doctor who is willing to do home deliveries and can care for you for the duration of your pregnancy. You are legally entitled to have another doctor perform this function, and you can find out which GPs in your area have the necessary obstetric qualifications by looking on the GP list at your local main post office or library. If you find a doctor who agrees to deliver your baby at home, he or she may want to have a second opinion from a consultant obstetrician to establish that your pregnancy is going well.

If you are unable to find a doctor, or decide after talking to your GP that you can do without one, your district health authority has a legal obligation to supply you with a midwife. Write to the district health authority (the address will be in the telephone book under the authority's name), addressing your letter to the District Supervisor of Midwives. Alternatively, you can hire a private midwife from a local nursing agency or via the Royal College of Nurses.

Attempting to find a doctor or midwife to attend you at home can sometimes be frustrating, but you should try to avoid getting into arguments. If you find it very difficult to obtain the right attendant(s), get

Equipment for a home birth

Women having a baby at home often surprise themselves by giving birth in a place other than the one prepared in advance. So be flexible – it may happen on your bed, on the floor, even in the bathroom. As long as the surface is firm, all you will need is a plastic sheet for protection. Other things you might need include:
* A telephone
* Adequate heating: the room should be between 21 and 24°C (70-75°F)
* Old sheets and towels
* An Anglepoise lamp so that the midwife can see in dim light
* A chair
* A large bean bag and some floor cushions
* A low stool to squat on
* A natural sponge
* Suitable soft drinks
* A mirror
* Music, candles, camera, food (for supporters)
* A fresh nightgown and sanitary towels for afterwards

For the baby
* Hot water bottle or electric heating pad to warm any clothes, shawls and towels that will come into contact with the baby's skin
* Soft towels and sheets for the birth and to wrap the baby in
* Soft towel for drying the baby
* Cotton wool
* Pure almond oil
* Nappies
* Soft cotton clothing
* A shawl

in touch with one of the relevant support associations, such as the Society to Support Home Confinements, the Association for Improvements in the Maternity Services (AIMS), the Association of Radical Midwives (ARMS) or the Independent Midwives Association (*see* p. 347).

Medical back-up

You do not need to attend ante-natal visits at a hospital, but it may be a good idea to go to one or two appointments in order to familiarize yourself with the hospital in case your plans for a home birth have to be abandoned. You may also wish to avail yourself of specific tests such as an ultrasound scan or amniocentesis.

When planning a home birth, it is essential to arrange medical back-up in case of unexpected complications. All midwives are entitled to call on the services of any doctor on the obstetric list and to use hospital facilities if this proves necessary. In addition, an emergency obstetric back-up unit – commonly known as the 'flying squad' – may be needed.

This is a mobile emergency unit directly linked to the nearest maternity hospital, and consists of an obstetrician and/or paediatrician and an experienced midwife. They will have the necessary equipment for emergency procedures, such as blood for transfusions, intravenous drips, drugs, etc. They are only required for a small minority of home births, the commonest reasons being retained placenta and haemorrhage.

You should, however, check that a flying squad will be available to you during your home birth, as in some areas they have been phased out because of increasing hospitalization.

The midwife

Although the progress of your pregnancy and the birth may be under the joint supervision of a doctor and a midwife, the midwife will be fully responsible for supervising labour and delivery. Your doctor may be present at the birth, but he or she will play a secondary part unless a difficulty arises.

You will have the opportunity to get to know your midwife well before the birth, and there should be ample time for discussion. Sometimes several community midwives are attached to a large family practice, and it may be difficult to know who will be there on the day. Try to meet the ones most likely to be present, as well as your midwife's deputy so that you are prepared if the former is away or off duty when you need her.

Although the emphasis at a home birth is on minimal intervention, this is dependent on the attitude, philosophy and sensitivity of your attendants. It is important to discuss your preferences with your midwife beforehand.

When labour starts, you will contact your midwife, and she will remain in touch by telephone until your labour is well established. Then she will join you at your home for the birth, having already arranged to have or bringing with her a sterile maternity pack containing all the necessary medical equipment and supplies. The following day, she will visit you twice, and then once daily for the next nine days. This continuing contact with the midwife is invaluable, and can be very enjoyable for you both.

C H A P T E R   9

PREPARING FOR BIRTH

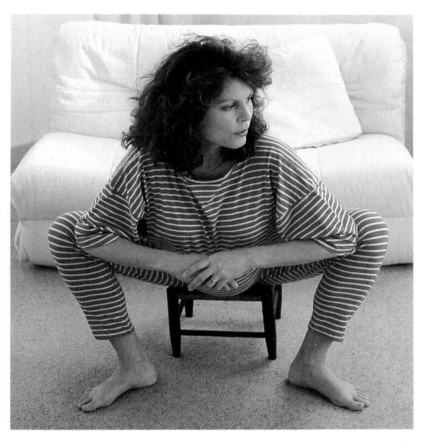

Squatting on a low stool is a good first-stage position.

Women use a variety of positions in labour, and your body will guide you instinctively at the time. However, in the last few weeks of your pregnancy, it is helpful to set aside some time to practise positions which may be useful in labour, combined with movement, breathing and massage.

The first stage: breathing for labour

Deep breathing is calming and relaxing, and will ensure a good flow of oxygen to you and your baby. Begin by practising deep breathing for a few minutes (*see* pp. 238-40). Try out each position on the next page and breathe through a few 'practice' contractions in each one.

Positions for the first stage

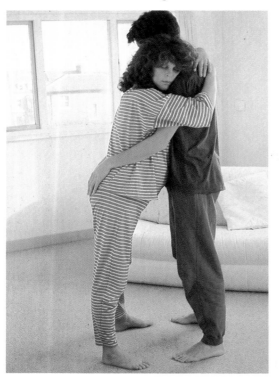

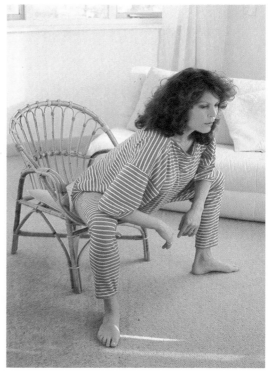

Standing and walking

Many women choose to stand up or walk about during the first stage. This will stimulate contractions, the downward force of gravity assisting the baby's descent and the dilation of the cervix. It will also help to make the contractions more efficient and less painful.

You may enjoy a combination of walking and some other position such as kneeling, squatting on a low stool or simply standing and circling your hips. You may like being held or rocked by another person, or having your lower back massaged rhythmically in harmony with your movements. During contractions, you may want to lean forward against someone else or on to a wall.

Some women prefer to stand or walk throughout labour, while others find that, as the contractions grow stronger, other positions are more comfortable.

Sitting

Sitting upright and leaning forward with your legs apart can be very comfortable. You can simply sit on the floor or on a chair or the edge of the bed. Many women enjoy sitting astride a chair, facing the chair back and leaning forward on to a cushion. In this position, your body is completely supported while vertical, your pelvis is open and you can relax and have your back massaged. Many women find sitting on the toilet very comfortable during labour.

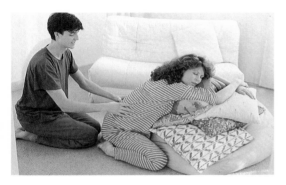

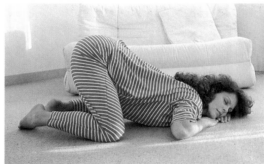

Kneeling

Kneeling in labour, as if in prayer, is an instinctive position, particularly towards the end of the first stage when the contractions are strong. There is a sense of being literally 'on top' of the contractions, and it is a way to increase your feeling of privacy and concentration, and to feel more grounded.

To kneel comfortably for several hours, you will need something soft under your knees – for example, a mattress or a folded blanket – plus a pile of cushions, a large bean bag or a few very large floor cushions to lean over. Make sure you have enough support to remain vertical. By going down on all fours, you will lessen the downward force of gravity and thus reduce the intensity of the contractions. If they are overwhelming, kneeling forward with your head down and bottom up will be a help. Many women find that moving their hips also helps to dissipate pain. This is especially useful if you are feeling the contractions in your back.

Some women find that kneeling is the most comfortable position to adopt throughout the first stage. However, it is often best to kneel later on, when contractions are stronger and closer together. If you have been kneeling for a long time, you will need to change position – to lift one knee or to stretch up between contractions.

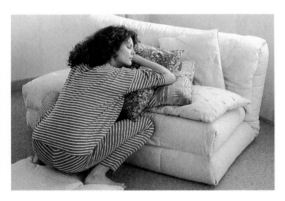

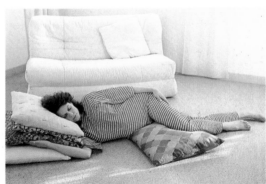

Squatting

In this position your pelvis is opened to its widest, and the baby's angle of descent is maximal in relation to the shape of the pelvic canal and the force of gravity. You can squat comfortably using a low stool or supported by another person, or holding on to something in front of you, or leaning forward on to a pile of cushions. A cushion under your heels may be helpful.

Squatting tends to intensify contractions, and you could squat between them and stand up as you feel one starting.

Lying down

It may be appropriate at certain times during your labour to lie down. If your labour is progressing well you may be most comfortable lying on your side, well propped up with cushions.

However, it is wise to avoid lying on your back for long periods (see p. 138). It will not harm your baby if you lie back to be examined, but this may be uncomfortable if you have been upright.

Whichever position you choose, once you are in labour you will find concentrating on your breathing very helpful in coping with your contractions. As you feel each contraction beginning, relax your whole body and centre your awareness on your breathing, concentrating on a complete exhalation; after it is finished, relax and then inhale slowly, breathing deeply into your belly. Stay focused on your breathing over its peak, and continue until the 'wave' of the contraction is over.

Move your body freely, circling your hips or rocking in harmony with your breathing. In this way, position, breathing and movement are combined to help you cope with your labour.

The second stage: breathing for bearing down

It is impossible to rehearse bearing down to give birth to your baby in the absence of the powerful expulsive reflex which occurs during second-stage contractions. Usually this reflex takes over spontaneously, and there is no need to try to 'do' anything at the time.

While you have no conscious control over your uterus, you can consciously relax your pelvic floor (see pp. 252-3). It is best to practise this first while squatting (see below) and then try out other positions.

As you squat, you might also try visualizing your baby being born, how her head will descend down into the pelvic cavity to rest on the pelvic floor. Imagine the force of a contraction bearing down on her body, and her head pressing down and beginning to emerge through your vagina. Try to imagine the vaginal tissues expanding as the head emerges.

As you are doing this, breathe deeply, releasing the pelvic floor each time you exhale. Try blowing out gently but firmly in a steady stream, puffing out your cheeks as you do so. This will automatically release the pelvic floor, and is useful during the second stage if you feel confused and do not know how to direct your energy. Breathing like this as a contraction begins will lead you into bearing down spontaneously.

It is never necessary consciously to hold your breath for long periods: your breathing will naturally adjust to the urge to bear down.

Positions for the second stage

This part of your labour can vary in length, and you may use several different positions until the final stages, when the baby is ready to be born. It is best not to have any preconceived ideas about which position you will use at the time; instead, practise all the possibilities beforehand.

It is easiest if you are free to move about during the second stage and give birth on the floor but you can use upright positions on a hospital bed.

Most of the positions suggested below are variations on the basic squatting position. This is optimal for birth as it opens the pelvis to its maximum, and promotes the descent of the baby's head at the perfect angle in relation to the downward force of gravity. The soft tissues of the vagina and perineum and the muscles of the pelvic floor are also at their most relaxed and can expand easily, lessening the likelihood of tearing. Squatting also ensures a good blood supply to the uterus and to your baby.

Several of the positions involve one or two other people working together as a team to support you. Anyone who acts as a supporter should feel comfortable because, if they are tense, their feelings may make it difficult for you to relax and let go. Equally, it will be easier for them if you relax completely and surrender to being supported.

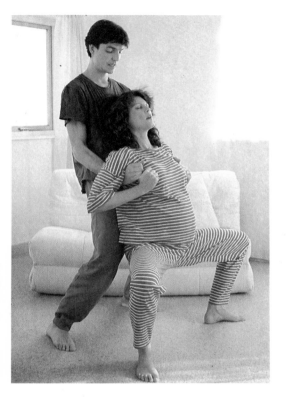
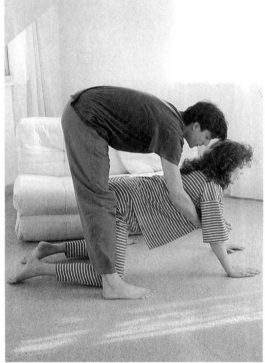

Standing squat with one supporter Between second-stage contractions, you can stand or kneel on all fours, but as a contraction begins, your helper should stand behind you while you allow your weight to be supported by his or her body and let go completely, surrendering to the contraction. Your knees will bend as your body becomes heavy with the downward force of the contraction, and your feet should be spread apart with your soles firmly planted on the floor so that your pelvis is open.

Your supporter, preferably barefoot, could stand with his or her feet comfortably apart, knees bent a little, leaning backward slightly while keeping thighs and buttocks firm, so that all the strength comes from there rather than the arms. This position will help the supporter to avoid straining the lower back, especially if care is taken not to stoop forward or tense the shoulders. If your supporter has a weak back, it is helpful if he or she rests the buttocks on the edge of the bed or a chair.

The position of the arms is important, too. Your supporter can pass his or her arms underneath your armpits and grip your thumbs. Your wrists should never be gripped as this can damage the nerves running through them and cause numbness.

Once you are comfortable in this position, both of you should relax and breathe deeply. If the support is right, you should be able to let go of your body completely without undue strain on your supporter. At first it may seem difficult, but with practice and if the dynamics are right, even a small person can manage it. Bear in mind that this position will not be used throughout the second stage but only once the baby's head 'crowns' (*see* pp. 155-8), and then only during contractions.

Once you are at ease with your supporter, you could try having him or her lift you up into a supported squat from the kneeling position, by placing his or her hands under your arms and holding on to your thumbs and then slowly taking your weight against his or her body as you stand up. Alternatively, you can try facing your supporter, placing your arms around his or her neck.

In this squatting position, the baby may be born very quickly, with the whole body sometimes emerging in one contraction. Generally, the midwife only needs to 'catch' the baby and place her on her belly face downward between your legs. This will allow the fluids to drain from her nose and mouth for a few seconds until you sit down and gather your newborn into your arms for the first time.

Because birth is usually rapid in this position, it is ideal if there is any reason to speed up delivery, such as in a case of foetal distress (*see* p. 311) or a long labour. It is particularly useful in breech births (*see* pp. 296-7).

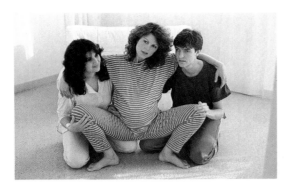

Squatting with two supporters Your supporters can kneel on either side of you, each placing one knee beneath your buttocks, thus giving you some support from underneath. You can then place your arms around their shoulders, while they each, in turn, put one arm around your back.

In between contractions, you can stand up or kneel forward, coming back to a squat once the next contraction begins. The knees and ankles of your supporters need to be quite strong and flexible if they are to adopt this position, and they will find it helpful to kneel on a flat cushion or a folded blanket, and to place a small pillow between buttocks and calves.

In this full squatting position, the pelvis is open to its widest capacity, and is also only a couple of inches above the ground so that your baby can, in fact, slip out unaided and will land in the perfect position on her belly in between your legs. You can use your hands to help your baby emerge.

Although this position is best used on the floor, it can easily be adapted to a hospital delivery bed. As both supporters stand on either side of the bed, squat with your arms around their shoulders, possibly with a cushion rolled up under your heels for support.

Unsupported squat Some women prefer to give birth independently with little or no support from their attendants. You can do this most easily if you have something stable in front of you to hold on to, or if you lean forward on to your hands. You may wish to hold on to one of your attendants, who can sit or kneel in front of you. Pressure on the perineum at the end of the second stage can be eased if you come forward and perhaps kneel right at the end of the birth. This will spread the pressure evenly throughout the vulva.

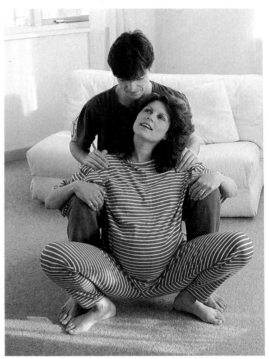

Squatting with one supporter This position, enjoyed by many couples, is similar to the last one, but you will need only one supporter – say, your partner – who can sit on the edge of a chair with his knees comfortably apart. Placing yourself with your back to him, squat down between his knees, leaning your trunk and head against his body, so that you are cradled between his legs and can use his knees for support. In between contractions, you can kneel on all fours or stand up and move around.

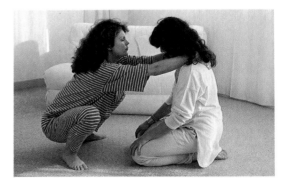

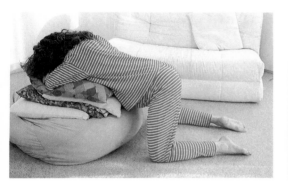

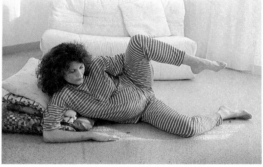

Kneeling on all fours This is an instinctive position used by many women, and is particularly suitable if the second stage is easy and progresses rapidly. It will give you a feeling of being 'grounded' and a sense of control if the contractions are fast and overwhelming. It will also help to lessen the pressure on the soft tissues of the perineum, giving them more time to expand as the baby is born because the tension is shared with the front half of the vulva.

The midwife will be ideally placed to protect the perineum if necessary. She can also receive the baby from behind and then pass her through your legs to be placed, face downwards, on a soft, clean towel in front of you. You can then sit down and welcome your baby.

Women often discover variations of this kneeling position intuitively during the second stage – e.g. half-kneeling/half-squatting or kneeling upright.

Kneeling positions can be used effectively either on the floor or on a bed. Many women adopt them on hospital delivery beds, holding on to the bars of the backrest. It is essential that a large bean bag or some large cushions are available to support your trunk, head and shoulders, and some women choose to take their own with them into hospital.

Lying down Some women feel happier or more 'earthed' giving birth while lying down – either in a semi-reclining position or on their sides in what is known medically as the *left-lateral position*. These positions do not make the best use of the effects of gravity, but if the birth is progressing rapidly, this is of no great significance. If this is the only way you can make yourself comfortable, there is no reason why you should not use it. It does allow birth attendants easy access to the vaginal outlet but sometimes reduces placental blood flow.

Lying on your side is preferable as this will allow more room for the perineum to relax, and the sacrum will be able to move to increase the size of the pelvic outlet. It also lessens the pressure on the blood vessels supplying the uterus, thus helping to avoid foetal distress. Compared to a semi-reclining position, the left-lateral position is less stressful for the perineum, so tearing is less likely.

Preparing emotionally

Childbirth is an unknown adventure. Although you may be looking forward to the event with great excitement, it is common to feel some fear and anxiety before any new and intense experience. The following describes some of the emotions that are commonly experienced by expectant mothers and fathers as the day of the birth approaches.

The mother's experience

In the last few weeks of pregnancy, you may find that you are calm, relaxed and confident as your expected due date draws nearer. It is also common to feel a sense of apprehension at the inevitable approach of the birth. Even though you are looking forward to having your baby, or have given birth before successfully, intense last-minute anxiety is possible. Many women experience these feelings, but they are usually temporary, and may leave you perhaps more ready to face the challenges ahead of you.

Expectations You may find that, as the time draws near, you are confronted with the fear of not being able to live up to your own and others' expectations. The best way to deal with this fear is to try not to expect anything in advance and to keep an open mind. Other than preparing as well as you can, you cannot make an unknown experience predictable. Becoming a mother is enough of a challenge in itself without setting yourself rigid standards to live up to. Whatever happens during labour and childbirth, producing a healthy baby is a great achievement.

Your body and giving birth There are many fears, normally unfounded, which women can experience just before giving birth. Sometimes there is anxiety about being physically capable of giving birth, particularly if this is a first pregnancy or if a previous birth was difficult or complicated. As the baby grows larger towards the end of the pregnancy, it may seem incredible that she will be able to fit through the pelvis and vaginal opening, especially if the mother is short or has been told that her pelvic size or shape is unusual or that the baby is large. However, nature generally ensures that the baby's size is appropriate for the maternal pelvis.

Many of these anxieties stem from hearsay, and the best way to overcome them is by understanding the physiological processes involved in giving birth (*see* Chapter 10), and by practising stretching exercises (*see* Part V) and the positions natural to labour and birth (*see* pp. 121-7). As your body becomes more loose and open, you will experience a growing sense of trust and confidence in your instinctive ability to give birth.

Coping with pain You may be worried about how you are going to cope with the pain during your labour. Some women feel that accepting all the sensations involved in giving birth will help them to accept and enjoy their babies and the many experiences – both pleasurable and painful – involved in being a mother. Knowing that their baby will be spared the side-effects of pain-relieving drugs can be an incentive. However, it is always helpful to allow yourself the option of using pain relief if you need it (*see* pp. 327-8). For some women who have a low pain tolerance or do not feel that experiencing all the sensations of labour is a necessary part of becoming a mother, this choice can help to make labour a positive experience.

Losing control Labour is a biological process which involves surrendering to powerful involuntary reflexes. This is a time when we cannot control what our bodies need to do.

Although it rarely happens, many women are concerned that, at the onset of labour, their waters might break in a public place or that, during labour, they might involuntarily urinate, vomit or empty their bowels – intimate body functions that usually require privacy. There may also be some fear of losing control emotionally: falling apart, letting yourself go or making too much noise. Women often need to cry, scream or release their feelings during labour, but may feel too inhibited to do so.

These fears are understandable, but it is helpful to come to terms with them beforehand because labour will progress better if you are able to overcome your inhibitions and allow your body to take over.

Bear in mind that midwives and doctors are familiar with these events and are likely to be understanding. Sometimes, however, hospitals expect women to be quiet or to use controlled breathing and pushing techniques. This may disturb the natural process and make things more difficult for you, and it is an important consideration when choosing the place of birth.

In many ways, losing control is precisely what you need to do. Although it may seem contradictory, this will help you feel at one with the intense sensations you will be experiencing.

Privacy and intimacy For some women, the loss of privacy and intimacy involved in giving birth in hospital can be very difficult to cope with. A woman having her baby in a large hospital with frequent changes of staff may feel anxious about whether she will be able to communicate well with her birth attendants.

If you value your privacy, you may consider a home birth, or else try to choose a hospital in which your needs are likely to be understood. Your partner may be able to help by supporting and protecting you at the time (see pp. 130-2). On the positive side, many doctors and midwives are now aware of the problems that occur in hospital, and often try to ensure that the environment is as pleasant as possible and that care is sensitive and considerate. Many hospitals try to give mothers privacy, and attempt to reduce the impersonal and clinical atmosphere.

Interventions Fear of medical interventions such as the use of forceps or episiotomy is also very common. It is essential that you find out well ahead of time the hospital's policy or that of your attendants regarding medical intervention, and to make your feelings and desires on these matters known to them and recorded (see p. 114).

You may be worrying unnecessarily. Your attendants may be able to reassure you that intervention will not be used unless it is really needed and then only with your consent. When appropriately used in the case of a complication or emergency, intervention may save a life or resolve a difficult situation. A hospital can be an amazingly supportive place if you need help during labour. In the unlikely event that this happens to you, you will then probably find that it is a great comfort to be surrounded by the expertise available.

Many pregnant women fear that they may need to have an emergency Caesarean section (see pp. 297-8). In fact, when birth is active only a very small percentage of births end up as emergencies. It is, however, reassuring to know that obstetric techniques are now so sophisticated that, when help is really needed, it is widely available and usually done skilfully, and that the outcome is almost always positive.

Looking forward to the birth Although some fear and anxiety is a natural part of preparing emotionally for childbirth, these feelings are generally overshadowed by the tremendous excitement and glowing optimism which many women experience as they approach the day when their baby will be born. In the last few days, apprehension often disappears, and a calm, quiet energy, confident expectation and a feeling of strength and well-being usually prevail as pregnancy reaches full term.

The father's experience

Becoming a father, particularly for the first time, is a momentous event. As the birth becomes imminent, expectations will build and you will anticipate seeing, hearing, feeling and touching your child. If you choose to be an active participant in your child's birth, it is likely to be one of the most meaningful experiences of your life.

Although you may be excited and joyous at the thought of the adventures that lie ahead, you are bound to have some fears which may not be easy to express. You have probably heard of difficult labours and births and may be afraid for your partner and the baby. While you should be prepared for problems, it is reassuring to know that the majority of labours are uncomplicated.

Preparing for the birth Many men approach childbirth and fatherhood knowing very little about the subject. There are many ways in which a baby can be born, and you may be involved in making important choices and decisions when the time comes.

You may find it helpful to attend a course of preparation classes if these are available for couples in your area. You will find that attendance at a couples' group can be entertaining and interesting as well as useful. You will learn about the physiology of birth and the events that your partner is likely to go through. This will make you feel much more knowledgeable and confident, and if any difficulties arise, you will feel far better equipped to deal with them.

At many of these classes, men are introduced to parents with very young babies, and this will give you an important insight into how you will actually handle your own baby later on. You will also come into contact with other fathers-to-be and have the opportunity to share your experiences and make friends.

Accompanying your partner to her ante-natal checkups, as well as arranging well ahead of time to visit the hospital or midwife, are other ways you can find out about the subject. There are also many books and films available.

Being there During the past 20 years, there has been a dramatic change in attitudes towards the father's participation in birth. In the early 1960s, it was unusual for a man to attend the birth of his child in hospital, whereas now it is the rule rather than the exception. This represents a great cultural alteration which in primitive societies would have taken generations or even centuries to occur.

In some cultures, the mother gives birth supported from behind by the father of the baby, while in others – for example, among Muslims – the men are excluded and labour and delivery are handled solely by women. However, in modern society, a woman may well feel closest emotionally to her partner, and it is now very common for the father of the baby to be the person that she chooses to support and be with her during the birth of her children.

When deciding if and how you would like to participate, it is important to base your decision on your own feelings rather than feel pressured by the current fashion. If you are not at ease, your presence may well be counterproductive as your partner is sure to sense your discomfort. You may, for example, find that you are happier to be present just during labour, preferring to leave the room for the actual birth.

For many men, attendance at the birth will represent their first foray into the 'female world'. They will witness the flow of amniotic fluid, the passage of blood and mucus and the birth of the baby. It is helpful to bear in mind that the fluid has comprised the 'miniature sea' in which your baby has floated for the past nine months, and that the blood is from the nourishing walls of the uterus, unlike the blood normally associated with injury or accident. In some hospitals, male partners are encouraged to remain present even in the event of a forceps delivery or Caesarean section, or might witness the incision made during an episiotomy. This can be disturbing, and you will want to consider this possibility and give yourself the option of leaving if you want to.

It is natural to be a little afraid of attending the birth, particularly if you have never witnessed one before. Although you are likely to *empathize* with what your partner is experiencing, it is helpful to remember not to *identify* with her. Remaining objective in this way will help you to relax.

It is also quite common to be apprehensive about feeling squeamish, to be unsure about how you will behave or react – whether you will be a nuisance or a help – or how you might cope if the going is difficult or a complication arises. The traditional joke about fathers fainting may lurk in the back of your mind. You may also be worried that watching your partner give birth will somehow affect your feelings for her. These concerns are natural and most men experience them in anticipation of the event. However, when the time comes, they usually disappear in the intensity of the moment.

Many men are afraid of feeling helpless as they witness their partner in pain. There is no doubt that the majority of labours are painful and that it can be difficult to watch a loved one go through this. You cannot stop the pain, but the presence of a loving and supportive partner is one of the most important elements in making it bearable.

Despite the fashion in many hospitals of inviting fathers to attend the births of their children, the attitude can be one of 'allowing' you to be a spectator rather than respecting your right to share actively in the experience, and you may feel uncomfortable. If you are familiar with the routine practices and medical language used in the labour ward, you can approach the situation with more confidence.

Your support can make all the difference to your partner, particularly if she is giving birth in a hospital where routine procedures may differ from her ideas. For instance, if she is hoping for an active, natural birth in a hospital where intervention is used frequently, the staff may be willing to assist her but may not be very familiar with ways in which they can support her or with changes of position. Your presence can then be invaluable, as you will be able to assist the staff to help her. If your partner chooses to have her baby at home, you may enjoy the freedom and intimacy which is possible when you are in your own environment (see pp. 115-120).

Some men prefer not to take part in childbirth, and their wishes should be respected. Some couples, who may have a very close and deep relationship, may feel that they do not wish to share the intimacy of the birth experience, preferring to keep this aspect of a woman's sexuality private and mysterious. There are also some women who have a strong need to be alone during childbirth.

The father's role at the birth There are many ways in which you can help, depending on your partner's needs. If you are to be present, it should be to *share* in the experience and respond to her rather than to instruct or 'coach'. By sharing, your emotional support can be invaluable as you are the person whom your partner knows best. You can also be helpful in a practical way, by supporting her physically or massaging her if it seems appropriate, and ensuring that she has the privacy and calm she needs in order to feel relaxed and undisturbed.

Many couples enjoy great closeness during the hours of labour, and express their tenderness and affection for one another. There will be many moments when your partner emerges from her inner world to share her feelings, fears, pain and, often, humour.

If you are an active participant, you may find yourself working almost as hard as she does to give birth to your child. Supporting her weight against your body, you will feel the tremendous power of the contractions while she gives birth. Being involved at a birth can be hard work. Long hours of intense concentration can be fatiguing, and it is important to look after yourself, taking regular breaks to eat, rest or have a breath of fresh air. It will help if you ensure that you are comfortable, staying relaxed and wearing light, loose summer clothing as the room is likely to be very warm.

Your partner may need you constantly during labour, to be held or massaged almost continuously. On the other hand, she may not want to be touched at all or may prefer this contact with the midwife or another woman. It is important to come to terms with both of these possibilities beforehand, to avoid disappointment.

Once the long first stage is over, you may begin to wonder during the second whether your baby will ever be born. Finally you will see the baby's head appear between your partner's labia, and as it 'crowns', it may seem as if the vagina will never stretch sufficiently to allow the baby to emerge.

Then, within moments, the baby is born and you are looking at your new child with an incredible surge of emotion flowing through your body. It is at this point that many men spontaneously cry. Witnessing the birth of a child as first the head and then the body emerge is bound to be one of the most powerful and moving experiences of a lifetime.

Now you and your partner can celebrate the fulfilment of the conception, pregnancy and birth that you have shared together. Any fears you may have had will disappear in the immediacy and intensity of what is before you. Even for men who do not wish to be present at the actual birth, it is wonderful to wait outside and then be witness to the first minutes of the baby's life.

PART III
BIRTH

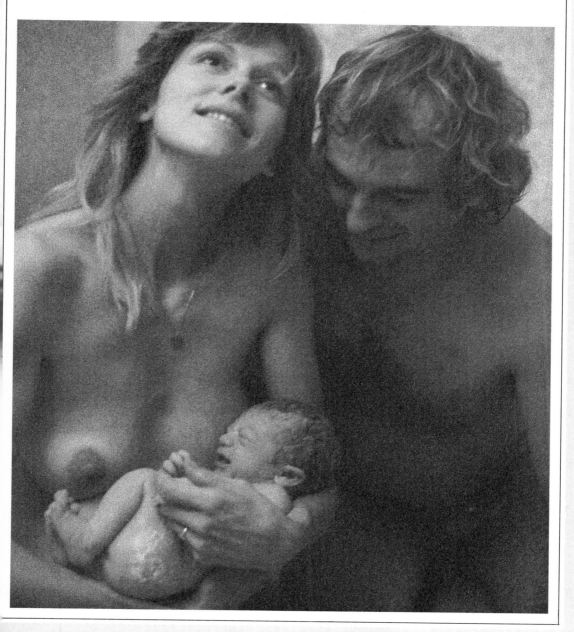

C H A P T E R   10

THE PHYSIOLOGY OF BIRTH

Birth is part of the continuum which begins with conception and carries on into your baby's infancy. It is, at the same time, a physiological process, the transition of a child from the womb to the world, the initiation of a woman into motherhood, a man into fatherhood and the start of a family. Birth is sacred, a time when we welcome and celebrate a new life and experience the tremendous power of creation and the regeneration of life.

During this extraordinary journey, the baby will leave the familiar environment within the uterus and will pass through the pelvic canal, to emerge into an entirely new world. This is likely to be a monumental experience for you both, during which your womb will gradually open to allow you to give birth to your child.

For you, these hours are likely to be among the richest and most meaningful of a lifetime. In giving birth and being born, both mother and baby are intimately linked in a process which unfolds with a marvellous synchronicity, starting with the first movements and contractions of the uterus and ending with your baby safely born and lying contented and at peace in your arms. Although mother and baby are at the centre of the drama, many fathers take an active part in the birth, sharing and supporting both physically and emotionally.

During the months of pregnancy, as the day of birth approaches, you are bound to wonder what it is going to be like. Memories of your own birth, stories and tales told by relatives and friends, dreams and imaginings will all be part of your expectations. Will it be long or short, easy or difficult, painful or pleasurable?

In this part of the book we attempt to answer these questions by trying to describe the wide range of possibilities and the many variables, some of which are likely to be part of your own unique experience.

The stages of labour

The birth process is usually described as occurring in three continuous stages:

● The *first* stage begins when your uterus starts to contract at regular intervals, and continues until the cervix opens, or dilates to about 10cm (4in) in diameter, wide enough for your baby's head to pass through. This is generally the longest part of labour.

● The *second* stage begins when your cervix is fully dilated and ends with the birth, and is usually much shorter than the first stage. Your baby's head and body move down through the dilated cervix and pelvic canal, to emerge through the vagina.

● The *third* stage follows immediately after the birth, when your baby takes his first breath and you experience your first contact together outside the womb. At the end of this stage, the placenta separates from the lining of the uterus and is expelled by more contractions. The umbilical cord is clamped and cut – either before or after the expulsion of the placenta.

However, the birth is not yet complete. During the first few hours, the baby is usually wide awake and alert, acclimatizing to life in the outside world. This is an important time, when you and your baby will begin to get to know each other. Many events take place – for example, the first sucking at the breast, eye-to-eye and skin-to-skin contact – and it is this early 'bonding' that marks the true end of birth.

How labour starts

Your uterus contracts throughout pregnancy, but in labour, the contractions are coordinated to become frequent and strong. The exact stimulus for the onset of labour is unknown, but there are a number of influences which originate both from your body and your baby's.

In the weeks approaching labour, both your pituitary gland and your baby's are active, secreting the hormone *oxytocin* which enters the bloodstream and stimulates the uterus to contract. The baby also secretes other hormones once a certain maturity is reached. Changes take place in his brain at around the 34th week of pregnancy, which stimulate the adrenal glands near each kidney to secrete cortisone. This hormone helps his lungs to mature in readiness for breathing air, and also stimulates the lining of your uterus to produce *prostaglandins* – hormones which, among many other functions, cause the uterus to contract as well as soften and ripen the cervix. If the membranes of the amniotic sac rupture – commonly called the 'breaking of the waters' – pressure from the baby's head on the cervix will also stimulate the release of prostaglandins.

These hormones affect your autonomic nervous system – the 'primitive' part of the brain – which controls all the most basic reflexes of the body, including those of the uterus. The autonomic nervous system acts as a fine-tuning mechanism throughout labour, coordinating and regulating uterine contractions, as well as playing a part in the initiation of labour. It is influenced by a variety of factors, including your thoughts and feelings and signals from your organs.

The initiation of labour is complex, involving a delicate interdependence between the endocrine and nervous systems of both mother and baby. The processes behind initiation build up gradually in the weeks prior to labour, which is set in motion when the baby reaches maturity and is ready to be born.

The length of labour

The length and pattern of labour vary quite widely from woman to woman, but in general, first births tend to be longest, and second, third and fourth births are usually shorter and may be easier. However, the length of labour is no indication of whether the birth is 'easy' or 'difficult': a short labour can be intense and difficult, while a longer one may be experienced as easy, or vice versa.

With a powerful uterine action, a small baby, a large pelvis, a ripe cervix and a conducive atmosphere leading to the secretion of the appropriate hormones, labour tends to be shorter. Generally, however, dilation at a rate of 1 cm ($\frac{1}{3}$ in) per hour is the measure of normal progress in the first

The following chart will give you some idea of what the average length of each stage is. Bear in mind that this is just the estimated average; variations are very common.

First birth
1st stage   4–24 hours
2nd stage $\frac{1}{2}$–2 hours
3rd stage   10 minutes –
          1½ hours

Subsequent births
1st stage   2–12 hours
2nd stage   10 minutes–
          1½ hours
3rd stage   10 minutes –
          1½ hours
The length the first stage lasts usually depends on a number of factors:

* how the mother feels.
* the presence or lack of disturbance.
* the strength of uterine contractions.
* the ripeness of the cervix at the start of labour.
* the size and position of the baby.
* the size and shape of the pelvic cavity.
* the maintenance of adequate fluid and nutrient intake.
* the balance of hormones.
* the use of upright postures during contractions.

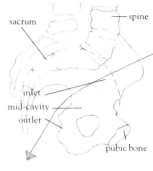

sacrum

spine

inlet
mid-cavity
outlet

pubic bone

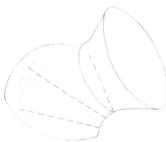

Above: The pelvic canal is surrounded by the sacrum and pelvic bones. It is funnel-shaped, and the baby's head engages through the inlet, passes through the mid-cavity and is born through the outlet.

Below: The baby's head descends through the pelvic canal during labour.

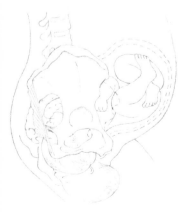

stage. It should also be remembered that sometimes dilation can be slow for hours and then progress rapidly towards full opening of the cervix.

The length of the second stage is dependent on similar factors. Provided mother and baby are well, there is no reason to accelerate labour, which could be considerably longer or shorter than outlined above.

Your pelvis

Your pelvis is a bony girdle which forms the base and outlet of your trunk. Shaped like a funnel with a curved inner canal, it is made up of four bones: the coccyx (tailbone) and sacrum at the back, wedged between two large hip bones. Each hip bone actually comprises three bones – the iliac (flank or side), pubic (groin) and ischial (buttock) bones – which fuse at puberty. The pubic bones meet together at the front, and the iliac bones are joined to the sides of the sacrum at the back.

These pelvic bones form the curved pelvic canal through which your child must pass to be born. The opening at the top of the canal is called the *inlet* and the opening at its base is known as the *outlet*. In a typical pelvis, the inlet is wider from side to side than from front to back; the outlet is just the opposite – that is, wider from front to back. A number of variations in the pelvic shape are possible, but provided the size is adequate, this will not affect the birth.

Before birth, your baby's head will probably enter into, or *engage* in, the pelvic inlet so that the widest diameter of his head is lying sideways, in line with the widest diameter of the inlet. During labour, the head will rotate through 90 degrees, encouraged by the hammock shape of the pelvic-floor muscles, so that, by the time the head reaches the outlet, its widest point will be positioned from front to back, in line with the widest diameter of the outlet.

As your baby's head descends into the pelvic canal and rotates, it negotiates the pelvic curve by pivoting under the pubic bones as the face sweeps along the back wall of the vagina; it then emerges beneath the pubis, under the pubic arch. Once the head emerges, the body will continue to turn, completing the spiral until the shoulders and then the rest of the body are born. Your baby's journey through the curved canal of the pelvis will be much easier if you are in an upright position – standing, kneeling, sitting or squatting – so that the angle of descent is in harmony with the downward force of gravity.

The pelvic joints Your pelvic bones are held together by ligaments (which prevent excessive movement) at four joints: the pubic joint in front; the two sacroiliac joints at the back; and the sacrococcygeal joint between the coccyx and the sacrum. These joints become more flexible during pregnancy due to the softening effects of hormonal secretions on the ligaments, and they are capable of considerable expansion during labour to make as much room as possible for your baby. The pubic joint can open as much as 1.3 cm (½ in), and the sacrococcygeal joint allows the coccyx to swivel out of the way as the baby descends.

The sacroiliac joints are also capable of some expansion sideways, but their most important movement during birth is a pivotal action which enables the sacrum to move to and fro and alters the size of the pelvic canal considerably. If you lean forward or squat, the top part of your sacrum tilts forward with your spinal column, the lower part tilts back and the pelvic canal opens wide. If, however, you are lying down or semi-reclining, your weight rests on your sacrum and forces the top part backwards and the lower part to tuck in and narrow the space within the canal.

The squatting position increases the area of the inlet by up to 25-30 per cent, and also expands the diameter of the outlet in all directions. When you squat, the pubic bones widen, the hip bones move apart, the sacrum moves back and the pelvis opens to its maximum, making the most of the flexibility and mobility of the pelvic joints, whereas in the semi-reclining position, up to one-quarter of the potential for expansion is lost. The use of upright postures and the squatting position will ease the progress of the baby through the birth canal, and may help to avoid the need for intervention, particularly if there is a slight disproportion between the size of the baby's head and the mother's pelvis.

Your uterus

The uterus is a muscular organ made up of three layers of criss-crossing muscle fibres, as well as blood vessels and nerves, surrounding a cavity which is connected to the Fallopian tubes above and, through the cervix, to the vagina below. (*See also* pp. 12–16.)

During pregnancy, the uterus grows, its main function being to accommodate, protect and nourish the growing baby. At this time, its lower segment is thick and firm, the circular muscle fibres of the cervix holding it closed, thereby providing a sphincter-like valve which will resist opening until the baby is ready to be born.

During labour, the cervix opens and the uterus expels the baby. After the birth, it contracts to expel the placenta, and then retracts to stop any bleeding and returns to its pre-pregnancy state within a few weeks.

Contractions These generate the tremendous power and energy which brings about the birth. Each contraction begins at the top of the uterus and then spreads downward towards the cervix. At its peak, the entire uterine muscle is contracted, and it then relaxes from the top down.

Every labour has a rhythm of its own, with the contractions following each other rather like waves in the sea which flow one after the other at regular intervals. Like a wave, each contraction has a beginning, in which it gathers strength, and a peak of full power, before it breaks and begins to ebb away. You can feel it coming on like a rush of energy which reaches full intensity at the peak and then slowly dissipates as the muscle fibres relax. Between contractions, there is a rest period until the next one begins. As labour advances, the contractions become longer and stronger, and the intervals between them shorter, until full dilation is reached.

The intermittent quality of contractions is of enormous value. In the intervals, the pressure on your child is relieved, you can rest and the blood flow to the uterine muscle and the placenta, which is slowed down at the peak of the contraction, is restored. The blood supplies the energy needed for the muscle to work, as well as oxygen for the baby.

Contractions have another important function. Throughout the pregnancy, the developing baby has become accustomed to living with them as they massage him through the fluid that fills the amniotic sac. In labour, the contractions stimulate all the sensory nerve endings in his skin, which in turn stimulates, via the autonomic nervous system, every part of the baby's body in preparation for life outside the womb.

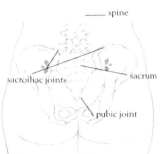

spine

sacroiliac joints

sacrum

pubic joint

The sacrum is able to pivot at the sacroiliac joints (above). In the squatting position (below) it tilts backwards, enlarging the pelvis, whereas in the reclining position (bottom) the tilt is forwards and the size of the pelvic cavity is reduced.

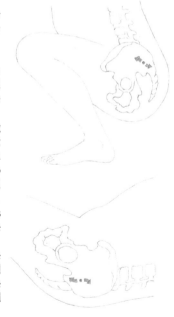

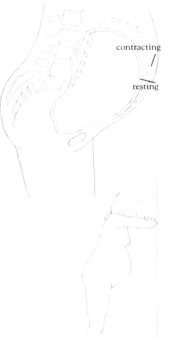

contracting

resting

As the uterus contracts, the muscle fibres shorten and the uterus tilts forwards. In an upright position contractions will be most efficient, whereas in the reclining position they must work against the pull of gravity.

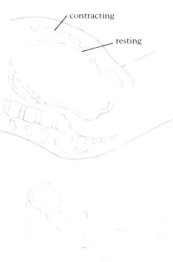

contracting

resting

Posture and the work of the uterus It is vital for the work of your uterus and for your baby that your body position during labour enhances both the circulation of blood to your womb and the effectiveness of contractions.

You can ensure that the blood supply to your baby is optimal by staying upright or kneeling forward on to cushions or on all fours. This will reduce pressure on the large blood vessels which supply blood to the uterus and placenta. In addition, the uterus tilts forward each time it contracts, and if your trunk is leaning forward, you will be helping your uterus to work against the least resistance.

Contractions are aided by the downward force of gravity to become stronger and more effective. When a woman is upright in labour, the uterus contracts less frequently, but during each contraction, the pressure within is greater. Each contraction will be more powerful, while each resting phase will be longer, and this will improve the overall flow of blood to the placenta.

Your baby's descent through the pelvis will also be helped by the downward force of gravity if you are in this position. The increased pressure from the baby's head on the cervix will hasten the speed of dilation, and in the second stage, when the baby is born, his weight will act in harmony with gravity, thus increasing the expulsive force of the contractions.

If, however, you lie down, this opposes the force of gravity. Any muscle that has to work against resistance will soon begin to ache, and therefore contractions will be more painful and perhaps less effective, as well as more frequent.

Your hormonal balance

During labour, a delicate and complex equilibrium of hormonal secretions is maintained which regulates the rhythm of the labour. Your brain will also secrete *endorphins* which will promote and enhance your labour. These substances, which are produced at other times – for example, when we sing or exert ourselves physically – play an important role in all aspects of sexual behaviour, including love-making and birth, by acting as natural relaxants and encouraging a sense of well-being which helps to reduce pain.

In deep states of meditation, our endorphin levels are at their highest. As labour intensifies, the level of endorphins rises, inducing an almost trance-like relaxation in which you are able to let go of your normal conscious, thinking mind and sink into the intense sensations within you. As you get closer to the moment of the birth, this concentration and turning inward increases, enabling you to surrender to the involuntary forces in your body. For many women, this is not unlike the letting go that takes place when they make love.

Labour and childbirth need to take place in a setting which encourages the release of endorphins, where the mother will have the freedom to be uninhibited. In this respect, she shares a common need with many mammals, who, when approaching the time of delivery, will look for a quiet, dark and secure corner where the birth can take place without disturbance. For humans as for other mammals the ability to give birth is instinctive. If you are able to relax and trust your instincts, your body will do the rest.

On the other hand, when you are anxious, frightened or cold, your body will produce stress hormones such as *adrenalin* – the 'fight or flight' hormone. Among other things, adrenalin stimulates muscles to tighten, increases blood pressure and, during labour, effectively reduces the power of uterine contractions in the first stage. However, in the second stage, adrenalin may help to stimulate the expulsive reflex as the mother's muscles gather strength to aid the birth of her baby.

The baby's position

The occipital bone at the back of the baby's head is used as a marker to describe two of the three positions that a baby may adopt in the womb.

Occipito anterior (OA) position At the time of birth, most babies lie head down, with their spine facing their mother's abdominal wall, lying slightly to the left or right, and their limbs adjacent to her back and to the other side. When the head engages, the occipital bone points towards the front and the baby faces the mother's spine. This position facilitates the baby's progress through the birth canal.

Occipito posterior (OP) position Babies in the womb seem to like to face the placenta, so if this has implanted on the front wall of the uterus, the baby is likely to lie, head down, with his spine next to his mother's spine and his limbs towards her abdominal wall. When the head engages, the occipital bone points towards the back. Another reason for a baby to adopt an occipito posterior position (*see* p. 325) may be the shape or size of the pelvic outlet. Such a position may prolong labour, and contractions may be felt in the back.

Breech position In this, the baby's buttocks or feet are nearest the pelvis, and the head lies under the ribs. (*See also* Breech birth, pp. 296-7.)

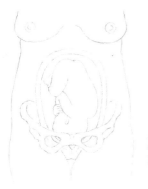

Occipito anterior
presentation

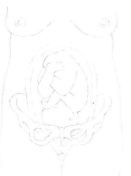

Occipito posterior
presentation

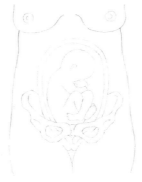

Breech presentation

C H A P T E R   11

APPROACHING BIRTH

During the last six weeks or so of your pregnancy, the uterus prepares for the birth. You will notice an increasing number of contractions, which are usually mild and painless and are felt as a hardening or tightening of the abdomen, quite different from the baby's movements inside the uterus.

These are *Braxton Hicks contractions* – named after the gynaecologist who first identified them – and in some women, they are infrequent, while others experience runs of powerful tightenings which can last for 15 to 30 minutes at a time.

During the last four weeks of pregnancy, the baby's head usually descends into the pelvis. In this process, called *lightening* or *engagement*, the widest diameter of the baby's head settles into the inlet of the pelvis. This occurs more commonly among Caucasian women, while many African, Afro-Caribbean and Asian women find that their babies' heads remain high until the onset of labour. Engagement prior to labour is also more common in women having their first child; this is because, in subsequent pregnancies, the uterine muscle is more elastic and so babies are under less downward pressure. Lightening is often accompanied by quite strong contractions and a noticeable lowering, or 'dropping', of the baby. You will now be able to breathe more easily, as there is less pressure on your diaphragm, but you will probably also find that you will have to urinate more often as the baby may press on your bladder.

In the days before labour begins, your baby may move less frequently, although some babies move more. If you are concerned that your baby is not moving enough, you will find it reassuring to be checked by your midwife or doctor.

Your changing consciousness

During labour and birth, as your womb slowly opens to give birth to your baby, it becomes the energy centre of your body, and the sensations you are likely to experience will be immensely powerful. There is an expansion of normal, everyday consciousness, so that, by the time you are ready to give birth, you will be at your most open. You will be deeply in touch with your inner, instinctive self, so that you will not be functioning from your logical, rational mind, but completely involuntarily from your basic, primitive roots. This can be extraordinary, comparable with the transcendent states of mind that may be experienced through meditation.

For some women, it can also be a frightening prospect, and the struggle to resist this is perhaps one of the causes of difficulties in labour. It is natural and even inevitable to fear such an awesome if marvellous experience.

The process of opening up to the depth and intensity of the birth

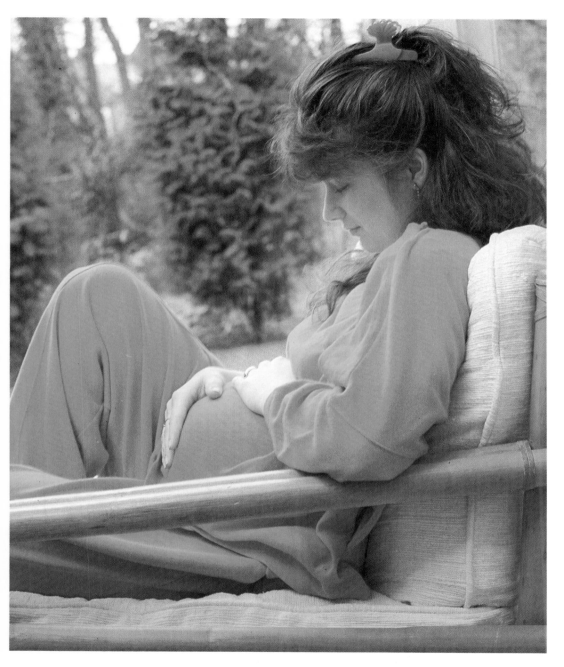

experience begins during pregnancy. There is a natural tendency for your attention and interest to focus inwards as your sense of harmony with your inner self increases. The release of hormones in your body makes you more sensual and instinctive and less intellectual; you will probably find it increasingly difficult to focus your mind, to study or read or to remember things. Your ability to do all these things will return after childbirth, but for the time being, the more psychic and intuitive aspects of your nature are most dominant.

For most women, it is easy to accept this change in consciousness and to flow with it. Practising deep breathing, yoga and meditation (*see* Part V) will help you to surrender to this unique experience and enhance its pleasure.

Waiting

Because the length of pregnancy is variable, very few women actually go into labour on the estimated due date. Although some go into labour unexpectedly early, for many there is a time of waiting at the end of their pregnancies which can seem to last for ever. This period can be fairly trying, particularly if you have passed your estimated due date and are anxious and possibly under pressure to have labour induced (*see* pp. 317-18).

Instead of becoming impatient, it may be a good idea to make the most of this period by doing stretching exercises, bathing, sleeping and generally relaxing, enjoying any quiet activity which prepares you for the birth. Some women have a last-minute rush of energy just before labour starts, and sudden urges to decorate, cook or bake are not unusual.

Labour can begin at any time of the day or night and may last for a relatively long time, so it is important that you and your partner have plenty of rest. Sleep may be more easily achieved if you do regular, gentle exercises during the day. Many couples find this waiting period a marvellously intimate time – for some, it is like a second honeymoon prior to the birth of their first child.

When labour is imminent

The uterus contracts throughout pregnancy, but during the last few weeks the frequency of these contractions increases, causing a change in the balance of muscle fibres. The cervix gradually shortens as it is drawn up, and the lower segment thins while the upper segment thickens. The thinning of the lower segment is known as *effacement of the cervix*.

'Ripening' and the 'show'

This change is accompanied by a softening, or 'ripening', of the muscle fibres caused by the secretion of hormones (prostaglandins) by the inner lining of the uterus, and oestrogen, progesterone and relaxin mainly from the placenta. If the cervix is fully effaced and ripe prior to the onset of labour, the labour is likely to be short.

As the cervix ripens and then begins to open (dilate), the plug of mucus which sealed the opening may be released. This is known as the 'show', and consists of a mucous discharge from your vagina. This can be either watery or sticky like a light jelly, and is usually stained brown, pink or bright red. There may be a slight discharge lasting several days or the show may appear suddenly, all at once. If the discharge resembles heavy bleeding, you should contact your midwife.

A show can be the first sign that labour is about to start, although in some women, the mucous plug does not come away until later, when contractions are well established. Alternatively, many days may elapse from the time of the show until labour actually begins.

'Breaking of the waters'

Another common sign that labour is imminent is the rupturing of the membranes of the amniotic sac which surround the baby in the uterus, with subsequent leakage of amniotic fluid – commonly called 'breaking of the waters'.

Once the baby's head engages, the amniotic fluid is contained both above and below it. The 'hindwaters' are above, surrounding her body, while the 'forewaters' form a cushion between the head and the cervix. Sometimes when the membranes rupture, there is only a small gush of fluid; this is usually the forewaters, the hindwaters remaining inside, kept in place by the snug fit of the baby's head in the pelvis. Other times, the waters may break in what may seem an enormous flood. Often, amniotic fluid leaks for days, but since the uterus is constantly replacing the lost fluid, its volume does not diminish, and thus the fear of a 'dry' birth is totally unfounded.

Although the waters sometimes break before labour starts, most commonly this occurs during the first stage, when the cervix is nearing complete dilation. It may even happen that the membranes do not rupture until the baby emerges. This is known as being 'born in a caul'.

Sometimes the waters break hours or even days before the onset of labour; this is called 'premature rupture of the membranes' (see p. 331). If this happens, the amniotic fluid should be clear and colourless; if it is stained green with meconium (the baby's first bowel movement), you should contact your birth attendants immediately. It is also advisable to have your midwife or doctor check the location of the umbilical cord to exclude a prolapsed cord (see p. 331).

As the waters usually break during the night, it is wise to protect your mattress with a waterproof undersheet as your due date approaches.

Bowel changes

In the days leading up to the birth, the bowel is stimulated by prostaglandin, a hormone released by the lining of the uterus, and it will empty more frequently in readiness for the birth. It is common for bowel movements to be loose when labour is imminent.

The natural tendency of the body is to empty the bowels before and during childbirth. This normally happens as a preliminary to labour, but pressure from the baby's head on the rectum may also stimulate the bowels to empty spontaneously during childbirth. If this happens, the midwife will protect your vagina from being soiled.

In the days approaching the birth, it is sensible to eat easily digested, light meals that contain a lot of dietary fibre – including raw salads and fruit – to encourage the natural emptying of the bowels.

Shivering

Occasionally, labour may be preceded by involuntary shivers. Although you may not feel cold, you may find yourself trembling uncontrollably. This is a common occurrence that can also happen during or immediately after childbirth, and is the body's way of releasing tension, but it can be alarming if you do not know that it can happen and why. The bouts of shivering usually last only a few minutes. Deep breathing, a calming massage down the spine, increasing the warmth of the room or having a warm bath will all help.

The first contractions: pre-labour

The first contractions are usually similar to intense menstrual pains and will be felt either in the lower abdomen or in the lower back. They may occur at intervals of anything between 10 and 30 minutes, and progressively increase in power and frequency. There are, however, variations: some women start and continue labour with contractions every five to ten minutes; others have periodic, irregular contractions over a few days before the onset of strong, regular ones; and a very small minority hardly feel the contractions at all. Occasionally, contractions are irregular throughout labour.

You may mistake your Braxton Hicks 'practice' contractions (see p. 140) for true labour. However, when the latter starts, the uterus usually contracts rhythmically at regular intervals, and each contraction starts off mildly, builds in intensity until it reaches a peak and then ebbs away. Once you are in established labour and your cervix begins to dilate, the sensations are undeniably strong, so if you are in any doubt as to whether you are in labour yet, you probably are not. Your midwife or doctor can help you to confirm true labour by assessing the contractions or checking to see if your cervix is dilating.

The uterus often begins to contract for a few hours or more in the days before labour starts, and then may stop for a few hours or even a day. It is quite common for this 'pre-labour' to continue for some days; it is as if the uterus is practising for birth. If the contractions keep you awake at night, try to sleep or rest in between them.

If you were not very aware of contractions in a previous pregnancy, or if you had a very short labour, you should stay close to home when your due date is near.

What you can do when labour is imminent

- Carry on with your life as usual.
- Take some exercise: go for a walk, swim or do some stretching exercises to keep your body relaxed and open. Be sure to avoid positions which involve lying on your back.
- Eat small, light meals that are easily digested. You need enough food to give you energy and keep your blood sugar in balance, but too much will be difficult to digest once labour starts.
- You may enjoy having a bath. Make sure that the water is not too hot; otherwise, you will feel drained.
- If you are too excited and elated to rest, try drinking some camomile tea, which is calming and soporific. Listening to music or having a good massage may also be enjoyable.
- If your labour starts gradually over a day or so, or if you have bouts of 'pre-labour', it is wise to ensure that you rest or sleep between contractions.
- If mild contractions begin during the night, it is best to try and sleep. However, you may find this impossible, in which case resting and dozing in a comfortable position can be a good substitute. Try one of the positions outlined on pages 122–3, using plenty of pillows.

CHAPTER 12

LABOUR AND BIRTH

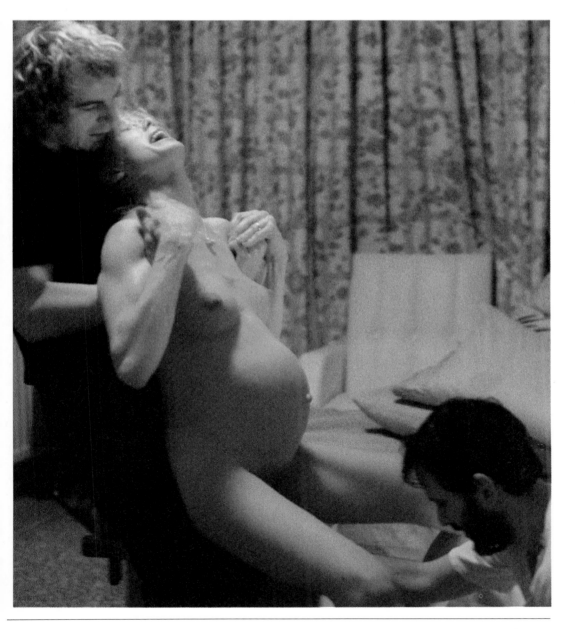

Labour is one of the most profound and deeply moving experiences you are ever likely to encounter. The range of feelings and sensations it includes are rich and varied, both physically and emotionally. Labour consists of regular uterine contractions which eventually cause the expulsion of the foetus and placenta, and can be divided into three distinct stages. Every labour develops a rhythm or pattern of its own as the waves of contractions slowly increase in frequency and become more powerful.

The first stage of labour

The first stage can be understood as consisting of three continuous phases. The *latent phase,* usually the longest part of the first stage, is concerned with the completion of the ripening of the cervix, and the first 4 cm (1 ½ in) of dilation. During this time, contractions may be mild or infrequent. During the *active phase,* the cervix dilates from 4 cm to 10 cm (4 in), progress is usually faster and the contractions are stronger, last longer and are more frequent. Towards the end, they become very intense as their power reaches a peak. The last phase of the first stage is called *transition,* which may last a few seconds or several hours.

In some labours, maximum intensity can be reached within one hour, whereas in others it may take as long as 36 hours to reach this point. The chart of dilations and contractions below describes what can occur in a 'classic' first labour:

Dilation	Contractions	
	Duration	*Intervals between*
Begins	20–30 seconds	10–20 minutes
3 cm	20–40 seconds	5–10 minutes
8 cm	40–60 seconds	2–3 minutes
10 cm	60–90 seconds	30–60 seconds

Not all women have such a predictable pattern: for example contractions can be 2–3 minutes apart throughout. However, once the cervix is in the final stages of opening, the contractions are usually very strong and occur at regular and increasingly shorter intervals.

How does it feel?

Excitement, joy and moments of bliss are as much a part of having a baby as pain, fear, anxiety and feelings of despair. There is no doubt that labour is usually hard work which will stretch you to your limits and even perhaps beyond, and there will be times when you are likely to feel intense pain. It is realistic to expect and prepare for this.

The first stage of labour can be compared to climbing a mountain. At first, it is uphill all the way, becoming steeper as you reach the top. It is natural to encounter difficulty *en route,* to reach a plateau now and again when you need to slow down and rest. You may even feel at some point that you are not going to make it, but after a rest, a change of position or a warm bath, you may then discover a fresh burst of energy, a new courage and the enthusiasm to carry on.

During labour, you will go through many moods and emotions. They can range from intimate feelings of affection towards your partner and blissful, joyful pleasure to moments of fear or panic, irritability, loss of faith, weakness and despair. You may need to express these feelings out loud, perhaps by crying, moaning, singing or laughing, and this may be vital to the progress of your labour. You will also be so intensely involved in the rhythm of the labour that time in its normal sense will be meaningless, and your attention will be fully absorbed by your bodily sensations.

Your body will work reflexively as it prepares to expel your baby, and all your systems will adjust to the great opening and emptying which takes place. Your bowels may spontaneously empty to make way for your baby, and you may need to retch or vomit. This will help you to release tension, and you will probably feel fine soon afterwards.

During the first stage, contractions are usually felt in the lower abdomen, although some women may feel them in the lower back or in the belly simultaneously. Occasionally, contractions can be felt along the inside of the thigh or up the spine.

How a contraction will feel is very subjective. Most women describe them as being similar to menstrual cramps, only stronger, but they may also feel like a rush of energy or like a sharp pain. Usually an intense contraction is painful at its peak, but as it ebbs away or in the intervals in between, the subsequent relaxation can be almost blissful, and the flow of energy released in your body can feel very pleasant. As labour progresses and contractions become more intense, pain tends to intensify too, so that the most painful contractions are usually towards the end of the first stage, when dilation is nearing completion.

The amount of pain felt varies from woman to woman. Some people hardly feel their contractions and will only begin to be aware of them once they are in strong labour and dilation is already well advanced; this is often the case when a woman has given birth several times before.

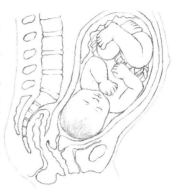

1. Before labour: the cervix is uneffaced and closed, and the baby's head is engaged.

What happens to your baby
Many babies become a little less active in the days leading up to the birth, although some continue to move quite a lot and can be felt moving and kicking throughout labour.

Your baby will be well prepared for labour, having experienced the contractions of the uterus during the previous months. During the first stage, he receives oxygen and nutrients via the placenta and perhaps even sleeps in the uterus, but as the intensity increases, he will feel the regular massage of contractions on his body and the pressure of the opening cervix on his head as it descends through the birth canal.

If the amniotic sac is intact, this pressure is cushioned by the amniotic fluid between the baby's head and the membranes. If it has ruptured, the head will exert a direct force on the cervix, helping it to open. Your baby may move and wriggle his head, which further assists dilation.

The bones of a baby's skull are still separate and able to overlap one another. This helps in the birth by reducing the size of the head.

As the first stage progresses, each contraction draws the cervix up over your baby's head like a glove. As soon as your cervix is fully dilated, his head is surrounded by the vaginal walls, which are in turn supported by the muscles and bones of your pelvis. While the cervix is opening, the head, continuing to rotate for birth, will descend into the pelvic canal.

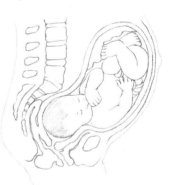

2. Early in the first stage: the cervix is effaced and about 1cm dilated.

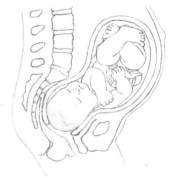

3. Late first stage: the cervix is now about 5cm dilated.

We can only imagine what the baby is experiencing through all this. He must be feeling all sorts of new sensations: the increasingly powerful contractions on his body; the vagina and cervix surrounded by the tight, bony walls of the pelvis compressing his head; the movement away from the familiar presence of the placenta. Perhaps he enjoys the rhythmic massage of the contractions, as well as experiencing fear, panic or pain as the pressure increases and he is propelled through the birth canal.

During birth, babies are active participants, both physically and emotionally. We have good reason to believe that babies are aware, sensitive and deeply responsive to what happens during birth and that the experiences that occur at this time become a part of us.

When to go to hospital or call your midwife

If you are having a home birth, you should inform your midwife when labour has begun. She will come and visit you to assess your progress and will then inform your doctor. If you intend to give birth in hospital, it is ideal if your birth attendants or your family doctor can visit you at home when you are in early labour to check your progress and help you to decide when to go to hospital. This is the case with GP units and the domino scheme (see p. 110), but if not, ring the sister at the labour ward.

Women vary as to when they want to go into hospital. Being at home until labour is well established is usually a good idea, since rushing into hospital earlier than necessary can make labour seem longer, and if labour is not well established, you may be sent home until things intensify.

No matter when you planned to go into hospital, you will need to leave home once your contractions are 40–45 seconds long and occurring at regular intervals of about four to five minutes. If this is your second or subsequent baby and frequent contractions quickly develop, you should go in as soon as possible. In the unlikely event of there being vaginal bleeding which is heavier than a 'show', or continuous severe pain in your abdomen or back, you should also go in right away.

It is wise to have your things packed well beforehand so that they are instantly ready (see p. 112). When travelling to the hospital, take your time, stopping to breathe through each contraction. Rather than sitting the normal way in a car, it may be more comfortable to kneel in the back seat facing backwards and lean over the top of the seat.

Changing your environment may be disturbing, and progress may slow down a little until you are comfortably settled in the labour suite.

At the hospital

Once you arrive in hospital, several admission procedures are carried out. You will be examined to check both your well-being and that of your baby and to assess the progress of your labour (see opposite).

At this stage, you may be offered a warm bath or an enema. However, there is no need for the routine use of enemas to empty bowel contents, as this usually occurs naturally before or during labour or during the birth itself. If you feel embarrassed at the thought of emptying your bowels during the birth, a small enema or the use of suppositories may be useful, although this is likely to be uncomfortable if you are in strong labour.

Rupturing the membranes artificially (see Induced labour, pp. 317-8) as a routine part of the admission procedure is also unnecessary and will increase the risk of infection and intensify contractions.

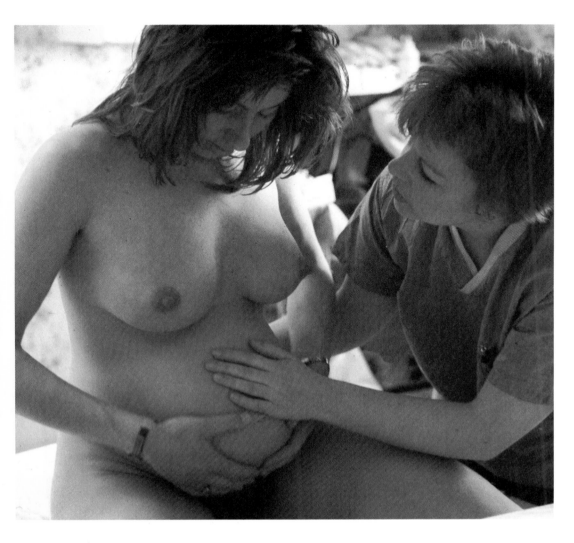

Progress checks and monitoring

Throughout labour, your well-being and progress, as well as that of your baby, will be observed by your birth attendants. Your own intuition is most valuable in assessing your progress, based on how you are feeling.

Your midwife will offer vital moral support during labour.

The Mother Your blood pressure, temperature and pulse rate will be checked from time to time, and your urine analysed. Observations will also be made of the strength, duration and frequency of the contractions.

Your midwife may examine you internally to assess the progress of your labour. Between contractions, she will gently introduce one or two fingers into your vagina to feel the cervix, to check how much it has dilated, its softness and its stretchability. She will also feel whether the membranes have ruptured and, if they have, will check the colour of the amniotic fluid. Through the open cervix, she will feel the position of the baby's head and how far it has descended into the pelvic canal.

During the first stage, vaginal examinations are usually done every four to six hours, or whenever the mother wants one. They usually take only a few minutes and should not be unduly uncomfortable if you relax completely and breathe deeply. However, they may hurt a little if you are tense and tighten your pelvic muscles, if the cervix is very high or if the baby's head is high and is thus awkward for the midwife to reach.

Comfortable positions for examinations include sitting on the edge of a chair, squatting, standing and kneeling on all fours. A skilled midwife or doctor may assess the progress of labour intuitively, and will require few if any vaginal examinations. The results of each vaginal examination are recorded on your chart. Some hospitals use *partograms,* a recording of the progress of labour on a graph.

The Baby The condition of your baby is assessed in a number of ways. Your birth attendants will examine the baby by feeling your abdomen and by vaginal examination. However, the most important check is the monitoring of your baby's heartbeat.

There are several methods for carrying this out. The simplest are the old-fashioned ear trumpet and the stethoscope, but today a variety of electronic heart monitors is used. The hand-held electronic heart monitor is ideal for an active birth as it can be used when the mother is in any position. A simple transducer is held against the abdomen in the proximity of the baby's heart. The rate of the heartbeat, and sometimes the contractions, are recorded on graph paper, and the sound of the heartbeat is magnified and can be heard.

Usually the baby's heartbeat is monitored at the onset of labour and then at intervals until the birth. The frequency will vary according to the progress of labour, and continuous monitoring may occasionally be used (*see* Foetal-heart monitoring, pp. 311-12). An abnormality of the heartbeat may indicate foetal distress (*see* p. 311).

Pain in labour

Women's experience of pain in childbirth varies enormously. While some do have painless labours, most women find that the pain of strong contractions surprises them with its intensity, and it may take them almost to the limits of their endurance. For some, it is completely intolerable and some form of pain relief is needed.

The attitudes of women towards labour pain vary, too. Some are ready to accept pain and feel that it is part of the experience, even though it may not be easy to cope with, while others choose from the outset to use pain relief. A woman's expectations and confidence during pregnancy can influence this decision.

Because it is impossible to know in advance exactly what the pain of your labour will be like, it is wise to know how to reduce the factors which may increase it and how to cope using your own resources, and also to know about the methods available for relieving pain if you need them.

Here, we will be dealing with ways in which you can cope with pain yourself. After reading this, turn to the section on pain relief on pages 327-9 for a guide to the various methods available if intervention is needed.

Coping with pain Your body is designed to be able to cope with pain. If the conditions are right, your brain will secrete *endorphins* – hormones which are natural painkillers and relaxants. The following are ways in which you can enhance the secretion of endorphins.

Through breathing, you have an amazing power to transform and dissipate the pain of labour. Like a surfer waiting for a wave to swell, you can catch each contraction as it arises, at the moment it begins to gather strength, and then, with your deep breathing, surf over the crest without being overwhelmed.

You can do this by relaxing your body in a comfortable position, and focusing your attention on your breathing as in the deep-breathing exercises for pregnancy (see part V). As each contraction begins, breathe slowly and deeply into your abdomen while the uterus does its work. Concentrate especially on the exhalation, keeping your attention focused on the breath until the contraction is over. With each exhalation, let go of all tension and open your body to the sensations you are experiencing, allowing yourself to accept and surrender to the contractions. Take each contraction one at a time, without thinking ahead, and use your energy economically by remaining calm and relaxed and centred on the rhythm of your breathing.

Along with breathing, you may need to make sounds in labour. This is a natural mechanism for releasing pain, and it is helpful if you can express this sound without inhibition.

Using your body well will make an enormous difference, too. Position yourself so that you feel comfortable, using positions that are in harmony with gravity and will allow labour to progress without resistance. Moving, rotating your hips, rocking and walking are all ways to reduce pain.

Massage may be invaluable for relieving pain. It can be done in any position and is easy to do; useful techniques are detailed in Part V. Some women need a lot of physical contact and will benefit from being held and supported by one of their birth attendants. For them, this fulfils a need to be mothered during labour, and may help them to let go.

Immersion in water is a very efficient way of stimulating the secretion of endorphins, and is thus an efficient way of relieving pain in labour. The water should be warm – just above body temperature – and as deep as possible to allow for changes in position. If a bath or pool is not available, warm water from a shower running down your back or on your belly can be surprisingly effective. Some women spend a lot of time immersed in water during labour, and are able to relax better, free from the effects of gravity. It is especially useful in a long labour or towards the end of the first stage. It may be wise to wait until contractions are strong before entering a bath or pool so as to keep this valuable resource until it is really needed. Often labour will progress rapidly once the mother relaxes in water. If the birth occurs in water, there is no need for concern: the baby is quite used to being in a fluid environment, and will not begin to breathe until you lift him out, when breathing will be stimulated by the air on his skin.

For some women, creative visualization is helpful. For example visualizing images of water or waves in the sea as the contractions begin, or creating mental pictures of flowers opening as if in slow motion, dolphins diving under waves or wherever your imagination leads can all be useful when combined with deep breathing, movement and massage.

Good preparation in pregnancy, both physical and emotional, may also help to reduce pain in labour. Relaxing stiff muscles and joints through exercise, resolving any fears, anxieties or problems in your relationships

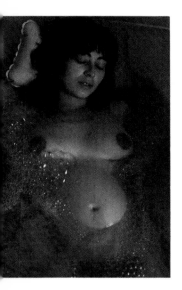

Lying in warm water helps to relieve the pain of labour.

with your loved ones, and cultivating the art of relaxation and meditation are all effective tools.

Also important is the right atmosphere, one of privacy, calm and intimacy, in which you can feel totally at ease and uninhibited, and where there are few distractions. Reducing sensory stimulation by darkening the labour room and making sure that it is quiet and peaceful can help to reduce pain. Your partner or a close friend or relative can be a great source of comfort. It is important that they should be able to share the experience unobtrusively, so that you have a feeling of security with the freedom to let yourself go.

Energy during labour

During the first stage, your breathing and movements should be slow to avoid diminishing your energy. You should rest and, if possible, sleep as much as you can in order to reserve your strength for the birth. Your body will also need fluid during labour, particularly if it is long.

Glucose provides the energy needed by the muscles during contractions. If your body is short of glucose, it will burn other fuel in the body such as fat, and if this goes on for a long time, you may feel low and labour may slow down. You may then become 'ketotic' – that is, ketones (acidic products of fat metabolism) will appear in your blood. Ketones will also be present as acetone in your urine. You can avoid this by making sure that you have a light, easily digestible meal when labour starts. If you have a long labour, you may need light snacks periodically, but food eaten during strong labour may cause vomiting.

You can ensure that your fluid balance and blood sugar level are maintained by drinking liquids such as grape or apple juice, honey in hot water or herbal teas such as raspberry leaf or camomile. You do not need a lot of sugar in labour; simply have a selection of sweet drinks and mineral water and follow your inclinations. If you feel low on sugar, glucose tablets are helpful.

Towards the end of the first stage, taking sips of water between contractions will be sufficient to avoid dehydration. However, at the end you may feel very thirsty and ready to drink a glass or more of water. Because a full bladder will hinder the descent of the baby's head, you will need to empty your bladder frequently during labour.

In some hospitals, drinking and eating during labour is not permitted because of the danger of inhaling acidic stomach contents should a general anaesthetic be required in an emergency. However, if the need arises, the contents of the stomach can be neutralized rapidly by drinking an alkaline solution, and careful induction of anaesthesia will prevent inhalation.

On rare occasions, fluid, minerals and glucose may need to be given intravenously by means of a drip. This will reduce your mobility, but if you are exhausted, the glucose can make you feel much better very quickly. If other medication is needed, it can also be given via the drip.

Positions and movements for the first stage

When labour starts, it is best to continue quietly with your usual activities until the contractions become strong enough to demand your whole attention.

It is natural and instinctive to want to move around during labour, changing positions from time to time, rocking or circling your hips or leaning forward during contractions. Many women discover a kind of birth dance and move their bodies to ease the pain of contractions. Others prefer to walk about, use one or two positions and remain quite still during contractions, or find it more comfortable to be immersed in water. Some relax completely and sleep between contractions.

To reserve your strength, it is wise to pace yourself by resting between contractions in early labour, and you should try to breathe normally until the contractions become really intense.

There are many ways to cope with the first stage of labour, and your own instincts will be your best guide. By following the urges of your body and trying to make yourself as comfortable as possible, you will discover for yourself the movements and positions most suitable for you and your baby (*see* pp. 121–7).

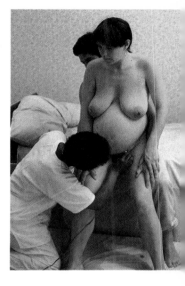

The midwife checks the baby's well-being with a hand-held foetal heart monitor.

Transition

Transition takes place at the end of the first stage, and is like a bridge between the final dilation of the cervix and the expulsive urges of the second stage when the baby is actually born.

The cervix is now almost fully open, and with the lessening of resistance, the downward expulsive force of the contractions begins to be established. Transition may be brief, lasting a few minutes, or it may take longer, sometimes several hours. Contractions tend to be long and intense, with very short intervals between them. The membranes of the amniotic sac often rupture at this point, followed by more intense contractions.

As dilation comes to completion, the cervix fully opens and your baby's head descends into the pelvic canal. The head now exerts pressure through the walls of the vagina on to your sacrum and lower bowel, which can cause a feeling of anal pressure similar to the urge to defecate. By the end of transition, the baby's head will have descended on to the muscular hammock of the pelvic floor, ready for birth.

Occasionally, as the cervix nears full dilation, the front rim, or *anterior lip,* may not open completely. If this is the case, when the midwife examines you she will feel a rim of cervix in front, between the baby's head and the pubic bone. Often, the first urges to bear down occur before this final rim has disappeared, but if you bear down too soon, the lip of the cervix may swell and delay the birth. It can be difficult to cope with the conflict of wanting to push but having to wait. However, if the urge to bear down is uncontrollable, the anterior lip will probably be taken up as the second stage begins.

4. Transition: the cervix is fully dilated (10cm).

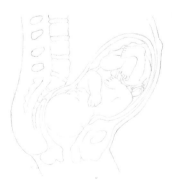

How does it feel?

No matter if your labour has so far been short or long, easy or difficult, this last part of the first stage is bound to be very intense. You will be deeply immersed in the powerful sensations taking place within you, and all your energy and attention will be absorbed by what you are experiencing.

This is an extraordinary time, when you are at your most open and vulnerable. Your concentration will be focused deeply inward, with contractions occurring involuntarily one after another as you prepare to give birth to your baby. Women react in different ways to transition. Although in the brief intervals between contractions the pain ebbs away and a deep, almost blissful serenity is experienced by some women, a feeling of exhaustion is also very common, particularly if it has been a long labour. It is not unusual for a woman who has been coping very well thus far to feel rather despairing, wondering how she will ever have the strength to give birth to her baby, and she may request pain relief. However, in most cases, it is wise to persevere and to avoid painkilling drugs which may have side-effects that could affect the baby or your ability to give birth spontaneously if given at this stage.

During transition, some women feel nauseous and need to retch or vomit, and they may also involuntarily empty the bladder and bowel as the expulsive reflex becomes stronger. Involuntary shivers are common, and can be eased by warmth, deep breathing and/or massage.

Some women also feel confused when the sensations of the expulsive reflex begin and the familiar (if intense) feelings of the first stage change. It is also very common to be irritable and at the end of your tether at this stage. In fact, midwives never take offence at this irritability but welcome it as a sign that birth is imminent!

It is also not unusual, especially if this is your first baby, for unexpected doubts or fears to surface. *Will the baby be able to fit through the birth canal? Will I tear or split apart? Will the baby be healthy and normal?* These feelings can be very intense and may need to be shared with your helpers. At this stage, fear also has a positive value in building up the level of adrenalin which will stimulate the expulsive reflex.

All these emotions are characteristic of transition, but usually, with the right kind of support and encouragement, soon pass, and a new energy arises with the expulsive contractions.

The key to a smooth transition is to concentrate deeply and to trust what is happening to your body, letting go of all physical and emotional inhibitions and allowing yourself to be completely instinctual. It is best to take each contraction as it comes – keeping to the moment rather than thinking of what is ahead. You may find relief in moaning or making any other sound that comes naturally. Contact with water can be very helpful: suck on a sponge; bathe your face with cold water between contractions; take a bath or shower if transition is long.

Positions and movements for transition

As always, it is important to make yourself as comfortable as possible. Any position that you found useful earlier in the first stage is suitable, but most women choose to kneel forward on to a pile of cushions. In this position, you will have a sense of control over the intensity of the contractions, and you will be able to rest and relax in the intervals between them.

You may also prefer to stand, squat or be held or supported. If you are very tired, simply sitting upright on the edge of the bed or a chair may be the most comfortable position for you. It is probably wise to avoid lying down as you are more likely to feel overwhelmed by the contractions.

If the anterior lip of your cervix is slow to dilate (*see* Transition, page 153), it is best to adopt the knee-chest position: kneel down on hands and knees with your head down and your buttocks up. This will lessen the intensity of the contractions, give the front rim of the cervix room to withdraw and help to bring the baby forward. If the urge to push is very strong, try blowing out firmly whenever you feel like pushing, as if you were trying to blow out a candle that is an arm's length in front of you.

The second stage of labour

The second stage of labour begins once the cervix is fully dilated and ends with the birth of the baby. Sometimes, especially in a first birth, there is a resting period between the first and second stages, during which contractions are infrequent or even cease for a while. If this happens, it is best to rest and gather your strength.

The second stage itself can last between a few minutes and a couple of hours, and occasionally even longer. In second and subsequent births it tends to be shorter, but in any birth the overall length of the second stage will depend on many variables such as the size, shape and position of the baby's head, the size of your pelvis and the strength of the contractions. If conditions are right and the environment is conducive, the baby may be born quickly. However, it is unnecessary to hurry or speed up the second stage, provided both you and your baby are doing well.

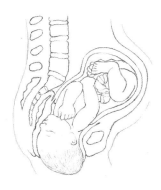

5. Second stage: the baby's head is visible.

Giving birth

When your cervix is fully dilated, your baby's head descends through the pelvic canal and the vagina. It may take some time before the expulsive reflex is established and the urge to bear down begins, or it may happen very rapidly. Bearing-down sensations occur once the baby's head makes contact with the pelvic floor. After it passes through this muscular layer, it will begin to emerge through the labia, stretching the soft tissues of the vulva as it 'crowns' – that is, when the top of the baby's head becomes visible at the vaginal entrance.

Sometimes the baby will be born very quickly – the head and body emerging in one contraction – or the birth may take place more slowly over several contractions, depending on your position and the size and position of the baby's head. It can occasionally be slow and painful, if the labia and perineum take a long time to stretch enough to allow the head to emerge. When this is the case, the midwife can help by protecting the tissues of the vagina and perineum and guiding you to breathe your baby out gently to avoid a tear. Usually the baby emerges easily as the perineal tissues involuntarily relax so that the midwife needs only to receive the baby.

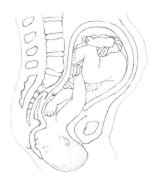

6. Second stage: the baby's head has crowned.

What happens to your baby

The contractions at the beginning of the second stage will bring the baby's head down on to the hammock-shaped floor of the pelvis. Contact with the pelvic muscle will encourage the baby to rotate his head so that it passes easily under the pubic arch and out of the pelvic canal. Usually the head turns to face backwards towards the sacrum – the occipito anterior position (see p. 139) – so that the widest diameter of the head is in line with the widest diameter of the pelvic outlet. Then, as the baby's head emerges under the pubic arch, the neck and spine extend to negotiate the curve.

Finally, the crown of your baby's head will show through the vaginal opening. If the membranes are still intact, they may rupture at this point. With the next few contractions, the head protrudes further and the baby's face will pass over the perineum. After the head is born, the body continues to rotate: first, one shoulder emerges, then the other, quickly followed by the rest of the body. The birth of the head can take much longer than that of the body, which usually emerges in one contraction. While the head is emerging, your baby will continue to receive oxygen from

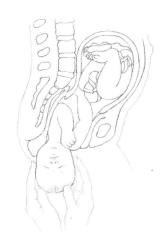

7. Second stage: the baby's body is being born.

Birth in the supported squatting position

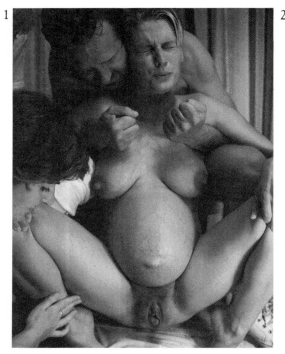

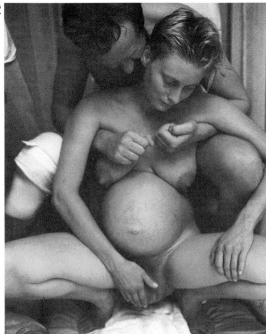

1. The second stage is well established. The mother bears down during a strong contraction and the baby's head becomes visible.

2. In between contractions, the mother feels her baby's head for the first time as it crowns.

3. The baby's head is born and the mother waits for the next contraction.

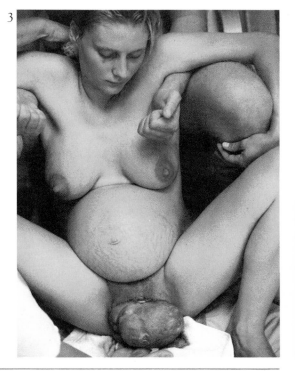

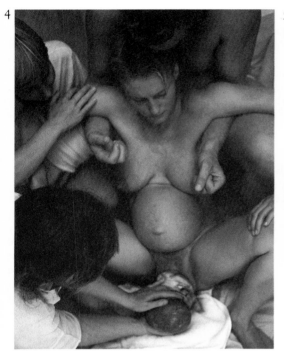

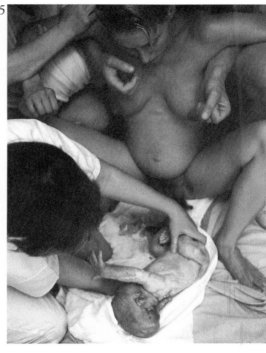

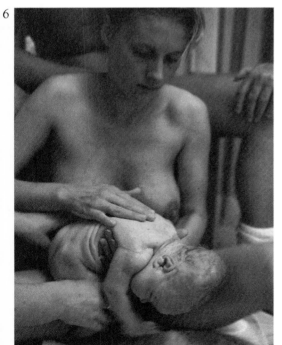

4. The midwife receives the baby as its body emerges.

5. The first moment after birth.

6. The mother strokes the baby's back to help clear the amniotic fluid from the lungs.

the placenta via the umbilical cord. Once the head emerges, your midwife may check the position of the cord: sometimes it is loosely wound around the neck, but this generally does not cause difficulty, the midwife simply slipping it over the baby's body as it emerges.

The second stage is probably very intense for the baby. As his head descends through the pelvic canal, it is likely that he feels a tremendous sense of compression and many other new sensations as his spine extends for the first time in many weeks. When the pressure is at its maximum, the experience may be quite frightening for some babies. Then suddenly the tension is released and a new world unfolds as the baby's head and then his body is born.

How does it feel?

The expulsive contractions of the second stage are often described by women as being like tidal waves. Most find them tremendously powerful, involving the whole body in a strong reflexive urge to bear down which is completely involuntary. This can come as quite a relief after the first stage, and you will probably find that the second stage brings with it new energy to help you give birth to your child. It often takes some time for the expulsive reflex to begin after full dilation, and there may be a period when you do not feel any urge to bear down. Once contractions begin, the intervals between them may be longer than in the late first stage.

Many women find the second stage less painful and more enjoyable than the first, but this is not always the case. For some, this stage can be difficult, especially if there is a fear of tearing or if the baby is very large. The use of upright or squatting positions (*see* pp. 124-6) will minimize these difficulties.

As the second stage begins and your baby's head presses against the back of your pelvis and the lower part of your bowel, you will probably feel a strong sense of anal pressure similar to the urge to defecate. As the head moves downward, rotates and reaches the pelvic floor, these sensations will change, being felt more in the actual tissues of the perineum and vulva as they stretch to allow your baby's head to pass through. You may feel a burning sensation, similar to what is felt when you stretch the corners of your mouth with your fingers. Many women instinctively reach down to touch the soft surface of their baby's head as it crowns. The actual birth may be a mixture of intense agony as the tissues of the vagina stretch to their limit and a tremendous orgasmic release as the baby's body slips out and is born.

In a long second stage, the burning, stretching sensation can be relieved if you breathe deeply, or if the midwife holds a warm moist compress against your perineum: the heat will bring blood to the tissues, helping them to expand. A fresh compress can be made every few minutes, using hot water that is just cool enough to touch. This is also an excellent way to prevent tearing.

Once your child is born, it is difficult to describe the complexity and depth of the feelings that may well up within you. Some women feel overwhelmed at first, and it may be some time before other feelings can surface. However, after a few moments of recovery, most women experience great joy, relief and amazement as they welcome their newborn for the first time. With these emotions, a new surge of energy usually arises, and the pain and tiredness of labour are quickly forgotten.

Positions and movements for the second stage

The best way to assist the second stage is to adopt an upright position in which your pelvis is open, your pelvic floor is relaxed and gravity can aid the descent of your baby. Many people assume that, during this time, the mother will remain in one position until birth. However, this is the exception rather than the rule: the majority of women, given the opportunity, will change position and move about throughout this stage, finding the right position for the birth once the head begins to crown.

Any of the positions described in Chapter 9 (*see* pp. 122-7) are suitable, depending on what seems right for you. It is best to follow your own instincts rather than to try to impose a particular position on your body, and it is not necessary to adopt the one you wish to use for the actual birth until the baby's head crowns. If progress is slow, bearing down will be easier if you use a supported squatting position.

Breathing and bearing down

The second stage of labour has a powerful rhythm of its own, each contraction bringing your baby closer to birth. Unlike the contractions of the first stage, the expulsive reflex which occurs as your uterus contracts will involve your whole body. As in other athletic activities such as running or swimming, your breathing will automatically adapt to the action of your body, and you will not need to think about it.

Until recently, women were encouraged to cope with contractions in the second stage by taking a deep breath, holding it as long as possible and pushing forcefully downwards with the diaphragm to assist the contraction. This approach went along with the use of the reclining position for childbirth, and involved a great deal of strenuous effort by the mother, who was usually strongly encouraged to 'Push!' by her attendants. Unless they were trained relatively recently, most midwives have been taught to encourage mothers in this way. With the use of an upright posture for birth, it is usually unnecessary to make these strenuous efforts, and in fact, prolonged holding of the breath may reduce the blood flow to the placenta and deprive the baby of oxygen. With the help of gravity, the spontaneous action of the uterus and the natural efforts of the mother are usually quite sufficient to ensure the baby's safe passage through the birth canal.

The rhythm of the second stage is one of directed effort and energy during contractions, with rest and relaxation between.

Many women give birth by simply adopting an appropriate position and then surrendering to the spontaneous urges of their bodies. This almost always involves releasing a primal cry which occurs naturally at the moment of the birth. For these women, instruction is unnecessary. However, some women do need help to direct their energy downwards, and others may enjoy making a conscious effort to work with their contractions. It is possible to bear down actively in a very similar way to the bearing-down used when defecating. It is not necessary to hold your breath for a long time while doing this; pushing can be done as you exhale, making a sound or holding your breath for short periods.

At the end of the second stage, as your baby's head crowns and passes through the soft tissues of the vagina, the perineum will stretch amazingly as the forehead and face gradually emerge. This process is aided by the natural secretion of lubricating fluids from the vagina.

At this point, some women may find any instructions intrusive and a

Birth in the kneeling position

1. The baby's head has emerged during the second stage of labour, with the mother on her hands and knees.

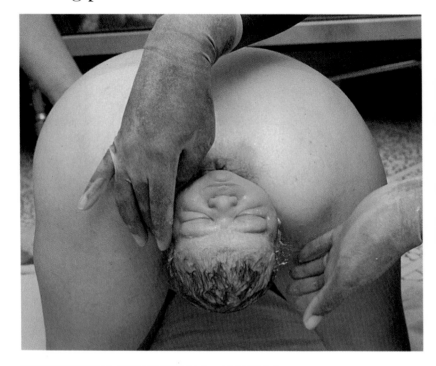

2. The midwife places the baby face down in the safety position on a soft towel between the mother's legs. The mother can then sit back to welcome the baby.

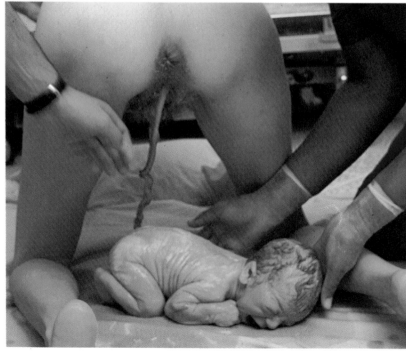

feeling of being watched may be inhibiting, while others need or prefer to have some guidance, particularly if this part of labour takes a little while. Your midwife can assist you by guiding you through the final contractions, encouraging you to bear down at times or asking you to go slowly to give the perineal tissues time to release. If you pant like a dog on a hot day, this will help you to slow down. Try to release the pelvic floor each time you pant, or alternatively, you could breathe deeply, releasing the pelvic floor with each exhalation. It is usually unnecessary to make any effort to bear down to help with the birth of the shoulders and the rest of the body: simply relax and allow your body to take over.

Occasionally, during these moments before the birth, women experience some fear and resistance. It is not uncommon to feel 'I can't do it' or 'The baby will never come', or to be afraid of tearing. Using upright postures which allow the vaginal tissues to relax and expand evenly will lessen the likelihood of a tear, and this is also less likely if you avoid strenuous bearing-down efforts and wait for the involuntary reflex to occur.

Usually these fears arise just before the birth. Then, suddenly, the second stage is over, your baby's head and then his body are born and, with a tremendous sense of relief, you realize that it is all over.

The third stage of labour

At last your child is born and lies, alive and vibrant, before your eyes. In these first indescribable moments, you will be recovering from the birth and seeing and touching your baby for the very first time. This is the moment you have waited for, when you can hold your baby in your arms, look into his eyes, stroke and caress his body as you welcome him and share the joy and emotion of the birth with those who are present.

While this first contact occurs, your baby begins to breathe and relaxes against the warmth and closeness of your body, the umbilical cord ceases to pulsate, and after a little while, the placenta separates and is ready to be expelled. The birth comes to an end when your child, contented after the first sucking at your breast and the first hours of life in the world, falls asleep beside you.

The baby after birth
Newborn babies are fully conscious and exquisitely sensitive, their perceptive faculties already well developed so that they can feel, hear, touch, smell and taste.

However, much of what the baby will now experience will be totally new. In the womb, his body was curled up in the foetal position, but during and after birth, his spine stretches and extends for the first time. At birth, there is a flood of new sensations: the feeling of the atmosphere on his body, new surfaces and textures, the effects of gravity, the experience of colour and light as he opens his eyes.

In these first moments, air is inhaled into the lungs, and cooler temperatures are experienced for the first time. Soon the baby will make contact with the breast and taste and swallow colostrum (the first breastmilk). He will be comforted by the warmth of your body, the smell and closeness of your breasts, the familiar sound of your heart beating, the features and contours of your face and the soothing tones of your voice.

Birth at home

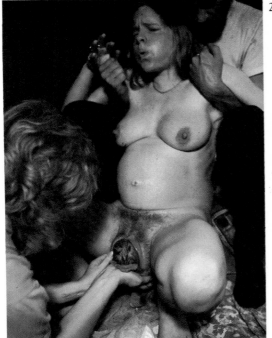

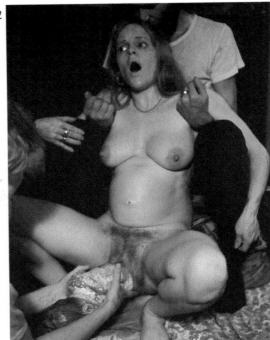

1. The baby's head has crowned and the face appears.

2. The mother cries out instinctively as the baby's body is born.

3. The first sucking takes place before the umbilical cord is cut.

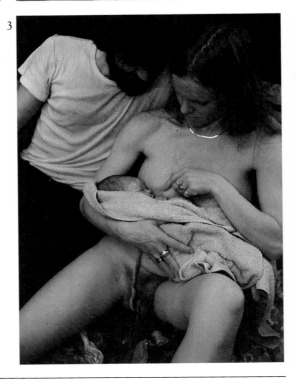

Birth the second time

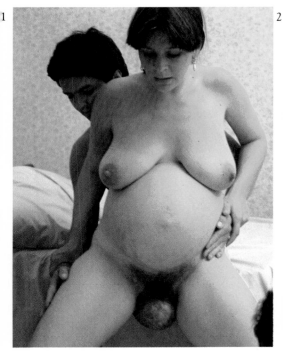

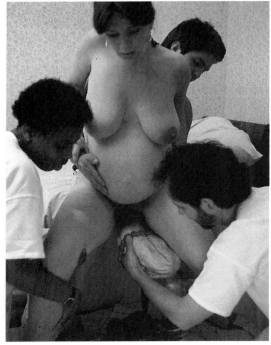

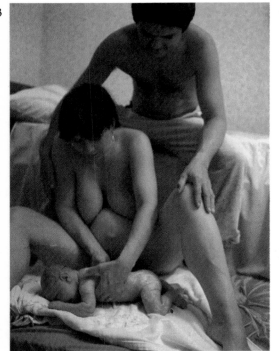

1. The mother stands as the head emerges without difficulty.

2. Since the cord was around the baby's head, it is slipped over the baby's body as the buttocks emerge.

3. Minutes later, the mother intuitively picks up her baby.

For everyone, these first impressions must be among the most important events of a lifetime. Whatever the birth has been like – whether it was easy or difficult, natural or Caesarean – there is much we can do to ensure that the baby is welcomed into the world in the best possible way, with respect and sensitivity. We can ensure that the first sounds the baby hears are soft and gentle, that the light is dim, the air warm and that the hands that help and caress are loving and sensitive.

The start of breathing Until now, your baby has relied on oxygenated blood from the placenta via the umbilical cord. At birth, the pathways in the heart through which blood flowed to avoid the lungs close (*see* p. 56), the placental circulation recedes and lung circulation takes over. With the first breath, the blood vessels in the lungs open dramatically, and blood flows through them to receive oxygen from the inhaled air.

The breathing reflex is well rehearsed, and after birth the contact with the relatively cooler air on his skin stimulates the baby to breathe.

If you have given birth while squatting, the baby will have emerged naturally face down from the birth canal – nature's way of ensuring the safe drainage of mucus and amniotic fluid from the baby's breathing passages. This will be assisted if the midwife lays the baby face down on an absorbent towel immediately after birth, or you could lay the baby on his belly over your thigh and stroke his back gently. Any remaining fluid will be absorbed through the lungs into the bloodstream over the next 12 hours.

Suction of the baby's nose and mouth to clear the mucus is not needed on a routine basis. If the baby seems to be struggling to breathe or if the amniotic fluid is stained with meconium, however, the midwife or doctor may need to use a small tube to suck fluid from the nose and mouth (*see* Meconium aspiration, p. 296).

The amount of crying a baby does after birth varies a great deal. Some give a single cry with their first breath and then begin to breathe quietly, while others cry lustily. Most babies are not ready to be put to the breast until breathing is established.

The umbilical cord The midwife checks your baby's general well-being soon after birth by feeling the umbilical cord to see if it is pulsating. There should be no hurry to clamp and cut the cord; the best times for this are after the delivery of the placenta or when the cord stops pulsating. The great advantage in waiting for the cord to cease pulsating is that it gives your baby a double lifeline as he makes the transition from the womb to the outside world – from obtaining oxygen via the placenta to using his own lungs. During this transition, the baby is intended to have two sources of oxygen, from both the placenta and the lungs.

Provided your baby is cradled in your arms or lies on your abdomen at more or less the same level as the placenta, there is no truth in the idea that his blood might flow back into the placenta, or that blood from the placenta might flow into the baby's circulation. Waiting for the cord to stop pulsating will allow the baby's circulation to adjust normally before the flow of blood to and from the placenta ceases.

Once the baby is breathing steadily, the cord will clamp itself automatically. It will change from being distended with the blood flowing through it, and become white and flaccid. It can then be clamped with a plastic clamp or tied and cut about 2.5 cm (1 in) away from the baby.

(Because this area contains no nerves, the baby will not feel the cut.) In the next few days, the stump that is left will become dry and leathery, and within ten days it will simply drop off, leaving the familiar 'belly button'.

Rarely, if the cord is wound tightly around the baby's neck at birth, causing the baby distress, it may need to be cut to free the baby quickly.

First movements Your baby may be fretful and need soothing and caressing and to hear the soft, familiar tones of your voice before he can relax in your arms. If the room is warm, there is no need to clothe the baby; a warm towel or a simple overhead heater will suffice. Your baby will also receive warmth from the skin-to-skin contact with your body.

Almost immediately, your new baby will begin to move and to explore your body and the environment. Babies usually go through a characteristic sequence of movements in the first minutes after birth. Beginning with eyes closed and fists clenched tight, they gradually open their eyes and then uncurl their fingers until the palms can be seen. Their hands search the air and touch their faces and their mother's body. Their heads will turn towards the sound of her voice, and their eyes will follow the movements of her hands and will gaze searchingly into her face.

The first sucking Some babies are interested in sucking straight away, while others want to look around, smell and sense the breast first.

When babies are ready to feed, the gentle touch of a nipple on one cheek will stimulate them to turn towards the breast and open their mouths to search for it. This automatic response is known as the *rooting reflex* (*see* p. 181). Once your baby's mouth is open and turned towards you, you can introduce your nipple into his mouth, making sure that he latches on, taking in all of the nipple as well as part of the areola, the dark area surrounding the nipple. You may be surprised by how strongly your baby can suck. Breastfeeding is discussed fully in Chapter 15.

This first sucking will stimulate your pituitary gland to secrete oxytocin, which will stimulate the milk flow and cause your uterus to contract.

Immediately after the birth, an Apgar test (named after Virginia Apgar, the anaesthetist who devised it) is performed to assess the baby's condition, and repeated five minutes later. In this, the baby's colour, breathing, muscle tone, crying and heart rate are observed and scored. An Apgar score of under 5 is often an indication of foetal distress (*see* p. 311).

Within a few hours a more detailed examination is done (*see* p. 187).

What happens to you

In the first half hour after the birth, most women experience a flood of emotion. The elation of actually seeing, touching and holding the baby after the work of labour is incomparable.

You may be surprised by the surge of energy and emotion that surfaces to greet the baby, even after a long labour during which you may have felt low, drained and even exhausted. However, it is also common to experience a kind of emotional vacuum, and it may take a while for feelings to arise. For some mothers, it can take a day or two before a feeling of love surfaces, although the protective instinct is usually strong from the start.

It is common to feel shivery after giving birth; an overhead mobile heater can warm you wonderfully until the shaking subsides.

Breech birth in the supported squatting position

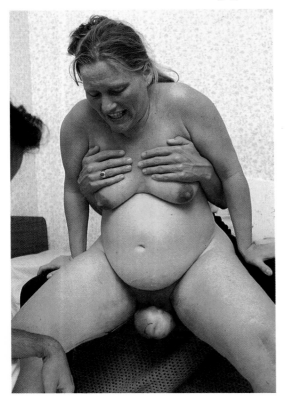

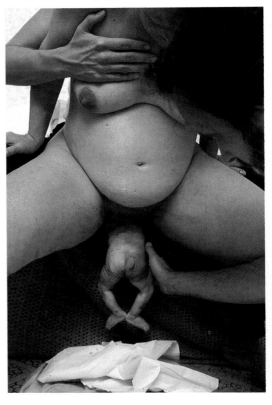

1. The baby's buttocks emerge, still covered by the intact membranes. The mother is supported by her partner as her instinctive efforts assist the birth.

2. The membranes rupture and the baby's legs and body emerge.

A breech birth

1. Before labour: the cervix is uneffaced and the breech has not engaged. The cervix dilates in the 1st stage as in a head presentation.

2. Second stage: the cervix is fully dilated and the feet have descended on to the perineum.

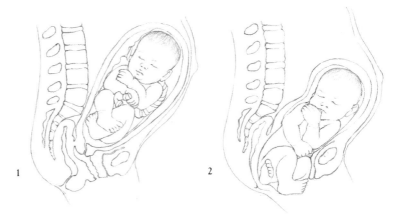

1

2

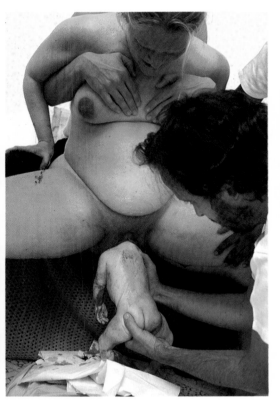

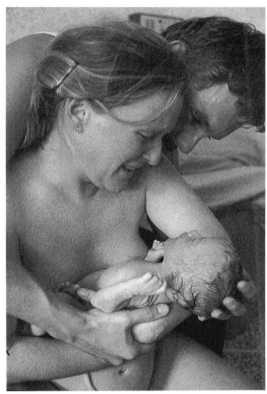

3. The baby's arms are out and the head is ready to be born. The mother squats to open the pelvis as wide as possible, and with the help of gravity the baby's head is guided out.

4. First eye contact between parents and baby in the moments just after birth.

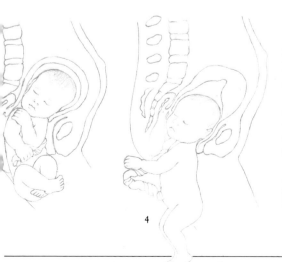

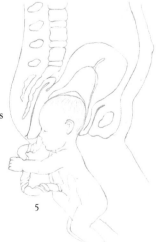

3. The baby's buttocks have been born and the chest has entered the pelvic cavity.

4. The head engages in the pelvis and the birth is assisted with the help of gravity.

5. The baby's body is supported as the head is born.

4

5

After the birth of your baby, the amniotic fluid will drain away and separation of the placenta from the wall of the uterus or vaginal tears causes bleeding. You will continue to shed the uterine lining over the next few weeks. This bleeding is called *lochia*.

Before the expulsion of the placenta, it is advisable to remain sitting upright for a number of reasons:

It is easier to hold the baby when you are in this position. The nipple is at the perfect height and angle for him to latch on, nestled as he is in the crook of your arm. The baby will also be able to see your face easily.

Sitting upright facilitates the separation of the placenta from the uterine wall due to the downward force of gravity, and ensures that the baby is at the same level as the placenta to provide optimal blood flow until the placenta circulation ceases.

This position prevents compression of the major blood vessels in front of your spine so that excessive bleeding is less likely.

You will need support behind you. A large bean bag is ideal or, alternatively, your partner or another supporter can sit behind you.

After the placenta has been expelled (*see below*), the midwife or doctor will check to see whether there are any vaginal tears and whether any stitching is needed (*see* Tearing and episiotomy, pp. 336-7).

Once the placenta has been expelled, it is no longer necessary to remain upright. Now is the time to relax and enjoy a well-earned rest with your new baby. Lie in any comfortable position, holding him in your arms or beside you in bed. You could try placing the baby on your chest so that he can hear the familiar sound of your heartbeat. It is perfectly safe to fall asleep with your baby in bed with you. He will benefit from your closeness and the warmth of your body.

Separation and expulsion of the placenta Between 3 and 30 minutes after the birth, when the baby's breathing is established, the cord will cease to pulsate and, stimulated by your first contact with your baby, the uterus starts contracting again. These contractions can be quite uncomfortable, especially if it has been a second or subsequent birth (when they are commonly called 'after-pains').

As this occurs, the placenta, no longer needed, will separate from the uterine wall, and will emerge through the cervix to be expelled from the vagina. Further contractions and retraction of the uterus will constrict the blood vessels of the uterus, to prevent bleeding.

Once the contractions of the third stage begin, you can stand up or squat to expel the placenta. Generally this happens spontaneously and help is not needed. Nevertheless, occasionally, once the placenta is fully separated, the midwife may gently pull on the cord with one hand while holding the contracted uterus with the other on the lower abdomen. This is called 'controlled cord traction', and it is done when the third stage is induced with drugs (*see* Prolonged third stage of labour, p. 333).

Once the placenta has been expelled, you may want to examine this amazing organ which nourished your baby throughout pregnancy. It is approximately one-sixth the size of the baby, weighs about 500 g (1 lb) and resembles a large piece of liver. Your midwife will be able to show you how the membranes of the amniotic sac are attached and where the baby was lying. If the cord has not yet been cut, this can be done now.

Many mammals eat the placenta, the hormones it contains being

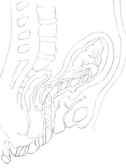

8. Third stage: the placenta has separated from the wall of the uterus.

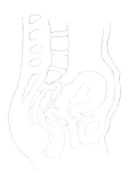

9. Late third stage: the placenta has been delivered.

absorbed back into the body to help regulate the hormonal changes that occur after giving birth. In many tribal societies, disposal of the placenta (usually by burial) is considered to be very important, in contrast to Western society where it is usually incinerated or sold to cosmetic companies for use in their products. Some mothers prefer to bury the placenta, and it is possible to ask for yours to be saved if you wish to perform this ritual yourself.

Bathing after the birth Soaking in a bath of warm water is a pleasure that both mother and baby can enjoy, and will soothe and relax the baby after birth.

If you take a full bath with your baby, make sure that the water is quite warm and as deep as possible, so that his body is completely immersed. It is best not to use soap or any other sort of cleanser in the water as this may remove the greasy vernix which coats his skin and which will be absorbed normally (see p. 179). Once in the bath, your child will need only a touch of support behind his head and shoulders, and you will find that he, like all other newborn babies, is completely at home in water.

Alternatively, a baby bath can be placed in front of you quite soon after the birth, and you can sit with it between your legs and lower the baby easily into the water. Partners often enjoy doing this together, and it is an opportunity for the baby's father to participate. Babies usually relax completely in the familiar watery medium, and look about themselves wide-eyed. This is a marvellous chance for both parents to enjoy handling and communicating with their newborn baby.

The main purpose of having a bath is pleasure, and if you do not feel like bathing after the birth, it is not necessary to do so; babies can go for several days without bathing. Sometimes nurses will give blanket baths to newly delivered mothers, and this can feel wonderful.

Early contact and bonding

The first few hours after your baby is born are very special, and the birth does not really end until he falls asleep some hours later. You, your partner and your baby will have been through a tremendously intense and powerful experience, and you will need time to integrate your feelings. Your baby will also be adjusting to an entirely new environment outside the womb. This is a time to be together undisturbed, to share in the wonderful glow and the sacred atmosphere which usually follows the birth. Through sight, touch, smell, sound and the expression and sharing of emotion, the first contact between you will be taking place in many ways.

This process, known as *bonding*, actually begins weeks before the birth, and is intensified once your baby is born and is lying, alert and responsive, in your arms. If for some reason circumstances prevent this occurring immediately after the birth, do not worry: make sure that, when the first opportunity arrives, you have privacy and time to enjoy your baby.

After this first meeting, your baby will fall into a deep and profound sleep to recover from the adventure of birth, and he is likely to spend a lot of time sleeping during the next few weeks. You may rest and doze as well, but often the high energy which occurs after childbirth is too intense for this. Many women stay awake at this time, to reflect on the extraordinary events of the birth. It is best not to interfere with this process by taking a sedative, even when labour has been long and exhausting. Sleep and recovery will come later.

The parents' experience

Whether your labour was straightforward or difficult, fast or slow, whatever you have encountered during the birth will soon fade into the past. After a few moments, you will probably have an irresistible urge to touch your baby's body and then to lift him up in your arms and to look at and hold him close to you. Then there is the marvellous moment when you first look into each other's eyes. As this happens, a flood of intense emotion is likely to overwhelm you.

However, it is also common, particularly for mothers, to feel a little dazed or awed and not to have an immediate rush of feelings, especially if the birth has been difficult or very fast. When you have rested and recovered, your feelings for your baby will emerge in their own time.

Although most parents are overjoyed and delighted with their new babies, not all feelings after the birth are positive. You may, for example, be nervous of touching and possibly hurting the baby, or disappointed at the sex or that he looks different from what you had imagined. If this happens, you will have to balance your expectations against reality. Love can come at first sight, or it can grow slowly, but however it arises, it is usually profound.

For the baby's father, this is generally the climax of the day. With the long hours of labour behind you and the baby safely born, you can now relax and enjoy the wonder of the first hours of your child's life outside the womb. The baby you have been waiting for is now a reality – alive and responsive, looking up into your face, responding to your voice, your touch and your facial expressions. In these moments, your relationship with your son or daughter begins with the first direct communication between you.

Holding your child in your arms for the first time is one of life's most moving experiences. Many fathers are hesitant at first, but very soon a familiar intimacy develops, as your child responds to your warmth, the tones of your voice and the strength of your arms. Some men like to remove their shirts so that they can have direct skin contact with the baby.

After you have had the pleasure of making the first announcements of the birth to family and friends, you and your partner should remain together with your baby for the first night if at all possible, especially if you have participated in labour and birth. However, if the baby is a second or subsequent child, you may need to be with your other child or children.

Older children

Many parents welcome the opportunity to include older children in the birth of a new brother or sister or as soon afterwards as possible, to reassure and cuddle them and help them accept the newcomer from the start.

If children have been present at the birth, the first few hours afterwards will be a marvellous time, with the whole family gathered together to welcome the new baby into their midst. Everyone can see and hold the baby, participate in bathing him and help the mother to settle comfortably into bed with her loved ones around her. Children who have witnessed a birth may need to ask questions or express their feelings, and there should be plenty of time for everyone to share in the joy of a birth in the family.

PART IV
AFTER THE BIRTH

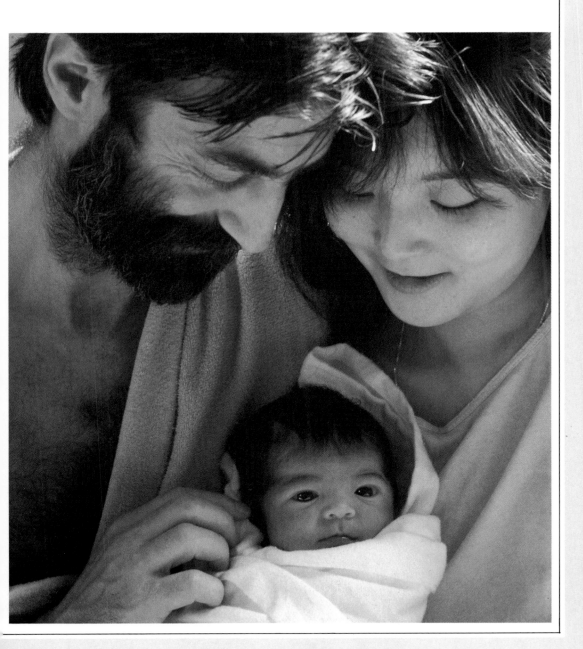

CHAPTER 13

YOUR BODY AFTER CHILDBIRTH

The first six weeks or so after giving birth are called the *puerperium* or the 'lying-in' period. At this time, your new relationships as a family will be established, and you will begin to learn about your baby's rhythms and needs. This is very much a time of exploration, and it is important for you and your baby to remain together and spend much of the time in close physical contact, so that she is protected by the warmth and familiarity of your body while she learns to adapt to life outside the womb.

This time is also important for you, for as well as recovering from the birth itself, you will be adjusting to your new separateness from the baby that has been inside and almost a part of you for so long. As well as celebrating the birth of your child, you will be adjusting to your new role, coping with interrupted sleep, starting breastfeeding, maintaining your relationship with your partner, learning to care for your baby – perhaps while looking after other children – and entertaining grandparents and visitors. It is essential to plan well for this, to ensure that you get enough rest, and to be sure of your priorities so that your own and your baby's needs are central at this time. A new mother needs to be looked after, and regular, nourishing meals and a calm and comfortable environment are essential. In some societies, a new mother is 'mothered' herself for up to 40 days after giving birth – a period when so many important things happen.

One of the great advantages of a home birth is that you are already together at home during this time. If your baby was born in hospital, you may enjoy a stay there after the birth, receiving support, reassurance and practical help from the staff. However, some women find hospital routines disruptive and prefer to return home as soon as possible, to learn how to care for their baby on their own.

Many fathers now make sure that they will be present for at least the first few days after their partner and baby arrive home, by taking part of their annual holiday; some more progressive unions and managements have agreements which allow for paternity leave. It is important to decide how to organize these first days at home and to plan ahead for this time. As well as resting and recovering your strength, you will be preoccupied with looking after and establishing a bond with your new baby. Your future relationship develops from ties formed in these early days, and so, if possible, someone else should do all the routine housework, shopping and cooking so that you can devote yourself to your baby. Your partner may, therefore, be the main organizer around the house – often for the first time. If he is not able to do all the chores, he should arrange in advance to get help from some other person, perhaps a friend or relative.

You will find that your baby wakes at odd hours and that you will need to adjust to an irregular sleeping pattern. The easiest way to cope with the new demands on your energy is to make the baby your first priority and to follow her pattern – sleeping when she sleeps and feeding her when she seems hungry. Within a few weeks, the baby's sleeping and waking pattern will settle down into something that is more or less predictable and more appropriate to life outside the womb.

Physical changes

After giving birth, many women feel radiantly healthy, but there may be some discomfort or pain in the early days and weeks as your body recovers and returns to normal. Generally, however, these aches and pains are minimized by the joy of having a new baby, and your body soon heals.

The genital area

During the first few hours, you are likely to feel some discomfort in the genital area when you sit, pass urine or empty your bowels. This may continue for several days, depending on whether you have had any stitches or are bruised or if you have piles (see p. 330).

A soothing herbal bath (see below right), which is antiseptic and healing, or the application of homoeopathic calendula tincture may help. Use the tincture sparingly after washing and drying the area, and apply it neat on a little cotton wool, or dilute it in warm water first. Salt baths are often recommended to promote healing. After bathing, keep the area dry.

Applying ice wrapped in a plastic pack will reduce any swelling. You may also find it more comfortable to sit on a rubber ring for a few days. For the aftercare of stitches, see pp. 336-7.

After pregnancy, the uterus gradually decreases in size – a process called *involution* – until it regains its non-pregnant size in about four to six weeks. This is assisted by breastfeeding, when the contractions of the uterus as it shrinks and retracts – i.e. *after-pains* – can be quite intense.

As the uterus involutes, its lining is shed. The resulting vaginal discharge, called the *lochia*, lasts for up to six weeks. Bright red at first, it turns reddish-brown and finally pale yellow or white as its quantity lessens. Use sanitary towels until the lochia ceases, not tampons. Your midwife will check your uterus and lochia to make sure that all is well; you should consult her or your doctor if your lochia remains bright red for longer than three weeks or becomes profuse, or if you find that you are passing clots (see p. 294). It should not smell offensive; if it does, this may indicate an infection which should also be brought to the attention of your midwife.

Urination and bowel function

In the first days after the birth, you will urinate more than usual as your body excretes the extra fluid that has accumulated in your blood and body tissues during pregnancy. At first you may find it difficult to urinate if you have had a tear or stitches (see above), or because the tissues around the vagina and bladder have been stretched during delivery. This should clear up within a day or so, but if it does not, check with your midwife to make sure that you do not have a urinary infection (see p. 342). Intense stinging or burning from a tear can be alleviated if you pour warm water from a jug on the area at the same time as you pass urine.

Urinary incontinence – the inability to control the flow of urine (see p. 341) – is an uncommon but distressing problem, caused by the stretching of

Herbal baths
A healing, antiseptic herbal hip-bath is wonderfully soothing and beneficial for the perineal area, and can be taken the day after the birth, even when there are stitches. It has a pungent aroma when being prepared.

For each bath, you will need: a large handful of each of shepherd's purse, bearberry (*Uva ursi*), comfrey; three heads of garlic. The herbs can be obtained from good herbalists and health food shops, and it may be a good idea to make up enough for a number of baths.

the pelvic-floor muscles. It is usually temporary, the muscle tone gradually returning over a few weeks. Recovery can be accelerated if you begin pelvic-floor exercises (*see* p. 253) and return to normal activity as soon as you can.

Before or during labour, you will have evacuated your bowels, and so for a day or two after the birth there will usually be no need to empty them. Because they have been stretched, the muscles around your anus may feel strange, and this, combined with any pain in the genital area or that caused by piles, can lead to constipation. A good diet containing plenty of fibre will help, as will pelvic-floor exercises. If you are constipated or afraid that a bowel movement will be painful, you could use a gentle glycerine suppository. Stitches will not be harmed by normal bowel activity.

The breasts

Breast changes after childbirth can be dramatic. These are discussed in full on pages 190–97.

The abdomen

Your abdomen, which has stretched so amazingly during pregnancy, may now feel floppy, and you may look at your bulging belly with dismay and wonder if it will ever tighten up again. You should prepare yourself for the fact that you are going to look as if you are about four months pregnant for some weeks yet.

The abdominal muscles may retract and firm up remarkably quickly and the skin tone improve as the underlying elastic tissue takes in the slack, but more often the process is gradual and it may be the best part of six months or even a year before you are completely back in shape. This will happen faster if you are breastfeeding, provided your diet is nutritious and well balanced. Start by gently toning and exercising your abdominal muscles after the birth, and following the exercise sequence recommended on page 264. This is not an appropriate time to diet: exercise will be a more effective way to regain your figure. It is both natural and becoming to be more rounded and somewhat voluptuous as a new mother. In due course, your body will recover its former firmness, strength and slenderness.

The joints and muscles

With the changes in hormone levels which follow childbirth, the softening of the ligaments ceases, and you may feel your body tighten up.

Until the ligaments completely firm up, and because of the new strain to which they will be subjected, your lower back and shoulders are the areas to protect. Your back has already carried a great deal of extra weight during your pregnancy, and it will be particularly vulnerable during the early weeks after the birth. Do some simple back-strengthening exercises (*see* p. 263), and when picking things up from the floor, take care always to bend your knees while keeping your back straight rather than stooping (*see* p. 261). Make sure that the surface on which you change your baby is at the correct height: while it is preferable to do this kneeling on the floor, you may find it easier on your back to use a table for the first week or two.

The muscles in your shoulders, neck and head can become very tense after hours of nursing and holding a young baby. Keep them relaxed by stretching frequently and attending to your posture when feeding and carrying your baby.

The hair and skin

Because of the decline in hormone levels, some hair loss is normal after childbirth, although it can be alarming if it comes out by the handful. However, there is no reason to worry as this is never permanent: replacement hairs are already growing, and your hair should be back to normal in a few months.

Any pigmentation that may have appeared on your skin during pregnancy will usually recede, and darkened areas will gradually lighten, although this may take months. Occasionally, when there is a tendency to develop moles the numbers of these may increase. It may be quite a time before pregnancy-induced acne clears, as the body first has to adjust to a new hormonal balance.

Any stretch marks will shrink and become pale and less noticeable, but it is unlikely that they will disappear altogether. Massaging them with a high-potency vitamin E oil may be helpful.

Varicose veins in the vulva usually go away completely, but those in the legs may not, although they will invariably become less apparent. In fact, it will be several months before you know how extensive varicose veins are going to be. Exercise will help, particularly the 'legs apart on a wall' exercise on page 270.

Swelling of the feet and ankles often worsens and can become quite marked for two or three days after the birth as the body redistributes fluid. However, it diminishes gradually as excess fluid is excreted, and you should be back to normal within about a week.

The blood

If you were anaemic during pregnancy (*see* Anaemia, p. 292) or if you lost an excessive amount of blood during the birth, your haemoglobin level may fall, causing you to remain or become anaemic. This will make you feel tired and drained. Once the demands of pregnancy are over, the level of iron in the blood increases quickly, but because it is essential to build up your store of this important mineral in preparation for breastfeeding and, later on, menstrual loss and perhaps another pregnancy, you may be advised to take iron supplements for the first three months, probably accompanied by zinc and multivitamin tablets.

Nutrition and weight

You should continue to eat foods rich in vitamins, minerals (particularly iron, zinc and calcium) and protein to replace the stores in your body following the demands of pregnancy and childbirth. The advice on nutrition during pregnancy, outlined in Chapter 7, is equally applicable now; in addition, there are a few specific aspects of nutrition that are especially important if you are breastfeeding (*see* p. 204).

You will have to wait for two or three weeks before you can judge whether or not you have put on extra weight during pregnancy. Many women are surprised to find that they actually look thinner than before, although the scales may show an overall increase in weight due to full breasts. Others will discover that they have accumulated some fat, but this can serve as an energy store, particularly if they are breastfeeding.

If you are breastfeeding, you should plan to get down to your pre-pregnant weight over a long period – say, no less than six months. If you are not, you should still not attempt to diet in the months after childbirth, when you will need a great deal of extra energy to cope with caring for your new baby.

Hormonal changes and mood

During the first week or so after the birth, your body will still be flooded with endorphins – the body's own painkillers – and a feeling of euphoria may continue for some time. Becoming a mother is generally so absorbing that, once you recover from the intensity of the birth, it may take a few weeks before you begin to come back to everyday reality.

With the birth of the baby and the expulsion of the placenta, the oestrogen and progesterone levels in your body fall rapidly. A similar event occurs before menstruation, but since the levels of these hormones are so many times higher in pregnancy, the effects of their decline can be much more intense.

Postpartum blues A few days after the birth – usually just preceding or coinciding with the milk 'coming in' (*see* pp. 191-3) – you may feel depressed. This is referred to as postpartum blues (or the 'baby blues' or 'third-day blues') and may reflect changes in hormone levels after the intensity and high of the birth, or may be a reaction to the reality of new motherhood. At this time you may find that almost anything triggers off a release of emotion and floods of tears, but this usually passes after a day or two and equilibrium returns. If you remain depressed, there may be underlying problems and you should consult your doctor, midwife or health visitor. (*See also* Depression and stress, pp. 306-7.)

The post-natal checkup

About six weeks after the birth, it is customary to visit the hospital or your family doctor for a checkup. Your blood pressure will be taken, you will be weighed and your urine will be analysed. Your abdomen and breasts will be checked, and advice on feeding and caring for your baby may be given if required.

You will also be given an internal examination, during which your uterus, cervix and vagina will be checked to ensure that everything has returned to normal. Your doctor may suggest exercises to strengthen the vaginal walls, and your perineum will be examined to ascertain that any tears and/or stitches have healed properly. If a cervical smear was not performed at your first ante-natal visit, one can be done now.

This is a good opportunity to discuss contraception if you have not already done so. The choices open to you are outlined in the chart on pages 304-5. If you had been using a diaphragm, it will need to be refitted in case the shape of your vagina and cervix has altered. While many women wait until after the post-natal checkup to resume love-making, this is not necessary (*see* p. 233), although you will need to use some sort of birth control method – even if you are breastfeeding – if you would prefer not to become pregnant again too soon.

You may also want to discuss your labour and the baby's birth with your doctor. It can help to bring a list of all the questions that will undoubtedly have accumulated since then. If the birth or post-natal events were complicated, you may want to talk over the details, as well as the outlook for future births.

CHAPTER 14

YOUR NEWBORN BABY

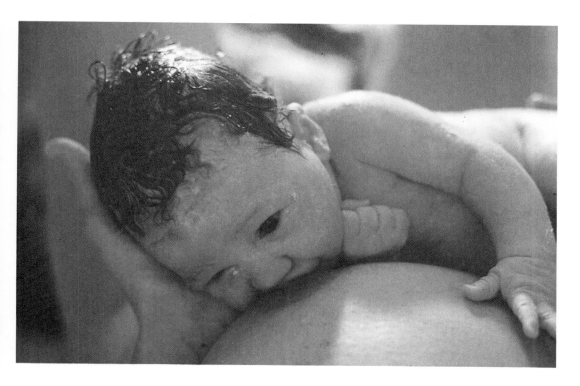

All babies are unique individuals. Some are calm and tranquil from the start, whereas others take some time to 'settle' after the birth. In the early days, you will be completely involved in getting to know your baby and learning to feed and take care of her. You will discover how to understand her signals, to communicate with her and to satisfy her needs. In time, your confidence will increase as your newborn child develops.

The head

A baby's head is the largest part of her body, in relative terms four times larger than an adult's. The bones of the skull are not yet fused but joined together by fibrous tissue. Because of this, the baby's head is more flexible than an adult's, and as we have seen, is capable of 'moulding' as it travels down the birth canal. After birth, the areas between the bones covered by the fibrous tissue can be felt as 'soft spots' known as *fontanelles*.

There are actually six of these, although most people are only aware of the two biggest: the diamond-shaped *anterior fontanelle*, which is located on the crown of the baby's head and about 4 cm (1½ in) across; and the

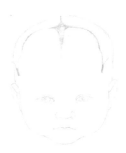

This drawing shows the position of the anterior fontanelle – the largest of the soft areas of fibrous tissue on a baby's head.

smaller triangular *posterior fontanelle* a little further back. If the baby does not have a lot of hair, you can see the pulse beating steadily through the anterior fontanelle.

Although they may seem terribly fragile, the fontanelles are in fact quite tough, and there is no danger of damaging them with normal handling. They need no special care – for example, the scalp over them can be washed in exactly the same way as the other parts of the head. However, if you notice that the anterior fontanelle is unusually sunken or bulges out, you should contact your doctor as this can be a sign of illness. All the fontanelles should disappear by the time your child is two years old, when the skull bones will have fused together.

After birth, your baby's head may not be perfectly rounded because of moulding, and it may be slightly pointed. Occasionally the pressure exerted during birth will cause the skin to swell, forming what is called a *caput*, but if the pressure is more extensive, the underlying tissue may bruise, causing *cephalhaematoma*, which usually occurs on one side of the skull. Caput disappears in a few days, whereas cephalhaematoma may take weeks. (*See* Birth injuries to the baby, p. 292-3.)

It is very common for a thick layer of brown crusts to appear on the scalp. When this appears in patches, it is called 'scurf', but when it covers a good portion of the top of the head, it is known as 'cradle cap' (*see* Skin problems in the baby, p. 335).

Some babies are born with a luxuriant crop of hair, while others are quite bald at birth. Most of the hair will usually fall out within three months after birth, to be replaced by fine new hair which may be a different colour. However, do not worry if this does not appear soon: it may take up to a year for a child's hair to begin to grow.

The eyes

A baby's eyes open soon after birth. The eyelids are sometimes swollen or puffy, a result of pressure in the birth canal; the swelling will go down in a few days.

Almost all newborn babies' eyes are bluish in colour, due to the absence of melanin (the body's natural pigment) in the irises. If your child is destined to have any eye colour other than blue, melanin will be produced as she grows, and the permanent eye colour will be fixed by the time she is about three months old. However, some babies, most frequently those with dark skins, will have brown eyes from the start.

It is quite common for newborn babies to have a mild infection of the eyes known as 'sticky eye', which produces inflammation and a yellowish discharge and crusting on the lids and lashes (*see* Conjunctivitis in the baby, p. 303).

You may notice that when your baby cries, there are no tears. This is because the tear glands only begin to function when most babies are between one and three months old.

The ears

The ears may have been somewhat flattened by the journey through the birth canal, but they will soon regain their proper shape. A waxy discharge is normal, but any other type should be reported to your doctor. You do not need to worry about getting water in your baby's ears when bathing: the eardrums completely seal and protect the inner parts of the ear.

The mouth

A newborn baby's tongue is anchored to the bottom of the mouth along a much greater proportion of its length than that of an older person, and may be fully attached. Growth of the tongue in the first year occurs at the tip, and there is no need to worry about your baby's ability to suck, or eat.

You may notice that your baby develops a blister in the centre of the upper lip. This is caused by sucking, is harmless and will disappear of its own accord.

It is normal for a baby being fed only milk to have a white tongue. However, white patches on an otherwise pink tongue or inside the cheeks, which cannot easily be wiped away, may indicate thrush (see p. 338).

Occasionally a baby is born with a tooth, but this is invariably loose and can be removed. Most babies do not begin to teethe until after the third month.

The skin and nails

Vernix At birth, your baby's body will be covered with *vernix* – a white, creamy substance which has protected the skin in the watery environment of the womb. Some babies have a lot of vernix covering their faces and bodies at birth, while others have relatively little. After birth, the vernix will help to protect the baby from the change in temperature, and will also protect the skin. It is absorbed or rubbed off within a day or two.

Body hair Some babies, and particularly those who are born early, have fine, fuzzy body hair, especially over the ears, shoulders and down the spine. This is called *lanugo* and has covered the baby in the womb. It is not a sign that your baby will be hairy, and it will disappear within a few weeks.

Dry skin It is common for a newborn baby's skin to appear to be dry and to peel during the first few days after the birth, particularly on the hands and feet. This is a normal adaptation of the skin from an aquatic environment to the relatively dry atmosphere, and will disappear in a few days. It may be helpful to rub a little pure almond oil gently into the baby's skin.

Colour Your baby's circulation may not yet be efficient at distributing the blood to the extremities. As a consequence, you may notice that her hands and feet appear pale or bluish, particularly after a long sleep. The lips and tongue will reflect the true state of the heart and circulation: a child with a pale or blue tongue requires urgent medical care. These colour variations will disappear within a few months.

Jaundice is the yellow colouring of the skin and the conjunctiva of the eyes which results from a build-up of bile pigment in the baby's circulation. It is very common and, if excessive, may require treatment (see p. 319).

Spots and marks It takes a while before the pores in your baby's skin begin to work efficiently. As she acclimatizes to life outside the womb, temporary blockages of the sweat and sebaceous (oil) glands can occur which appear as little white spots (particularly on the nose and the rest of the face) called *milia*. These disappear by themselves, and should never be squeezed.

Babies also often develop *neonatal urticaria*. In this, red spots or weals with white or yellow centres flare up and then disappear. This condition too clears up of its own accord and, like dry skin, may be the reaction of the baby's skin to a change in environment. New babies develop spots of many kinds, and most of these are completely harmless. However, if you are worried, consult your midwife, health visitor or doctor.

There are also many different kinds of birthmarks, some of which will fade and others which will remain throughout life. Among the most common types are red marks on the body which disappear within a few months, called 'stork-beak marks'. They are usually seen on the eyelids, forehead or the nape of the neck (*see* Skin problems in the baby, p. 335).

Particularly common in dark-skinned babies are blue patches known as 'Mongolian blue spots' which are often located on the lower back. Although they look like bruises, they are, in fact, caused by the accumulation of pigment under the skin. They are harmless and will fade; they have nothing to do with Down's syndrome ('mongolism').

Nails A baby born at the end of a 40-week pregnancy will have fingernails that reach the ends of the fingertips. If they are longer than this, it may indicate a gestation beyond 40 weeks.

The breasts

These often appear swollen at birth in both girls and boys, and a few drops of milk may even be secreted via the baby's nipples. This is due to the hormones which have circulated in the mother's body during pregnancy and entered the baby's bloodstream. It is perfectly normal and the breasts should be left alone. After a few days, the baby's system will clear itself of the hormones, and the swelling will subside.

The genitals

The genitals of both sexes are normally disproportionately large. The vagina of a baby girl may appear a little red or inflamed, and there may be a white discharge or even a few drops of blood. All this is also a result of the baby's response to maternal hormones during pregnancy. It will clear up naturally in a few days, and is no cause for concern.

In boys, the penis and foreskin, which have developed from a single bud, may be partly fused at birth and the foreskin is not able to retract fully. However, there is no need for any special cleaning of the penis in a young baby, and no need to pull back the foreskin.

Circumcision is hardly ever necessary for medical reasons (*see* pp. 300-1).

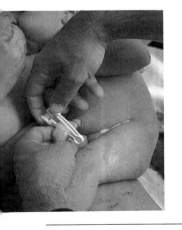

After the placenta has been expelled, the cord is clamped and cut.

The umbilical cord

Within a few minutes of birth, the umbilical cord stops pulsating and becomes limp and white as the walls of its blood vessels stick together in a spontaneous clamping action. To aid this, the cord is usually clamped or tied about 2.5 cm (1 in) from the baby's abdomen and then cut. The clamp or tie will be left in place for about 48 hours before it is removed – a painless procedure.

The cord stump then dries and shrivels up, the action of skin bacteria softens the tissue at its base, and within three to seven days it will drop off. The stump should be kept clean by washing it twice a day with warm water. Antibiotic or antiseptic creams and powders should not be used routinely because they inhibit the bacterial action, so that the stump may take weeks to drop off. The shape of the resulting navel (*umbilicus* or 'tummy button') depends on the structure of the muscle of the abdominal wall.

Basic body functions

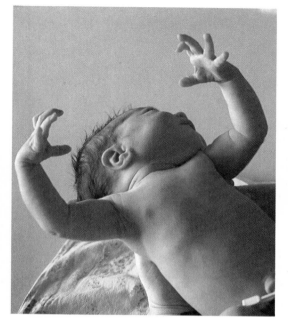
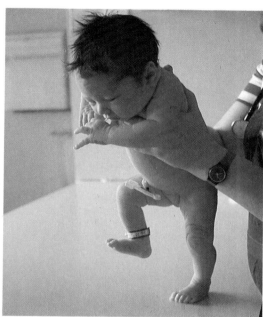

The early reflexes

By the time of birth, your baby will have already developed a number of vital reflexes.

Rooting reflex: a baby will instinctively turn her head towards the touch of a breast or finger on her cheek near the mouth. In this way, she searches for food.

Sucking and swallowing reflexes: your baby will have already practised these in the womb; some babies even suck their thumbs before they are born.

Grasp reflex: babies will automatically grab hold of a finger placed in their palms, and their grasp will be amazingly strong. This reflex is a relic of the days when our prehistoric ancestors needed to hold on to their mothers or to branches of trees for survival.

Startle reflex: also called the *Moro reflex* after the doctor who first described it. A baby will fling out her arms and legs and throw back her head when startled or if she experiences a sudden change of position. This can be seen as an attempt to regain balance and/or to grasp on to the protection of the mother's body.

Stepping reflex: if babies are held upright with their feet touching a firm surface, they will automatically make stepping movements, although they will not be strong enough to support their own weight or to walk.

Babinski's sign: when a hard object (such as a finger or an instrument) is firmly stroked down the sole of your baby's foot, her big toe will bend backward and the other toes will spread out. After the age of about two years, this reflex will disappear, and if the sole is stroked then, the toes will automatically curl down towards the sole.

In addition to the above reflexes, most of which will disappear within three

Left: the Moro reflex.
Right: the stepping reflex.

months as your child grows and increasingly develops voluntary movement, there are others which remain to perform vital functions needed for survival.

The *breathing reflex* is fully functional seconds after birth. Your child will *blink* or *close her eyes* if the light is too bright. She will *react to smells* and will *withdraw from painful sensations.* She will also be born with an instinctive *hunger reflex* and a *need to expel urine and to defecate* – all of which become increasingly voluntary with time.

Breathing

Babies breathe almost twice as rapidly as adults, because of their relatively small lungs. They also breathe very shallowly and, particularly when they lie on their stomachs, may seem to be hardly breathing at all. Babies breathe abdominally, their bellies expanding each time they inhale.

Many babies make a variety of snuffling noises when they breathe, caused by the air moving through the tiny nasal passages. These become larger after a few weeks, and the noisy breathing will then subside. Babies also sneeze frequently – a natural reflex to clear the sensitive linings of their noses. Hiccups are very common too; you may have noticed your baby hiccuping even before birth. Caused by sudden contractions of the diaphragm, hiccups do not seem to bother babies and do not indicate that there is anything wrong with the way they are being fed. You only need be concerned about your baby's breathing if you notice that her chest is being sharply drawn in with each breath or that the breathing is laboured or very noisy (*see* Breathing problems in the baby, pp. 295–6).

Bowel function and urination

In the womb, mucus from glands in the digestive tract and bile from the liver will collect in the baby's bowel. This sticky blackish-green substance resembling liquid tar is known as *meconium,* and it will be eliminated as stools when your baby starts to feed.

The meconium gradually becomes lighter until, after a few days, the baby's stools completely change colour and character. If the baby is being breastfed, they will be a mustard-yellow colour, fairly runny and quite pleasant to smell. Those of a bottle-fed baby will be darker and more solid, and will have a more pungent odour.

Babies normally begin life by passing several bowel motions a day for the first few weeks, but this will change. The milk drunk by breastfed babies is almost completely absorbed, and they may pass a relatively loose motion only every few days. This does not mean that they are constipated, a condition that is virtually unknown in breastfed babies. However, those raised on formula made from less easily absorbed cows' milk will usually pass one motion a day. If stools become infrequent and seem hard, the child probably is constipated (*see* p. 303). If your baby has watery or green motions, report this to your doctor as their appearance probably indicates diarrhoea (*see* p. 308).

Once urine flow is established after birth – sometimes up to 36 hours later – babies urinate very frequently. Occasionally, the first urine may be a reddish colour resembling blood. This is due to the presence of urate crystals and is harmless, but it is a good idea to keep the nappy to show your midwife or a nurse. All babies commonly urinate or empty their bowels while feeding: this is perfectly normal and healthy behaviour.

Growth and weight

During the first year, your baby's body will grow so rapidly that her head will eventually appear to be more in proportion. In fact, in the first six months, she will grow in height more quickly than at any other time.

Your baby will develop continuously, but sometimes you may not notice much change for weeks until she reaches the next growth 'spurt'. Sometimes advances take place where they are not obvious, such as in teeth formation and visual acuity. As babies grow, their need for nourishment increases, and sucking will increase when growth is rapid.

Most babies lose some weight in the first week. In fact, it is not unusual for there to be a loss of up to ten per cent, but this is usually quickly regained. Some parents associate health with weight gain, and are anxious to have their babies weighed frequently. However, a check once a month or so is all that is necessary, provided your baby regains her initial birth weight, grows well and develops normally. The way your baby looks and behaves is much more important than her actual weight.

If you are unsure that your baby is gaining weight or developing normally, discuss this with your doctor. (*See also* Low weight gain after birth, p. 323, and Obesity in the baby, p. 325.)

Getting to know your baby

The abilities of newborn babies are often vastly underrated. Their capacities are impressive and develop far earlier than has previously been believed. From the moment of birth, they show the ability to respond to their environment and can clearly discover, learn and remember, beginning with the very first exchange of communication with their mothers and fathers.

Immediately after birth, babies can express emotion – by crying, frowning and smiling. Crying is particularly important: it is their way of communicating, the means by which their needs are understood and met (*see* pp. 210-12). Very soon you will learn to distinguish between cries of hunger, pain, discomfort, loneliness and the need to express emotion or release energy. While smiling, too, begins very early, it does not become fully developed until about six weeks.

In the early weeks of life, babies have a great capacity for learning. Every cuddle and kiss as well as the simple act of feeding teaches them awareness and trust, love and pleasure. In fact, most early communication takes place during feeding, when a pre-verbal language of touch and sensation happens instinctively on an unconscious level between mother and baby. During this early communication, babies get their first ideas of the world.

After the first six weeks, a new social awareness will begin to blossom in your baby, and her responses to you will become more complex and direct. By this time, most parents have 'fallen in love' with their babies, especially when their children express affection and love in return.

Your baby's senses

Your baby's nervous system has been developing since the time of fertilization. As early as 20–28 weeks' gestation, circuits of nerve cells are present in the brain's cortex which are necessary for the development of consciousness. By the time of the birth, the nervous system has been

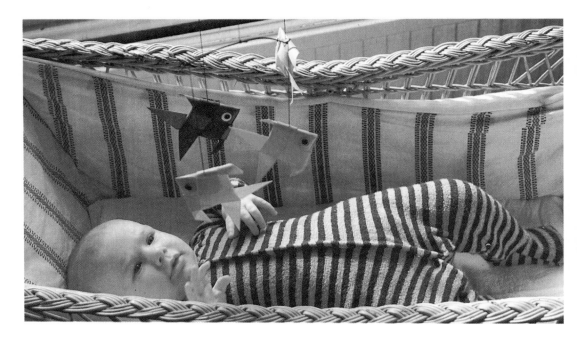

functioning and carrying messages efficiently throughout the body to enable the baby to make reflexive movements, swallow and suck, excrete waste, see, hear, taste, smell, sleep and dream. All sensory systems are functional, including the vestibular system in the inner ear by which your baby will orientate herself in space.

Vision A few decades ago, it was thought that, at birth, infants could not see at all but were only sensitive to light and dark. However, now it is known that their eyes are well focused at a distance of approximately 30 cm (12 in) – the perfect distance for your baby to see your features clearly when you hold her in your arms – and that their eye movements are purposeful and well coordinated. They usually interact with their parents by deep and intent gazing, but their vision will not be fully developed until they are between three and six months old.

The ability of babies to distinguish fine detail improves very rapidly, and they also respond to colour. They can perceive form and pattern, and prefer curved to straight lines, colours to black and white, three-dimensional objects to flat pictures, complex patterns to simple ones, and human faces to other forms. In fact, they can see and imitate the facial and hand gestures of an adult when they are only one hour old, and will soon develop remarkable lip-reading skills.

Accustomed to the darkness of the womb, babies are very sensitive to light in the days following birth. Some need to be protected for the first few days and acclimatized gradually to the brightness of normal daylight.

In the early days, you may notice that your baby appears to be squinting (*see* p. 335) – that is, she looks persistently cross-eyed – but this is usually an illusion created by the presence of little folds of skin on the inner sides of the eyelids. If you are in doubt after your child is 12 weeks old, bring this to the attention of your doctor.

Stimulating your baby

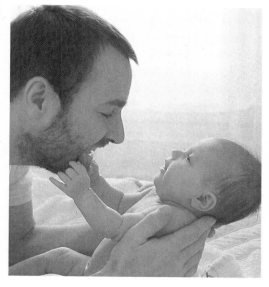
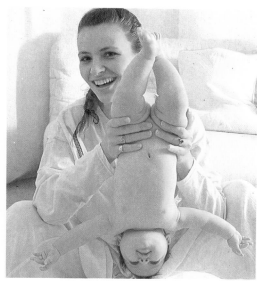

In each of the rooms in your home where your baby is likely to be, you could arrange a safe corner where she can sit propped up as well as lie down, and include toys and other objects of interest. This, together with the use of a sling to carry your baby around, will make it easier for you to attend to household tasks and still be involved with your baby.

Hang interesting coloured mobiles near where you change nappies or sit with your baby.

Include your baby in everyday household activities and introduce her to older children, allowing her to be held carefully and talked to by an older child.

Talk, coo and sing to your baby, and play beautiful music. Babies enjoy many sorts of music and songs, however simple, improvised or off-key they may be!

Take your baby outside to experience simple movements such as crossing her arms, 'bicycling' her legs, holding her up as if standing or walking. Support her as she enjoys stretching and extending her spine and neck. (See pp. 282–8.)

Encourage your baby to enjoy playing in water: bathing with her and/or taking her swimming from an early age is an excellent idea.

Taste and smell The taste buds are acutely sensitive at birth, having developed since the eighth week of pregnancy. Newborns seem to prefer sweet tastes, and they can also discriminate between 'good' and 'bad' ones. They also have an acute sense of smell, and are attuned to their mothers' body smell; they will turn away from an unpleasant odour.

By one week after birth, a baby can recognize and tell the difference between the taste and smell of her mother's milk and that of other women.

Touch and sensitivity to temperature The skin is not only the largest of your baby's sense organs, it is also the most primitive, having developed from the same part of the embryo as the nervous system about six weeks after conception. Many of the messages you send your baby are transmitted via body contact and touch when you hold, carry, nurse and care for her, and she will also be very responsive to massage which can be a very pleasurable and relaxing activity (*see* pp. 282-8).

Learning
Babies are particularly receptive to learning when they are in a quiet, alert state, and the time spent in this way will increase progressively as the hours of sleep lessen. They will learn faster if they are happy than if they use a lot of energy crying, and their learning will be enhanced if they are able to interact with an adult or child (*see* box above).

A baby will respond to hot or cold by withdrawing, radiating heat or shivering. Many parents are surprised to find how resilient older babies are to variations in temperature.

Hearing and vocalization In the womb, a baby hears a cacophony of sounds, among which are her mother's heartbeat and voice. After birth, these sounds will be familiar, and your baby will be soothed when held near your heart.

By the time she is a few weeks old, your baby will be able to identify the characteristics of the voices of different people, and recognize a vast range of sounds. She will react to different intonations of sound, preferring low, soothing tones to high ones. She will turn towards a pleasant sound, seem to react to other babies' cries and, during the first two months, will be startled by sudden noises (see 'Startle reflex', p. 181). It is important to get your baby used to general household noises – infants generally thrive with activity surrounding them and learn to sleep in the midst of familiar sounds.

At five to eight weeks, your baby will begin to associate hearing with looking. One day she will simply look into space as you talk to her, and the next will concentrate intently on your face as you speak and may even move her lips in time with yours. The first smile is often a response to your voice, as may be the first attempt at speech.

Babies begin to form speech patterns influenced by and synchronized with their parents' voices. Indeed, it is now thought that the 'mother tongue' has its origins in the womb, and its development is also very apparent in early infancy as children imitate the facial movements and sounds made by their parents.

The classic hearing test for a newborn baby is to stand behind her head and clap your hands loudly, first on one side and then on the other. Her head should turn towards the noise. If you have any doubt about your baby's ability to hear, you should have this checked as soon as possible (see Deafness, p. 306).

Motor control and coordination

Motor development begins in the womb, and at birth, your baby's reflexes allow her to step and make crawling movements. Conscious motor control increases throughout childhood and follows the same pattern: from the head down to the feet, and from the centre of the body out to the extremities.

From the start, control of the head is stimulated by the rooting reflex, when babies learn to turn their heads from side to side. By one month, they are able to lift their heads when they lie on their stomachs, and head control gradually improves from then on. This will expand a baby's world by allowing her to see surrounding activity.

During the first six to eight weeks, babies usually keep their hands clenched tightly into fists, only opening them for part of the time. Controlled movement of the arms comes next, as they begin to examine and play with their fingers and hands. By the time they are three or four months old, they will begin to reach for specific objects, and will grasp and play with rattles and other toys given to them.

Hand-to-eye coordination follows, as babies see things that they want to touch and feel and so reach out to grasp and put them in their mouths.

From this time onward, babies begin an intense exploration of their environment, and you should allow your child the freedom to do this, while watching carefully to make sure that she does not come to any harm.

In the next few months, your baby will learn to roll over, sit, crawl, stand and walk.

All babies learn basic motor skills more or less in the same sequence, but they vary widely in the age at which they reach various physical landmarks. This variation depends not only on innate ability but also on the amount of stimulation the child receives. In addition, babies often learn in spurts, and great significance should not be attached to the age at which landmarks are achieved. Often a baby who is concentrating on one area may be slow in another. If you are worried about your baby's development, you should consult your doctor.

The well baby

Shortly after the birth, your baby's breathing, heart rate, muscle tone, crying and colour will be assessed by your doctor or midwife, and an Apgar score will be given (*see* p. 165). Within a day of the birth, a more extensive paediatric examination is usually made (*see* right). At six weeks, babies are usually seen by their paediatrician or by a doctor at a local 'well baby' clinic (*see* below), when the paediatric examination will be repeated.

Community midwives, health visitors and clinics

If you have a home birth or leave hospital before your baby is ten days old, a community midwife will visit you every day to make sure that all is well and to help you to care for your baby. She will also attend to you physically by examining your breasts, uterus, lochia and any stitches you may have.

On the tenth day after the birth, the midwife makes way for the health visitor, a specially trained nurse who is interested in the physical and emotional well-being of both mother and baby. The number of visits she makes depends on your needs and her schedule, but you can also ring her and ask her to visit. Health visitors also go to the homes of childminders.

'Well baby' (child health) clinics are run by family doctors or by health authorities, and health visitors are often based at these. There you can discuss anything that may be bothering you, and your baby may be weighed and examined; you will also have an opportunity to meet other mothers in your area. A doctor will be in attendance to make developmental checks at appropriate times. You can also purchase vitamin supplements and formula milk at low prices, and immunizations can be carried out there.

Illness

Babies are generally very resilient and healthy, and not nearly as delicate and vulnerable as they appear. They can cope very effectively with such minor ailments as colds and coughs (*see* p. 301) and most of the common children's illnesses. However, if you suspect that your child is not well, it is wise to get in touch with your doctor as soon as possible.

An unwell baby may not feed, and may need to be held most of the time. This physical contact is the best cure for most ailments, but it can be very tiring for the parents. See Part VI (pp. 290-346) for information on individual problems.

The first examination

* Your baby's weight, length and head circumference are measured and recorded.
* The head and the fontanelles are examined.
* The chest is examined, and breathing and the heart are listened to with a stethoscope.
* The abdomen and genitals are checked. A boy's testes are examined to make sure that they have both descended into the scrotum (*see* p. 341).
* All the joints are examined. Special attention is focused on the hips to make sure that there is no sign of dislocation (*see* p. 308).
* Pulses and reflexes are checked. In addition, your baby's general condition is assessed, and there is an opportunity for you to ask any questions you may have.

When your baby is six days old, a drop of blood will be taken from her heel for a Guthrie test which detects *phenylketonuria*, a rare genetic disease (*see* p. 330); and part of the blood sample may also be used to check thyroid gland function (*see* p. 338).

Many paediatricians routinely give newborn babies vitamin K in a few drops of liquid or by injection; this vitamin assists the blood-clotting process. There is some controversy as to whether this is really necessary, and the decision to give vitamin K must be made jointly by the paediatrician and the parents.

CHAPTER 15

FEEDING YOUR BABY

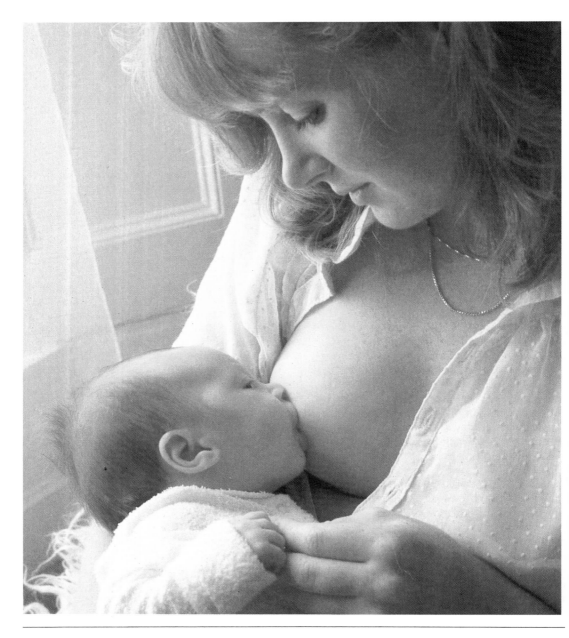

After birth, your child's digestive tract begins to function independently. He will experience hunger for the first time, and will have a powerful instinct to find the breast, suck and swallow. Breastfeeding is the ideal way to feed your baby during the first year of life, your body producing the perfect food to complement his appetite, and its many advantages make it the first choice if at all possible. However, in some circumstances, it may be more suitable to bottle-feed a baby, or a combination of breast- and bottle-feeding may be the best solution.

Feeding is an intimate experience between you and your baby, and it is essential that, in choosing your method of feeding, you follow your own preferences and choose what is best for you, your baby and your family.

Considering breastfeeding

Breastfeeding, although primarily for nutrition, has many dimensions. In the rich texture of the exchange that takes place between mother and baby, both are nourished in a unique way which is at once physiological, psychological and sensual.

The milk itself is the ideal food for babies' development and future health. It is impossible to duplicate: there is no formula or 'humanized', milk which provides all the nutrients and protective factors found in breastmilk, nor is there one which suits the digestion of babies so well. Breastfed babies are far less likely to develop digestive problems like colic, infections such as diarrhoea and gastro-enteritis, or respiratory disorders. This is because breastmilk enhances the defence mechanisms in the intestinal wall that prevent the entry of micro-organisms.

During pregnancy, your baby received antibodies – protective proteins – from your blood via the placenta. These are produced by your immune system in response to infections to which you have been exposed. When babies are a few weeks old, their bone marrow begins to produce their own antibodies, which are then released into the blood. These form a protective lining in the lungs and the gut which acts as a defence against bacteria and viruses. Although babies do not produce enough antibodies for complete protection until they are about three months old, your child will receive an adequate supply from your breastmilk. The more completely a young infant is breastfed, the greater will be his resistance to infective disease.

Allergic conditions such as eczema, asthma and hay fever are also far less common in breastfed babies. Many people are actually allergic to cows' milk, and this may be immediately apparent in infancy, or symptoms may appear later in life. Where there is a significant family history of allergies, breastfeeding is the effective way of reducing the risks of these in a baby.

There are other, more practical reasons for choosing to breastfeed. It is much cheaper than bottle-feeding: you do not need to buy formula, bottles, sterilizing equipment or supplies. It is also a great deal more convenient – no mixing, sterilizing, washing up or having to take lots of equipment when you travel or go on holiday. Night feeds are particularly easy, and you will never have to worry about whether or not your baby's food is sterile or the right temperature or whether he is getting enough.

During breastfeeding, a vital exchange takes place: while the baby receives the nourishment needed for basic survival and growth, both mother and baby experience pleasure and deep contentment. The repeated satisfaction of hunger and the comfort and security which babies experience while feeding are vital to their future emotional health.

Considering bottle-feeding

Breastfeeding has so many advantages that it is certainly worth a good try for the first weeks at the very least. It is particularly important that the baby should take the colostrum (*see* p. 193) in the first days after the birth. However, sometimes breastfeeding is not possible, and it may be preferable to bottle-feed. Babies can certainly grow and thrive when they are bottle-fed, and sometimes this is the best way to nourish a child successfully.

The most important factor of all is that feeding times should be a pleasure for you and your baby. It is better to bottle-feed comfortably and happily than to struggle with breastfeeding if you are really not enjoying it or if you have some other important reason for preferring bottle over breast. There are many reasons why women choose to bottle-feed:

• A mother returning to work may need to bottle-feed, or to combine breast- and bottle-feeding.

• She may plan to breastfeed but finds that things do not go as she had hoped or that there is a lack of good guidance at the start. This can be avoided by contacting a breastfeeding counsellor (*see* p. 197).

• For a few women, the idea of breastfeeding is unacceptable. For example, the strong physical sensation of a baby sucking at the breast, which many mothers enjoy, may be disturbing.

• Breastfeeding may be impossible due to illness (although this is rare).

• There may be deep emotional reasons, such as a woman's need to protect herself from her baby's hunger, a feeling of wanting her body to herself or anxiety about physiological changes to her breasts or figure.

• She may have a lack of confidence in her ability to produce sufficient milk to nourish her baby properly.

• There may be a failure to overcome initial difficulties.

Some of these reasons may be unavoidable, and if you are sure that you would prefer to bottle-feed, it is important to trust your own intuition and feelings. The final decision is best made once your baby is actually born. As long as the formula you offer is properly sterilized, nutritionally acceptable and given with plenty of body contact, cuddles and love, bottle-feeding can be a successful and enjoyable choice.

Breastfeeding

Successful breastfeeding depends, first, on an understanding of how the natural process takes place, and then on everyone concerned – mother, father, birth attendants, health visitors, relatives, friends and society at large – providing a setting in which this process can flourish. As with labour and birth, this will involve patience as well as trust in your natural instincts and body processes. There may be difficulties at first, but you will be giving your baby the best possible start if you decide to breastfeed your baby.

The breasts

During pregnancy, the levels of the hormones oestrogen, progesterone and prolactin in the body increase markedly, and the breasts react by enlarging in preparation for lactation.

The breasts themselves are made up of 15–25 segments, or lobes, each of which consists of several clusters of glands known as *alveoli*. These resemble bunches of 10–100 grapes, and each 'grape' – or *alveolus* – is lined with cells which produce milk. Surrounding each alveolus is a layer of muscle cells that are stimulated by the hormone *oxytocin* (*see* below) to contract and squeeze the gland so that the milk is forced out into tiny canals which converge to form the lobe's milk duct. There are 15–25 of these ducts, one for each lobe, and they open into the nipple, where they can be seen as little crevices. Once feeding begins, the milk is ejected through these openings, often flowing quite fast in fine sprays when the breasts are full.

Just before the ducts reach the nipples, they widen to form small balloon-like milk reservoirs called *ampullae* which are situated just behind each areola (the dark skin surrounding each nipple). They are capable of storing quite a lot of milk, and their capacity increases after a few weeks.

Surrounding and between each lobe are layers of fat which determine the shape and size of the breasts. Size does not have much bearing on the breasts' ability to produce milk, as small breasts contain the same number of milk-producing cells as larger ones and function as effectively.

The size of the nipples and surrounding areolas also does not make much difference during breastfeeding, but the ability of the nipples to protrude does. During pregnancy, the nipples will become larger and will usually lengthen so that the baby can take hold of them more easily. (If your nipples do not protrude, they may be 'inverted' – *see* page 318.) Although they are usually flat, the nipples will become erect when the baby is about to feed, just as they do when a woman is sexually aroused or cold. They have delicate nerve endings which make them very sensitive to touch, and after childbirth, this sensitivity is heightened. The baby's sucking will also stimulate the production of milk.

Each areola is surrounded by small glands called *Montgomery's tubercles* which secrete a natural lubricating fluid that keeps the nipple soft and supple. These glands become more active and prominent during pregnancy but will be less evident once lactation is over.

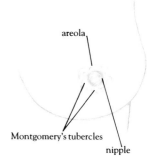

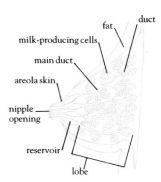

Each breast contains clusters of milk-secreting glands arranged in lobes and opening into the nipple via milk ducts. The reservoirs are where the milk is stored.

How breastmilk is made

From the beginning of pregnancy, the hormone prolactin from the pituitary gland, oestrogen and progesterone from the placenta, and also thyroid hormone stimulate the development of the milk-producing cells in the breasts. In late pregnancy, these produce colostrum, a yellowish fluid that is the baby's first food until a few days after the birth when the first true milk is produced, or 'comes in' (*see* below).

After the birth, when the placenta is expelled, oestrogen levels drop dramatically, and the release of prolactin increases. This is stimulated by contact between the baby's mouth and the sensitive nipple and areola. When the prolactin reaches the delicate network of blood vessels that surround the milk-producing cells in the breasts, the production of milk begins. All the constituents used to make the milk are also brought to the alveoli through the mother's bloodstream.

Milk is produced in a cycle that is entirely dependent on the baby's needs. The more the baby sucks on the nipple, the more the pituitary gland will be stimulated to produce prolactin, which in turn stimulates the production of milk in the breasts. In this way, nature has provided an ideal self-regulating mechanism to ensure that your body will produce just the right amount of milk to meet your baby's requirements, provided he is

How milk is produced.

The baby's sucking stimulates nerve endings in the mother's nipple, which transmit messages to the pituitary gland in the brain. Prolactin, produced in the anterior lobe, stimulates further milk production. Oxytocin, produced in the posterior lobe, causes the muscles lining the alveoli containing the milk cells to contract and 'let down' the milk.

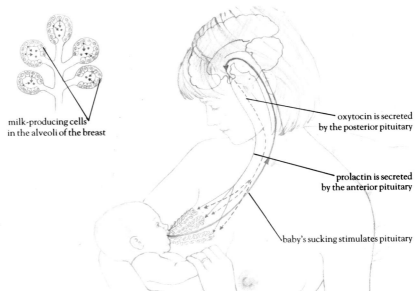

milk-producing cells in the alveoli of the breast

oxytocin is secreted by the posterior pituitary

prolactin is secreted by the anterior pituitary

baby's sucking stimulates pituitary

offered the breast whenever he indicates that he wants it (*see* pp. 198-9).

The increase in prolactin levels in the blood also has the effect of suppressing ovulation, and a woman who is breastfeeding fully may not ovulate for months. This is a natural birth control, but because you cannot tell exactly when the first ovulation will occur, it is necessary to use some other form of birth control to ensure that you do not become pregnant unexpectedly (*see* Contraception, pp. 304-5).

Breastmilk

Your body manufactures breastmilk from the nutrients and other constituents in your blood, and like blood, it is a living substance; in fact, if resembles blood but without the red blood cells. For example, breastmilk contains *leucocytes*, protective white blood cells which defend the body against infections and disease. It also contains many antibodies, enzymes, hormones and other active cells, all of which promote good health.

The milk of each mammal is unique, and is particularly suited to the specific developmental needs of its young. Human milk, similar to that of all primates, is low in protein because our growth rate is slower than that of most other mammals, while it is relatively high in lactose (milk sugar) to provide energy for our brains to develop faster to their larger size. Cows' milk, on the other hand, is quite different from human milk and is intended for the specific needs and characteristics of calves: it has, among other things, a much higher protein content and less sugar.

Modern formula manufacturers try to 'humanize' cows' milk to make it as similar as possible to human breastmilk. They do this by diluting it, adding more sugar and processing it to make it more digestible. Although the result is reasonably good and babies can certainly survive and thrive on formulas, it is as impossible to re-create breastmilk as it is to manufacture artificial blood. There are certain elements in breastmilk that, so far, have proved to be incapable of analysis, and new properties of this remarkable fluid are continually being revealed.

The composition of breastmilk is also not consistent, changing according to the stage of lactation or the time of day; in addition, the rate at which it flows alters throughout each feed and over the lactating period. This also happens to the milk produced by cows, but by the time it is 'humanized' and turned into baby formula, it loses this dynamic quality and the baby will receive milk with a consistent composition and an even flow at every feed. This ability to meet a child's changing needs makes it impossible for babies nourished on breastmilk to be overfed and lessens the risk of obesity in childhood and later in life.

Colostrum During the last few months of pregnancy and just after birth, the breasts begin to produce *colostrum*, the baby's first food. This highly nutritious fluid is much richer in protein – some of it in the form of valuable antibodies – than later milk, and because of this, the baby may sleep for long periods between feeds; thus both mother and baby can rest after the birth. There is also less sugar in colostrum than in mature milk, and less fat. It also contains vitamins A, B complex and E, as well as minerals such as zinc.

An important function of colostrum is its laxative effect. It helps to clear the digestive tract of the *meconium* – the baby's first sticky, greenish-black stools – which are contained in the bowel before birth and excreted during the first day or so.

Proper sucking of the colostrum will stimulate the milk-producing glands and the let-down reflex (*see below*), prepare the baby's system for digestion and protect him against various harmful organisms in the outside world. It is all your baby needs during the first few days of life: supplementary bottles of water, glucose or formula are almost never necessary and may interfere with the production of milk by quenching the baby's thirst and therefore diminishing the essential stimulation of his sucking. Restricting the amount of time that the baby feeds to one or two minutes on each side may also inhibit this natural process and reduce the amount of colostrum that he receives.

Colostrum plays an important part in your baby's adaptation to life outside the womb and in setting the tone for good health in the future.

Transitional milk When the first true milk 'comes in', it is still mixed with colostrum and looks rich and creamy compared to the more watery milk you will notice a week or so later. As it becomes thinner, the protein and antibody content decreases, and after about two weeks, the transitional phase is over and the breasts produce mature milk.

The transitional milk comes in some time during the first few days after the birth – usually on the third day – and there are various factors which can influence when this occurs:

● Early bonding with your baby and being together most of the time in the early days – including during the night – will stimulate milk production. If your baby is allowed to suck whenever he wants, this will promote the secretion of oxytocin and prolactin.

● Some drugs used for pain relief in labour (*see* pp. 328-30) may depress the baby's sucking reflex, and this can delay the production of breastmilk. However, as soon as his body begins to eliminate the drug, the sucking reflex will return, and once the breasts are stimulated, they will make enough milk and you can settle down to normal feeding.

Being relaxed and at ease and having enough privacy are also important. For this reason, many mothers arrange to leave hospital within 48 hours, provided the birth has been normal. However, it is essential to ensure you have enough help at home to allow you to rest and concentrate on caring for your baby. If a longer stay in hospital is necessary and early feeding is unsettled, do not worry – just do your best, knowing that, once you are at home with your baby, you will be able to come to terms with this new relationship in your own time.

For some mothers, the opposite applies: staying in hospital an extra day or two may help to establish breastfeeding securely, particularly if the staff are supportive and helpful and you are able to rest (see p. 114).

When the milk does come in, it usually does so gradually. If it comes in rapidly the breasts will feel very full and the baby should be encouraged to feed frequently.

The 'Let-down' reflex When feeding starts and the baby sucks, the rhythmic action of the jaws presses the milk stored in the ampullae out towards the nipple. At the beginning of a feed, they contain about a third of the volume of the whole feed; this is known as the *foremilk*, which has a low caloric and fat value, but does provide fluid.

As the baby begins to suck the breast – or even in anticipation of a feed – the nerve endings in the nipples send messages to the pituitary gland, this time stimulating the secretion of another hormone, *oxytocin*. This causes the muscle cells around the milk glands to contract, and the milk that they have produced descends – i.e. is 'let down' – through the milk ducts to the ampullae, and from there to the nipples.

This milk is known as the *hindmilk* and is rich in fat, containing approximately 30 calories per ounce as compared to 15 calories in the foremilk. It comes down very rapidly and is ejected with considerable force; in fact, the jets of milk can spray out a distance of several feet. The let-down reflex occurs in both breasts at once, and while the baby sucks at one breast, milk may spurt out of the other one. Pressing your hand firmly against the nipple will help to stop the flow.

In some women, the let-down reflex can occur as soon as they think about feeding their babies or if they hear them cry – as the milk-producing mechanism is set in motion, blood rushes to the breasts, which become warm and tingle. Generally, though, it usually takes about half a minute or so after the baby starts sucking for the milk to be let down, and it is not uncommon for two or three minutes to elapse before this occurs. This can be difficult for a baby, who may finish the foremilk quite quickly and then cry with frustration until the let-down occurs. A little perseverance and trust in the natural mechanism will result in milk flow in a moment or two.

If the baby is to be adequately nourished, the let-down reflex must occur to release the hindmilk. For this reason, it is important not to restrict the baby to only a few minutes of sucking each breast as the let-down reflex may be missed altogether and the breastfeeding process will be disturbed. If babies feed only on foremilk, they will be hungry, may cry often and may even develop diarrhoea because the foremilk is so watery.

Sometimes the let-down occurs without the mother being aware of it. On the other hand, it may be uncomfortable or even painful for the first few days until the milk begins to flow.

Both the milk-producing and let-down reflexes are delicate mechanisms involving the mutual interaction of mother and baby. If the mother is worried, anxious, embarrassed, in pain or afraid, this can inhibit the secretion of hormones so that she is unable to produce or let down milk. Given a conducive and supportive environment, virtually every mother can produce milk.

Mature milk Mature milk is white or bluish-white in colour. The more watery foremilk quenches thirst, while the hindmilk, with its increased fat and protein content, satisfies hunger. However, after the let-down has occurred and the baby has sucked the first of the hindmilk, the rate of flow slows down, so the baby has to work to get the most nutritious milk and cannot be overfed.

Mature breastmilk is primarily made up of water in which all the other ingredients – fat, protein, sugar (lactose), vitamins, minerals – are suspended or dissolved. It is interesting to compare the composition of breastmilk with that of cows' milk and formulas made from it.

Fat On average, breastmilk contains approximately 4 per cent fat, which contributes almost half the calories in the milk. It is an important source of energy and is needed for your baby's growth.

One of the important functions of fat is to help the development of the coverings of the nerves. In early infancy, your baby's brain and nervous system are growing faster than at any other time.

The enzymes which break down fat are called lipases, and breastmilk contains some of its own so that, by the time the milk enters the baby's stomach, it has already been partially broken down. Because of this, the fat in breastmilk is more easily digested and absorbed than that in cows' milk. Breastmilk also contains fatty acids which assist the absorption of calcium, needed for the development of strong bones and teeth.

The fat in breastmilk is mainly unsaturated and is quite different from that in cows' milk. Formula manufacturers add unsaturated vegetable oils and skimmed milk to cows' milk to make it more like breastmilk.

Protein The proteins in breastmilk have a number of nutritional functions. Some types act as enzymes, to set off chemical reactions throughout the body; others transport minerals. However, the most important property of proteins is that they can be broken down into amino acids, which are the basic elements of body tissue. In addition, the protective antibodies contained in breastmilk (*see* p. 189) are proteins.

Cows' milk contains about three times more protein than breastmilk, including much more of a type known as *casein*, which is bulky and hard to digest and will be excreted by the baby. Formula manufacturers process cows' milk to alter the casein to make it more digestible, but despite this, the curds remain in the baby's gut for about four hours. You can see the difference in the stools: those of a breastfed baby will be very liquid and mustard-coloured, while a bottle-fed baby has harder, darker stools.

Breastmilk contains proportionately more of another type of protein – *lactalbumin* – which is broken down much more easily and faster and is almost completely absorbed. This is why breastfed babies hardly ever become constipated, and it is also the reason why they become hungry more quickly and so need to feed more often.

Cows' milk proteins can also be the source of allergies in sensitive infants. (*See also* Allergies and hypersensitivity, pp. 290–1.)

Lactose The milk of all mammals contains sugar in the form of lactose. Human breastmilk has almost twice as much as cows' milk.

Lactose is a source of quick energy, but it also has a number of other functions. For example, it has a special effect on the micro-organisms that live in the baby's gut. Since only a proportion of the lactose in milk is digested, the remainder is fermented in the large bowel. This promotes the growth of a special group of bacteria known as *Lactobacilli* which reduce the incidence of diarrhoea. They are also responsible for the difference in the smell of the stools: those of breastfed babies have a sweet odour, whereas those of bottle-fed babies have a stronger, more foul smell.

Because cows' milk contains less sugar then breastmilk, manufacturers of formulas usually add other types of sugar such as sucrose (simple table sugar) or fructose (fruit sugar) to match the sugar level of human milk.

Vitamins If your own nutrition is good, your baby will receive all the vitamins he needs from your milk and in just the right proportions. Breastmilk contains larger quantities of vitamins A, C, B_{12} and E than cows' milk, but less vitamin K.

Because it takes a baby's bowel 48 hours to make vitamin K, which is vital for adequate blood clotting, some are given the vitamin after birth (*see* p. 187). Other vitamin supplements are unnecessary if you have a good balanced diet yourself.

Until the early 1970s, it was thought that breastmilk was lacking in vitamin D, which is essential for the absorption of calcium and phosphorus by the body. Researchers then produced evidence that vitamin D in breastmilk is water-soluble, and contained in its water molecules. In addition, cholesterol in the skin is turned into another form of vitamin D by the ultraviolet rays of the sun. A few minutes of sunlight each day is enough to ensure that supplementation is not needed.

Vitamins are sensitive to changes in temperature. In the constant temperature of breastmilk they are well preserved, but when milk is heated they may be destroyed, and bottle-fed babies may need to be given vitamin supplements.

Minerals The mineral content of breastmilk will depend on the mother's nutritional state and diet. In general, it has a much lower mineral content than cows' milk, but those it does contain are in just the right quantities. If babies are fed on untreated cows' milk, their immature kidneys come under a great deal of strain coping with the higher quantities of minerals.

In particular, sodium and potassium play an important role in the balance of fluids in the body, and an excess or deficiency of either one can cause serious problems. If formula contains too much, or is made up with too little water, the sodium level could be too high and make the baby thirsty. This can lead to a vicious cycle: more thirst, more formula, too much sodium, more thirst – and the baby's kidneys could be damaged. This is impossible with breastfeeding. Formula manufacturers do demineralize cows' milk, but it is likely that other valuable constituents in the milk are also eliminated in the process. Goats' milk contains even higher levels of minerals than cows' milk.

Babies absorb iron from their mothers in the last months of pregnancy and have enough stored in their livers at birth to last until they are about six months old. This reserve supplements the iron in breastmilk, the levels of which are more or less the same as in formula. However, breastfed babies are able to absorb iron more efficiently due to the presence of greater amounts of *lactoferrin*, which is a protein that binds with the mineral.

Breastmilk also contains copper and zinc, although less than in cows' milk. However, these too are much more easily absorbed from breastmilk.

Preparing for breastfeeding

The best way to learn how to breastfeed is to spend time with women who are breastfeeding, and it is also well worth contacting a breastfeeding counsellor before you have your baby. These specially trained women who have themselves breastfed their babies will advise on problems. Breastfeeding counsellors are usually available at any time on the telephone and may be able to visit you personally if a crisis arises. Contact the La Lèche League or the National Childbirth Trust (*see* p. 347) to find out if there is a counsellor in your area. Counselling is also available through your community midwife and health visitor.

You will begin to notice changes in your breasts from the earliest days of your pregnancy, as altering levels of hormones cause them to become more tender and perhaps heavier and larger than they were before.

The tiny glands which surround each nipple produce a natural oil which lubricates them, and it is also helpful to massage the breasts and nipples gently with a light vegetable oil such as almond, sesame or olive oil after bathing (*see* p. 279). If you enjoy having your breasts touched, the normal caressing that occurs during love-making is an ideal way to prepare for breastfeeding your baby.

Your breasts may begin to produce colostrum during the last months of pregnancy, but do not be concerned if you do not notice any before your baby is born. Expressing a little colostrum from time to time is sometimes recommended to 'unplug' the milk ducts, but is not necessary, as they will open spontaneously when you feed your baby. However, it will not harm you and may be helpful in making you familiar with handling your breasts.

As your breasts become heavier and increase in size, it is important that they are adequately supported by a well-fitting bra (preferably a cotton one), even if you do not usually wear one. Firm support during pregnancy will help to prevent stretch marks and sagging, which tend to occur then rather than as a result of breastfeeding.

After your baby is born, you will need some good nursing bras. There are two types available: those with flaps which open to reveal the nipple and areola; and those which open completely in front. Many women prefer the latter as they are more comfortable to wear and allow the baby to nestle against the naked breast and to explore it with his hands while feeding.

It is also a good idea to ensure beforehand that you have suitable clothing to wear when feeding your baby – i.e. clothes that open easily in front or can be lifted up from the waist, and which are comfortable, look attractive, can be easily laundered and do not require ironing.

Starting to breastfeed

If circumstances allow, the ideal time to begin breastfeeding is within the first hour or so after the birth, when your baby is at his most alert, taking in the first sensations of life outside the womb.

The way in which feeding begins will set the pattern for the future, and it will help if this encounter is satisfying to both mother and baby. If the first feed must be delayed for some reason, or if the first attempt is not as successful as it could be, begin afresh at the next opportunity.

It is important to have privacy and a relaxed, calm atmosphere in the room where the first sucking takes place. If it is warm enough, it is best if both you and your baby can be naked or at least partially so, so that direct skin-to-skin contact is possible. It is helpful if you sit upright, and you may find it helps to put a pillow on your lap to support the baby.

Once your baby latches on to the breast (see pp. 200-1), the sucking and swallowing reflex will begin. Some mothers are surprised at the strength of their babies' sucking and the powerful sensations of the vacuum created by the suction and of the milk being drawn out. However, contrary to what many people think, babies do not actually suck to get the milk. Rather, they move their jaws rhythmically to 'milk' the ampullae behind the areola. They do use some suction to keep the nipple and areola in their mouths, but once these are well drawn in, the action of their jaws stimulates the let-down reflex and the milk is ejected in fine jets, so that all they have to do is swallow. This action produces the typical look of a breastfed baby – i.e. prominent cheek and jaw muscles. Your child may suck steadily without pausing, or may suck for a few minutes, stop with the nipple in his mouth and then start again a few moments later.

Soreness of the nipples (see p. 199 and pp. 203-4) can be caused by the way you remove the baby from the breast. Never attempt to pull the breast away before breaking the suction; rather, first gently press down on his chin or insert your little finger gently into the corner of his mouth.

After the baby has sucked on one breast for a while, offer the other one so that both breasts are evenly stimulated. The next time you feed him, first offer the breast you finished with the last time, so that each breast benefits from the more intense sucking at the beginning when the baby is hungry. Some women prefer to offer only one breast at each feed, alternating sides each time.

How often should I feed my baby?

The many hours spent at the breast are among the most important and absorbing experiences of a baby's early life. The need for satisfaction and comfort when feeding is so great that his future emotional security depends on adequate fulfilment of this.

Many people are under the illusion that if babies are given the breast whenever they indicate that they want it, they will become dependent and clingy. However, in reality the opposite is true. Babies who are fed immediately whenever they are hungry tend to be calm and contented, developing later into remarkably independent, secure and healthy children. The feelings of satisfaction and pleasure at the breast are so blissful that constant repetition of these experiences imprints itself indelibly on a child's personality.

Breastfed babies absorb breastmilk quickly, and become hungry at frequent intervals. In fact, in the early days, weeks and months, they need to feed almost continuously when they are not asleep, usually within two hours or so of the last feed.

The easiest approach to breastfeeding is to be prepared to feed your baby whenever he wants, and to expect that there will be some times of the day when he will seem to be almost continuously hungry, and others when he will seem satisfied and will sleep for long periods. During the first few months, his eating pattern is likely to be quite irregular, the times of great hunger occurring both day and night, and you may find that, no sooner do you get used to one pattern than his needs seem to change. Although some infants are remarkably 'easy', sleeping mainly at night and feeding a lot during the day, it is equally usual for the opposite to be true.

Generally, the line of least resistance is the easiest one to take, allowing your baby's needs to lead the way while making sure that you are well nourished and get the chance to rest or sleep – if possible, whenever your baby does. Eventually, things will settle down to a pattern.

How long should each feed be?

Mothers are often told, when starting to breastfeed, to limit the baby's sucking time to three to five minutes on each breast for the first few days and then to increase the time gradually to about ten minutes on each side. The reason given for this is that, if the baby feeds too long or too often, you will get sore nipples.

However, very often the let-down reflex does not come into operation during the first five minutes, and if the baby is prevented from sucking before this occurs, the breasts will not be sufficiently stimulated to make more milk. If this happens often enough, it can result in failure to breastfeed. Because the baby is hungry, he will suck hard whenever he gets the opportunity, and your nipples may become sore. Frequent unrestricted feeding, with the baby sucking in a relaxed way for as long as he wants, is, in fact, much easier on the nipples and will stimulate milk production.

Some babies simply love sucking, even after they have drunk all the milk on offer. This can be enjoyable for both baby and mother, but it is probably wise to break the suction gently after a time in the first week or two to prevent nipple soreness – provided you are sure that the feed is over. Prolonged sucking (i.e. longer than an hour) every few hours occasionally indicates that the baby is not getting enough milk. This is usually due to the baby not latching on properly, so that he is sucking mainly on the nipple and not emptying the breast.

Comfortable positions for breastfeeding

It is essential to be comfortable when holding and feeding your baby. Choose a spot where you have everything you may need and will be undisturbed. It can be helpful to have a pleasant drink to hand, as many women feel thirsty while feeding. You can feed your baby either sitting up or reclining, and you will probably find both positions useful.

Sitting up The traditional nursing chair is low so that you can sit with both feet flat on the floor with your back well supported in an upright position; it also has no arms to restrict the way you hold your baby. However, any comfortable armchair can be used, provided you can sit up straight and the arms are at a comfortable height. Some women are happy simply to sit cross-legged on the floor, with their back against a wall.

To avoid backache, it is important to have your back well supported and your head and shoulders relaxed, and not to lean forward to place the nipple in your baby's mouth. To achieve the right height, you might find it helpful to place a pillow across your legs and then lay your baby across it.

Once you are comfortable yourself, simple hold the baby with his head cradled in the crook of one arm and his body turned to face towards you, with enough room for him to move freely or turn away for a rest. His head should naturally be a little higher than his body; this will allow any air that is swallowed with the milk to bubble to the surface.

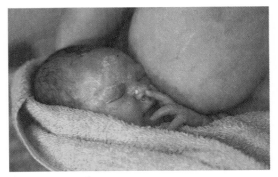

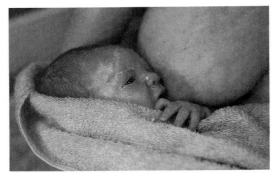

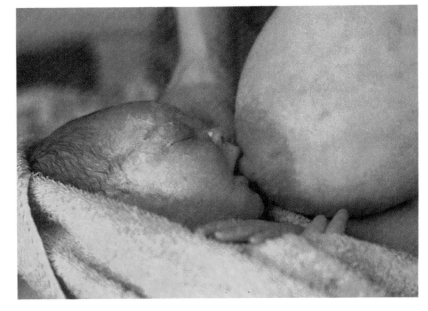

The rooting reflex
You can stimulate your baby's natural 'rooting reflex' (see p. 181) by gently touching his cheek near the corner of his mouth closest to the breast. You could also gently squeeze the nipple behind the areola to express a few drops of colostrum which the baby can smell and taste, or touch the baby's cheek with the nipple itself (above right).

Helping your baby to suck
When your baby has his mouth wide open (right), introduce the breast into it, making sure that he takes in both the nipple and part of the areola, not just the nipple which, if sucked on its own, will become sore. You can help him do this by making a U-shape with the thumb and fingers of your free hand, placing the nipple and areola between them and pushing the nipple outward.

Successful breastfeeding

Latching on Ensuring that your baby latches on to the breast correctly is one of the most important aspects of feeding. Many problems are caused by the baby not latching on properly, which produces stress and sore nipples.

Getting started There is no need to rush to introduce the child to the nipple. Wait until he is breathing comfortably and shows signs of searching for the breast or begins to make sucking movements indicating an interest in feeding. Some babies are initially more fascinated in exploring the new world of space, light, colour and sound, and others need time to recover from their experiences during birth before they are ready to begin feeding.

Some, however, seem to have an urgent need to begin sucking at once and search eagerly for the breast. Often their excitement is so great that the first attempts to latch on to the nipple are unsuccessful, and they may become frustrated and need to be soothed before trying again. Do not worry if it takes a while before you get started – the important thing is for your baby to be close to you and to begin to discover the breast.

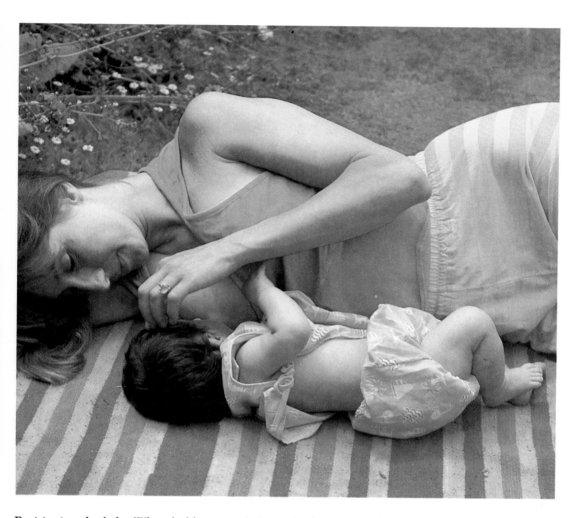

Positioning the baby When holding your baby to the breast, turn him so that the front of his body is *facing* yours, belly to belly, his head is just below your breast and he is at a comfortable angle for feeding. If the baby has to turn his head to suck the breast, he will pull on the nipple and this will soon produce soreness. Make sure that you are comfortable yourself, take a few deep breaths and relax, letting go of any tension in your body, especially in the neck, arms and shoulders.

Reclining Alternatively, you can feed your baby while lying on your side. You should be well supported by pillows, and your body should be gently curved so that your baby can fit next to you comfortably. He should be on his side facing towards you, his mouth in line with your nipple and his head supported in the crook of your arm. Draw his feet in close to your body, and hold his body at a slight angle, with his chin closer to your breast than his nose. In this position, he should be able to grasp the nipple easily while breathing freely. Make sure that he latches on to the breast correctly each time.

Caring for your nipples

Breastmilk contains natural antiseptic agents so there is no need to wash your nipples before each feed – this will simply remove the natural oils. Soap and nipple sprays (especially ones with an alcohol base) are to be avoided as these encourage dryness and a tendency towards sore nipples. Bathing them once a day with water only is sufficient to ensure that your breasts are clean.

Allow your breasts to dry in the open air after feeding. Then apply a small amount of a mild pure oil such as almond oil, or a good nipple cream such as one made from calendula (available from homoeopathic pharmacies, see pp. 315-16) to prevent tenderness. After a few weeks, when your nipples are used to feeding, there will be no need to apply any oil or cream.

You may find that, particularly in the first few months, the breast not being used leaks as the baby sucks. You can protect your clothing by using a soft cloth or nappy to catch the drips. It is important that you keep the nipples dry to prevent soreness, so avoid waterproof or plastic-lined breast pads, which may keep the breasts moist.

Breastfeeding in hospital

When it was common for women to be heavily sedated during labour, new mothers were generally unable to look after or feed their babies during the first 12 hours after the birth, and it became routine practice in many hospitals for babies to be taken to nurseries and given formula or glucose and water until their mothers were able to feed them. Today, however, with more women choosing to have natural and more active births, mothers and babies are alert and in intimate contact with each other immediately, and these practices are no longer appropriate.

When hospitals first came to recognize this change, and some began to encourage mothers to keep their babies near them at all times, they were surprised to discover that, although the wards were large, they were very peaceful and both mothers and babies seemed quite contented. However, there are also many hospitals in which the old-fashioned approach still prevails – where babies are kept in nurseries at night and sometimes during the day as well, and are brought to their mothers for feeds on a rigid four-hour schedule. In others, it may be up to the mother to inform the hospital officially that she intends to breastfeed on demand.

Many women find that, if they discuss their wishes with hospital staff beforehand or as soon as they are admitted, the staff are often willing to be flexible. Nevertheless, you may only feel at ease once you are home.

You will need peace and privacy, especially in the early days when you are still getting to know your baby and exploring a new and very intimate relationship. This can be difficult when you are in hospital – for example, visiting time may coincide with your baby needing a feed. You may want to limit visitors during the first few days, asking them to wait until you have settled in at home.

Another problem that women encounter is the conflicting advice given to them by well-meaning staff. Midwives, doctors, health visitors and breastfeeding counsellors may all have different opinions about breastfeeding, and you may find all the information confusing, not knowing whom to believe or what to do. This is best overcome by discussing it with one person – perhaps a midwife or breastfeeding counsellor – whom you feel understands your needs and the subject of feeding.

Common difficulties in the early days and weeks

For some women, breastfeeding starts quite effortlessly and, from the very beginning, proceeds without any problems. However, for many – especially first-time mothers – breastfeeding takes some getting used to.

Sometimes the first week or two can be quite difficult, as the milk supply is being established, your nipples are becoming accustomed to the baby's frequent sucking, you are adjusting to a completely different sleeping pattern and the sudden changes in your body and you may have a period of 'postpartum blues' (see p. 176). Women often do not realize there may be difficulties and become discouraged by the problems that can occur at the beginning, most of which, with a little perseverance and patience, will soon pass. The following is a guide to coping with the most common; others that occur less frequently are discussed on pages 294-5.

Engorgement When the milk comes in, you will probably find that your breasts fill up and feel enormous. The full milk glands will make them very firm and warm due to the increased blood supply, but if they become very distended, hard and hot, this is known as 'engorgement'.

Engorgement develops within a day of the milk coming in. The breasts can become very uncomfortable, and if they are very large, there may be pain on their sides and in the armpits. In addition, they may be so full that it is difficult for your baby to latch on to the nipple and areola. Engorgement should diminish within 24 hours as the 'supply and demand' system becomes established and production adjusts to your baby's appetite.

What you can do

- It is important to carry on feeding the baby, to relieve the fullness in your breasts and to ensure that enough milk continues to be produced.

- To enable your baby to latch on to your nipple and areola, it will help to express a little milk just before feeding. This can be done with a gentle breast massage (see p. 279), and will be easier if you first gently warm the breast in warm water in a bath or shower. Try lying on your belly in the bath and massaging the breast towards the nipple.

- If you do not already do so, wear a comfortable cotton nursing bra.

- A very effective (if unusual) method of relieving breast engorgement is to take white cabbage leaves that have been chilled in a refrigerator, roll them with a rolling pin to soften them and then place them in your bra against the skin. This will draw the heat out of the breast and reduce fluid in it. After an hour, expose the breasts to the air. Repeat every four hours.

After-pains Oxytocin, which stimulates the let-down reflex, simultaneously causes the uterus to contract. These contractions, known as 'after-pains', occur rhythmically each time the baby feeds. They help the uterus to return to normal after the birth, and this generally happens faster if the mother is breastfeeding. After-pains may hurt at first, especially if this is a second or subsequent baby: try breathing deeply and relaxing while they occur. Avoid painkillers: they may pass via the milk to your baby.

Sore nipples Many women develop sore nipples during the first few weeks of breastfeeding, and this is the most common reason why some give up. Contrary to popular opinion, they are not more common in fair-skinned women. With patience and perseverance, soreness can easily be overcome

How to avoid sore nipples

- Make sure that the baby is latching on to the breast properly.

- Try using a variety of feeding positions to distribute the sucking pressure to different parts of the nipples – e.g. sitting, lying down, holding the baby under your arm or across your lap.

- Ensure that your baby sucks until the let-down occurs and then continues. Removing the baby before a feed is properly established will be as hard on your nipples as it will be on your baby. You will find that the soreness you felt at the start of the feed will become less as the milk begins to flow.

- Offer your baby the least-sore breast first, and expose your breasts to the air as much as possible, particularly after feeding. Mild sunshine will be helpful.

- Some women find that rubber nipple shields, which protect the skin during feeding, are effective.

- Avoid using soaps, nylon bras and plastic-lined pads.

- When your nipples have dried after feeding, you can apply a little oil or a suitable cream – e.g. almond oil or calendula cream sparingly around the base of the nipple and on the areola, avoiding the top of the nipple. The application of antiseptic aerosol sprays is not recommended.

as the breasts get used to the baby's sucking. If you want to continue to breastfeed, do not put your baby on to the bottle to give your nipples a rest; the milk supply may dwindle. Care over how the baby latches on is the most important consideration.

Nutrition for breastfeeding

Nutrition at this time is more important than ever, and it will be worthwhile to re-read Chapter 7 to refresh your memory about what you should eat to achieve a well-balanced diet. You will need 500 calories more each day then you did during pregnancy, but with a normal diet and a healthy appetite, there is no need to go to any special lengths to ensure that you take in this extra amount. However, there are three areas which do need special attention: fluids, vitamins and minerals, and possible substances that you should avoid.

Fluids You will require extra fluid and may need to drink frequently, but you should let your thirst be your guide. It may be a good idea to have a supply of mineral water and a variety of herbal teas available throughout the day. Fruit juices should be diluted with water and drunk sparingly.

Vitamins and minerals Try to eat unrefined foods rich in vitamins and minerals. Ensure that you take in enough calcium to replace that lost in your breastmilk. Eating plenty of iron-rich foods is important.

Things to avoid A proportion of all the things you eat, drink or smoke finds its way into your bloodstream from there to your milk, to be absorbed by your baby. Because of this, there are certain things that are best avoided while you are breastfeeding. You should cut down on or eliminate alcoholic drinks, cigarette smoking and coffee (including decaffeinated varieties), and try to do without drugs. If you are taking medication for a chronic condition, check that this will not affect your milk.

In addition, your baby may react to certain foods that you eat, and show symptoms such as 'wind', diarrhoea, colicky pains which make him draw his knees up towards his chest, vomiting and inconsolable crying. It can be very difficult to pinpoint the food causing the problem, but you can try by eliminating one or two suspicious items from your diet for a while and then, later, introducing them one at a time to see how your baby reacts.

Expressing milk

You may need to express milk from your breasts occasionally, especially if you need to be separated from your baby for a time or plan to return to work (*see* Working mothers, p. 346). There are several ways to do this.

Expressing milk by hand Before you begin, wash your hands well. Lean forward so that gravity can enhance the let-down reflex.

Support your left breast with your right hand, with the heel of your palm against your ribs. Make 'scissors' of the first and second fingers of your left hand, and place them about 4 cm (1½ in) behind the nipple. Squeeze together and release your fingers a few times to compress the ampullae behind the areola (felt as little lumps) and to stimulate the flow of milk. Avoid using strong pressure or pinching. Rotate your hand so that you can squeeze and release another area of the breast, until you have pumped the

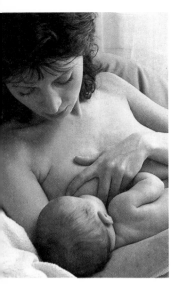

To make sure that your breast is not blocking your baby's nasal passages, press down the part of the breast that is above his nose with a finger of your free hand to let him breathe easily.

Food allergens

It is impossible to give a comprehensive list of all the foods that may cause upsets in some babies, but the following are the most common:
- Cows' milk and cows' milk products: milk, butter, cheese, chocolate
- Spices: curry, chillies, pepper
- Brassicas: cabbage, broccoli, cauliflower, Brussels sprouts
- Onions and garlic
- Fruit and fruit juices: prunes, grapes (including raisins and wine), citrus fruits (oranges, lemons, grapefruit)
- Wheat products: bread, biscuits, pastries

entire breast. Then pump the other breast. Change breasts every few minutes to allow the milk to collect in the ampullae of the resting breast.

Once you become accustomed to expressing your milk, you can pump the unsupported breast using thumb and middle finger while, with your other hand, you hold a sterile container to collect the milk. You must treat expressed milk in the same way as formula, sterilizing the equipment you use and storing it carefully (see p. 207).

In the beginning, you will probably only succeed in expressing very little milk, but with practice, it is possible to express as much as 250 ml (about 8 fl. oz) each time.

Hand pumps There are many types of hand pump, available from most good chemists, but the most popular variety is the cylindrical 'piston' type. With some, the milk is pumped directly into an attached feeding bottle.

Electric pumps The advantage of electric pumps is that the process of emptying the breasts becomes virtually effortless. They can be useful for a variety of reasons – for example, difficulty in feeding or a health problem – and some working mothers keep one at work to express milk at the times when the baby would normally have fed, in this way collecting enough milk for the next day. Electric pumps are expensive, but can be hired from the National Childbirth Trust and the La Lèche League (see p. 347).

Weaning from the breast

Although it is preferable not to do so during the first year, sometimes there are reasons for weaning a baby off the breast and on to a bottle. This should be done gradually so that both you and your baby can adapt successfully. It may be a good idea to start with expressed breastmilk and then change to formula once the baby is used to the bottle.

Start weaning your baby by dropping a feed in the evening when your milk supply is low, substituting a bottle of formula. After a few days, eliminate another feed, adding another bottle, and continue in this way until your baby is having approximately five bottle-feeds and only one breastfeed. If your breasts feel uncomfortably full or your baby becomes unhappy at any time during this process, wait a few days before dropping another breastfeed. Keep offering the breast once a day until you sense that your baby is ready to give up.

While you are weaning your baby, your hormonal system will be adjusting to the diminishing breast stimulation, and if this is done gradually, painful engorgement can be prevented. If your breasts do become full, having your baby suck for a minute or two on each side will relieve any discomfort while not really stimulating milk production. Other suggestions for coping while suppressing lactation can be found on page 206. If any lumps or signs of infection or mastitis appear (see Breast problems after childbirth, pp. 294-5), urgent treatment is necessary.

Weaning a baby may not be easy, and even if you are firm in your decision to do so, you and your child may be a little depressed for a while.

Many children, if their mothers are willing, will continue to breastfeed for anything between one and four years, eventually weaning themselves away. This is quite natural, and a child fulfilled and breastfed in this way is likely to be very healthy, independent, confident and secure, with a strong emotional and psychological foundation for the future.

**If you don't want to
breastfeed:**

**If you don't want to
breastfeed:**
- Wear a good bra
providing firm support.
- If the milk comes in
and your breasts become
engorged, you may need
to increase support by
wrapping a towel firmly
around your trunk and
breasts and tying it in
place. This will prevent
the accumulation of
milk, and is usually only
necessary for about 24
hours.
- Engorgement can also
be relieved by placing
chilled cabbage leaves in
your bra against your
breasts (*see* p. 203). You
should only need to do
this for 24–48 hours.
- If engorgement is
severe, a prolactin
inhibitor – *Bromocryptine*
– can be given in tablet
form. This has to be
taken for 14 days;
otherwise rebound
lactation may occur.
Bromocryptine is a
powerful drug which may
have side-effects.

Bottle-feeding

Before your baby is born, you may have strong ideas about how you are
going to feed him. Whether you intend to breastfeed or bottle-feed from
the start, it is always a good idea to keep an open mind, inform yourself
about all the alternatives and, when the time comes, discover which
method of feeding is best for the two of you.

Even if bottle-feeding is most suited to your circumstances, it is advisable
to try to breastfeed for the first few days so that your baby can benefit –
immediately and in the future – from the nutrients and antibodies
contained in the colostrum you will produce (*see* p. 193). You may surprise
yourself and enjoy the experience more than you thought you would, or
you may become confident in your decision to bottle-feed and feel ready to
introduce the bottle to your baby.

Once you have decided to bottle-feed your baby, you should inform your
midwife following the birth. Without stimulation, the production of
breastmilk will eventually cease, and so it is usually possible to stop
lactating without drugs, although this may involve a few days of
discomfort.

Choosing a formula

Bottle-feeding usually means giving a baby modified cows' milk, although
special soya products are occasionally prescribed if a baby is allergic to this;
in fact, soya milk formula is the first choice of many women. It is not
advisable to give fresh cows' milk to a baby under the age of six to nine
months. Goats' milk is very salty and should not be given to newborn
babies. Both unmodified evaporated milk and sweetened condensed milk
are also unsuitable.

If you began to bottle-feed in hospital, you probably fed your child small
prepared bottles of formula which are not available in shops. If this
particular brand seems to suit your baby, the formula powder can be bought
to be made up at home.

If you need advice, check with your health visitor or doctor. Study the
list of ingredients on packets if you have any special dietary requirements –
e.g. vegetarian or kosher diets. Not all brands suit all babies, and it is quite
common to try out a few before you find the one that your child thrives on.
When your baby is about 12 weeks old, you should give him supplements of
vitamins A, C and D to make up for the lack of these in formula.

Equipment and supplies

You will need equipment and supplies both to feed your baby and to ensure
that all teats and bottles are sterile.

Some types of teat have been designed to be as close as possible in shape
and texture to the feel of the breast. These are said to be better for the
development of the baby's jaw, as the muscular action needed in feeding is
similar to that of breastfeeding. In addition, the holes in teats are different
sizes. What you want is one that, when the bottle is inverted, allows a
steady stream of droplets to emerge. If the hole is too small, there will be
too few droplets, and the baby will have to struggle to feed; as a result, he
may become exhausted, or may take in large amounts of air with the milk.
If the hole is too large, the milk will flow too quickly and he might choke.
Bottles can be either glass or plastic. Glass ones are easy to see through

to check that they have been cleaned properly, but they are heavy and can break. For this reason, plastic ones are often preferable. Whichever type you buy, make sure that they come with caps that will allow the teats to be inverted and covered for storage.

As well as the more common bottles, you can now buy pre-sterilized plastic bags which have to be attached to a bottle-shaped holder. These do not need sterilizing, and they may reduce the amount of air sucked in, thus reducing wind (*see* pp. 212-13). They also have nipple-shaped teats.

Cleaning and sterilizing

Bottle-feeding requires strict hygiene to prevent the growth of bacteria in the milk. There are two methods of sterilizing bottles, teats and equipment: immersion in sterilizing solution or boiling.

Before sterilizing, bottles and teats must be scrupulously cleaned. Rinse bottles with cold water, then wash in hot soapy water, using a bottle brush to clean all the corners, and rinse clean. Teats and all equipment should be washed in hot soapy water and then rinsed.

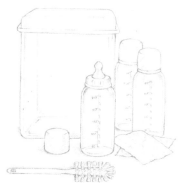

The basic equipment and supplies for bottle-feeding
- Formula powder
- 8 bottles (preferably plastic) *or*
- Supply of pre-sterilized bags and holders
- 10 teats
- Sterilizing tank
- Sterilizing solution or tablets
- Bottle brush
- Measuring jug
- Funnel

Immerse all feeding equipment in a tank of sodium hypochlorite (e.g. Milton) sterilizing solution, made by adding the required amount of sterilizing liquid or tablets to warm water. The equipment must remain in this for the length of time recommended by the manufacturer, usually at least one hour, and fresh solution will have to be made daily. It is best to rinse the equipment in previously boiled water after sterilization.

Rather than using sterilizing solution, you may prefer to boil your equipment instead. After washing and rinsing, place all items in a large pot, making sure that everything is immersed in the water (you might have to trap teats in an inverted strainer to keep them down). Boil for at least ten minutes. This is quicker than using sterilizing solution, and can be done in any kitchen. However, if you have other small children, you may want to avoid having this quantity of boiling water in your home.

Frequent sterilizing or boiling can change the shape and texture of a teat, and can also alter the size of the hole. The latter should be checked daily; you should always have replacements to hand.

Preparing the formula

Before beginning, always wash your hands and the surfaces on which you will be working, and dry them with a clean towel.

You should always strictly adhere to the manufacturer's instructions on the package of formula, mixing together precisely the stated amounts of formula powder and water. Use only the measuring scoop provided and, after breaking up any lumps, pour in the powder and use the back of a knife to level it off. *Never* overfill the scoop, compress the powder or put additional measures into the feed: this will make the formula too rich and can result in indigestion or overfeeding; more seriously, the high levels of sodium and phosphate can damage your baby's health.

You can make up each feed just before your baby needs it, or you can fill up the number of bottles that he will drink in one day (plus an extra one or two in case his appetite suddenly increases) and store them in the refrigerator until they are needed. Any left over at the end of the day should be thrown away, as should any amounts left in a bottle after a feed.

Some babies are quite happy to drink cold formula straight from the refrigerator, but you may want to heat it up first in a bottle warmer or in a

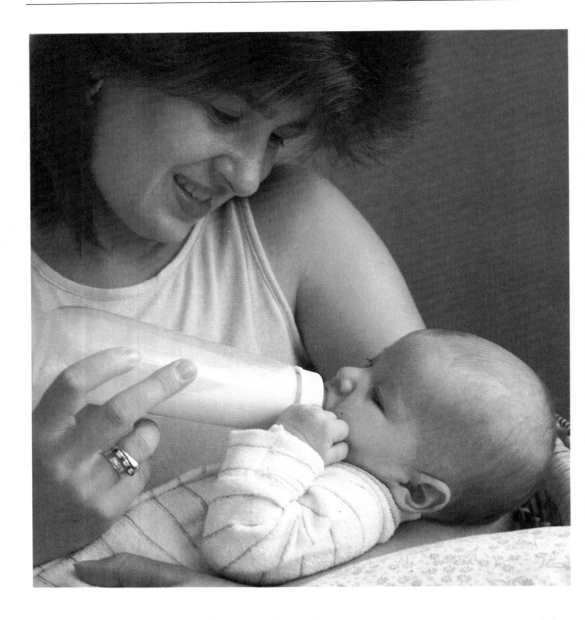

bowl of hot water. To check the temperature before giving it to your baby, shake a few drops of formula on to your wrist: it should feel neither hot nor cold. Warm formula should never be stored in a thermos – there is no more ideal environment for bacteria.

If you are travelling and proper facilities are unavailable, make up some formula beforehand and store it in bottles in a refrigerator until it is cold. Then place it in a cold-storage box to carry with you until your baby needs to be fed. It is not advisable to carry an unrefrigerated feed for more than six hours. You can, however, buy bottles of pre-sterilized formula from chemists, which will be perfectly safe for long periods.

When should I feed my baby?

On average, most bottle-fed babies will begin with five or six feeds spread throughout the day and night. Try to feed your baby when he wants it, rather than restricting the number of feeds.

One of the advantages of bottle-feeding is that, once the very early, irregular period is over, you should be able to predict feeding times, and bottle-fed babies tend to give up middle-of-the-night feeds sooner than breastfed ones. However, as with most things concerning newborn babies, there is no right or wrong schedule, each child being unique, so some flexibility on your part can be a great help.

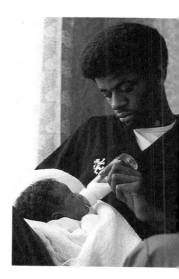

How much should I give?

Babies up to about five months old require approximately 120 calories a day for each kilogram they weigh (or 55 calories per lb). To receive these many calories, they will need about 200 g of made-up formula per kilogram per day (or 3 oz per lb).

The above is simply a guide; many babies will differ. You will find out how much your baby needs by trial and error: if he finished all the formula during a feed, he may need more next time; if some is left each time, less is probably required.

Enjoying feeding your baby

A great advantage of bottle-feeding is that partners can share not only the work involved in sterilizing equipment and preparing feeds, but also, and more importantly, the closeness and joy that should accompany feeds.

Feeding is more important than just food – it is a very basic way to show your love for your child. Sit down comfortably, cuddle the baby close and talk or sing as you offer the bottle. Touch his cheek with the teat or with your finger to make him aware of the bottle so that he turns towards it. Make this a gentle time when you can be close and enjoy the warmth of being together.

When the teat is taken into your baby's mouth, make sure that the bottle is tilted enough so that air is not swallowed. However, the teat needs to be released from the baby's mouth quite frequently to let air into the bottle; otherwise, sucking will be difficult. (This is not necessary if you are using the pre-sterilized plastic bags.)

Spend time stroking and caressing the baby. His changing expressions and seemingly unblinking eyes cannot fail to fascinate you. Do not always hold him in the same way: change positions so that he gets to see you from another angle and does not always have to lie on the same side.

Never leave your baby alone with a bottle propped up so that he can drink unaided. Not only is there a very real danger that he could choke and suffocate, but you will be depriving him of absolutely vital physical contact, caresses and a sense of security.

Combined feeding: breast and bottle

Many mothers who, through practical necessity, decide to bottle-feed do not realize that it is possible to breastfeed as well so that the baby can thrive on a combination of breastmilk and formula. As long as the baby sucks the breast regularly, even if it is only once a day – say, in the evening – milk will continue to be produced in a quantity that corresponds to the amount of sucking. This is particularly suited to many working mothers.

C H A P T E R   1 6

EVERYDAY CARE

Young babies have a few primary needs that are essential to their survival and happiness. As well as being kept warm, dry and clean, a baby needs to feel loved and wanted, and the ways of showing this are infinite. Close physical contact is vital; a baby needs to be held, hugged, caressed and carried in order to thrive, and he will continue to require such contact and the expression of affection throughout childhood and later life. Repeated and immediate satisfaction of hunger is the way a baby learns to trust. Food is needed not only for nutrition, but also for the nurturing, affection and stimulation the baby receives while being fed. Finally, a baby must have plenty of opportunities to enjoy the world around him and, as he develops, to be stimulated and encouraged to explore and learn.

If these needs are satisfactorily fulfilled in infancy, a baby will grow up healthy, both physically and emotionally.

Crying and colic

Young babies express their emotions directly and immediately, and crying is the main way in which they communicate their needs to those who are caring for them. Babies' emotions are not hidden like those of adults: if a baby is in either physical or emotional discomfort, this becomes immediately apparent as he begins to cry.

A baby's cry has been designed to be powerful and penetrating so that it is difficult to ignore. This is important to every baby's survival. A crying infant should not be left to 'cry it out', because not only is there the possibility that something vital is being overlooked, but you may also find that the original cry for food or warmth turns into a cry of frustration that becomes progressively more difficult to soothe.

Why babies cry

While every baby is a unique individual, all babies have a common 'language' when it comes to crying. There are many reasons why babies cry, and you will soon become skilled at interpreting your child's signals.

Hunger This is the most common reason, and this cry is the one most likely to compel a mother to respond immediately. In general, it is a good idea first to see whether your baby wants to be fed before looking for any other cause.

Need for security Your baby may want to be picked up and held. Do not forget that, until very recently, he was securely contained inside your womb where all his needs were automatically met, and where he was carried and gently rocked as you moved and was constantly comforted by your body. From time to time, he will want to return to a womb-like feeling of security.

A feeling of security is almost as vital as feeding, and if this need is satisfied as much as possible in infancy, your baby will probably be very contented. This is clearly evident in infants who spend much time carried on their mothers' bodies as they go about their daily activities. Babies who have had a difficult birth, were separated from their mothers or are unwell may be particularly sensitive and need to be held a great deal.

Indigestion and colic Occasionally very young babies find the powerful sensations involved in the digestive process disturbing. Some may cry prior to emptying their bowels, and need to be reassured, held and comforted. 'Wind', too, can cause discomfort and make a baby cry (see pp. 212-13).

Colic occurs when the bowel wall goes into spasm and the sustained muscular contraction causes pain in the baby's abdomen. True colic – in which the pain is so severe that the baby usually draws up his legs and the abdomen feels tense and hard – is rare, but crying for other reasons is often mistakenly attributed to it. If it does arise, it is usually related to feeding. A breastfed baby may be only getting the foremilk due to the mother's poor let-down reflex (see p. 194), or something in her diet may be passing into the breastmilk and upsetting the baby's system. A bottle-fed baby may be on a formula that does not suit him.

Discomfort A baby who is too hot or too cold may cry to let you know. A soiled or wet nappy or nappy rash may be another reason.

Illness If your baby is ill, he may communicate pain or discomfort by crying, although babies tend to be quiet when extremely unwell. If your child cries in a sharp or otherwise unusual way, contact your family doctor.

Venting emotion Like adults, babies need to vent their emotions, and this generally takes the form of crying. Some babies take several months to 'settle' and may cry more than others. Many need plenty of physical exercise and may cry to release pent-up energy; these babies respond very well to massage and physical games.

Infants usually cry and fret most in the evening – say, between five and ten p.m., when their parents' energy may be at its lowest – and some simply want to feed almost continuously then. This restless period will probably disappear after a few weeks, and almost certainly by about 12 weeks.

It will help if you can arrange to rest in the afternoon, and make sure that you have a nourishing lunch and a snack at tea time. If you can, do most of the preparations for the evening meal in the morning. Try bathing or massaging your baby before the fretful time, or go out for a walk.

Mother's mood Mothers and babies are closely linked, and sometimes your mood can be contagious. If you are unhappy, worried, tense or irritable, your baby may come to feel the same way and express it by crying, and a vicious circle can be created. If this happens to you, make a conscious effort to breathe deeply and keep calm. If possible, give the baby to someone else and take a break for a while. Contact with other mothers can be invaluable.

Coping with crying
First of all, make sure that your baby is not hungry, in need of a cuddle or winding, too hot or cold, wet and/or soiled or unwell. If you have a baby who just seems to cry a great deal, there are quite a few things you can try.

  Put him in a baby sling (see p. 218) and walk around with him.

  Try taking a bath together (see p. 219).

  Some mothers find that, if they wrap both themselves and their babies in a large shawl and sit in a rocking chair, their babies settle quite quickly.

  Try singing to your baby or playing some calming music.

  Some babies, when they are overtired, do not want to be held at all. Try placing your baby on the floor or in a carry cot, cover him with a blanket and gently pat or rub his back.

  Introduce him to massage (see pp. 282-9) at a time when he is not crying and is likely to enjoy it.

  One time-honoured solution is to take him for a ride in a car.

  Perhaps your partner can give you a break by taking the baby.

  A consultation with a qualified homoeopath who specializes in this problem may be useful.

  Cranial osteopathy is a new technique which, some say, does wonders to calm fretful babies.

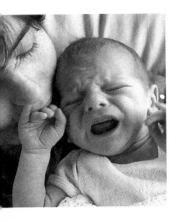

When crying becomes a crisis

The incessant crying of a small infant can make the most well-meaning and loving parent feel desperate. There are bound to be times when your baby continues to cry inconsolably even after you have tried everything. If you are tired and run down, a bout of incessant crying can make you feel desperate, frustrated and inadequate, all of which may well turn into anger at the baby. These are feelings that all parents discover when they are at their weakest, but it can come as a shock when baby battering suddenly seems frighteningly possible.

The best thing to do in this situation is to hand over the baby to someone else and take a break. If you are on your own and there is no one you can call on to help, put the baby in a separate room for a little while (making sure that he is safe), and try to calm yourself, focusing on your breathing, putting on some soothing music and reminding yourself that this can happen to anyone; alternatively, try going out for a walk or a car ride with your baby. If this happens frequently, get some help before you reach breaking point. Talk to your health visitor or doctor, or telephone a support group such as your local branch of the La Lèche League or National Childbirth Trust (*see* p. 347).

Generally, babies have a good reason for crying, and if this happens frequently, it is important to seek help in order to discover the underlying causes. However, every baby is bound to have the odd difficult day and be inexplicably out of sorts at times. If you can weather the storm, it will pass.

Winding your baby

Sometimes babies swallow air along with breastmilk or formula, and the resulting bubbles in the digestive tract may cause discomfort so that they cry or become fretful or fussy. This tends to happen more with bottle-fed babies, especially if the hole in the teat is too small or if the bottle is not held at the correct angle and air is drunk in with the milk; the baby may then require winding midway through a feed.

However, air swallowing can also happen when a baby is being breastfed: if your breasts are very full and the milk comes streaming out very rapidly at first, the baby may have to gulp in order to swallow fast enough and can easily take in some air at the same time. You can help to slow down the flow by placing a finger on either side of the areola and pressing upward, away from the baby's mouth, until the flow slows down.

Babies who cry for a long time before feeding or become very disturbed are likely to be difficult to calm as the feed begins and may swallow air as a result. Sometimes this can be avoided if you anticipate feeding times and start the feed before your child begins to cry.

To relieve any discomfort, simply hold the baby upright so that the air bubbles will rise up the digestive tract and be expelled. Try holding him against your chest with his head over your shoulder and pat his back gently. Alternatively, place him face down across your knees and rub his back. Sitting him upright on your lap while supporting his chest and head can also be helpful. Sometimes the baby will bring up a little milk at the same time and so may be hungry again. If he has not brought up any air after three minutes, do not worry about it. Carrying your baby close to your body or in a sling after feeding is an ideal way to expel any air bubbles.

The need to wind all babies by thumping them vigorously on the back after every feed is undoubtedly exaggerated. In fact, many of the things often ascribed to 'wind' are actually due to inadequate feeding. The necessity for winding can be avoided if a baby lies with his head a little higher than his body when feeding. Many babies need no winding at all.

Posseting and vomiting

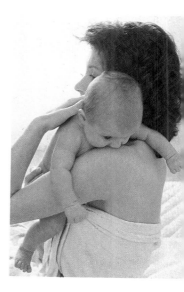

All babies bring up a little milk from time to time, and some do so more than others. The milk is usually mixed with saliva and is quite a small quantity, although it may look like a lot. This is called 'posseting', and is the baby's way of expelling any overflow.

Because an almost inevitable part of parenting a small baby is the endless milk stains on your shoulders or sleeves, it is a good idea to wear clothes that are easily washable and do not need ironing. Keep a cloth handy to wipe up dribbles of milk as they occur.

While every baby brings up some milk, frequent vomiting accompanied by a fever or diarrhoea could mean that your child has developed an infection (see Diarrhoea and gastro-enteritis, p. 308). Contact your doctor as soon as possible, and in the meantime, make sure that your baby drinks as much milk or formula as possible to replace lost fluid.

Very occasionally, babies vomit out the entire contents of their stomachs, the partially digested food often shooting out with great force and landing a good two or three metres away. This is called 'projectile vomiting', and if it occurs frequently the baby will lose a lot of nourishment. If it does happen often, you should see your doctor, who will check that the outlet to your baby's stomach is not narrowed – a condition called *pyloric stenosis* (see Vomiting in the baby, p. 345).

As long as the baby is obviously gaining weight and urinating frequently and your doctor has assured you that he is well, there is no need to be concerned about the occasional bout of vomiting. Try feeding him more frequently and, if possible, make sure that he is calm before each feed.

Warmth

Babies are happiest and most comfortable when they are warm, and from birth onward, they use their muscles to release energy in the form of heat. However, because of the relatively large surface area of their skin, they are unable to conserve their body heat efficiently. In particular, a great deal is lost through the scalp, so cover a baby's head outdoors in cold weather.

At a normal room temperature of about 20°C (68°F), a baby will be warm enough if dressed in, say, a vest, nappy and stretch suit. When he is naked – if you are, for example, undressing, massaging or bathing him – the room should be heated to about 29° (85°F). The ideal way to keep your newborn baby warm is through such direct contact with your body. Going out of doors for walks in lower temperatures will not harm your baby, provided he is well wrapped up with head, feet and hands covered. However, young babies should not be left outdoors in cool weather.

By the time babies are about three months old and weigh 5–6 kg (11–13 lb), their ability to conserve body heat will have improved.

How can I tell if my baby is cold?

This can be done very simply by feeling your child's abdomen: if it feels cool, your baby is cold. He will also probably let you know that he is uncomfortable by becoming restless, breathing faster than usual (to create more heat) and perhaps crying.

It is dangerous to allow babies to become really chilled. When this happens, the chest and abdomen will feel cold, and the baby will become pale and will not waste energy by crying. In the unlikely event of this happening, hold your baby right up against your body under a warm blanket or shawl until he warms up; and seek medical assistance (*see* Hypothermia in the baby, p. 316).

How can I tell if my baby is too hot?

Babies are fine even in temperatures over 32°C (90°F), as long as they are dressed only in very light, pure cotton or left naked. When it is very hot, keep your child out of nappies if possible, and try not to use plastic pants as these will encourage the development of nappy rash. Overdressing babies in hot weather will increase their body temperature, make them uncomfortable and possibly cause a heat rash (*see* Skin problems in the baby, p. 335). A baby's skin is very sensitive, and so exposure to direct heat or sunlight should be gradual.

A baby who is too hot looks flushed and may be irritable and cry. Babies radiate heat as adults do, but sweating only develops later. You can help cool a hot baby by fanning him, and it may also be useful to immerse him in a bath of lukewarm water or to sponge his body with warm water to reduce body temperature. These methods can be used to lower a fever (*see* Fever in the baby p. 310), but always consult your doctor before doing so.

Nappies

Your child will begin to develop awareness and control over the processes of elimination some time in his second or third year. Until then, these functions occur involuntarily, and your baby will need to wear nappies.

You can choose between fabric nappies (which need to be sterilized and laundered) and various types of disposable nappies. Your choice will depend on your lifestyle, laundry facilities and personal preferences.

Fabric nappies

Some mothers feel that terry-towelling nappies are the most comfortable for a baby to wear, in addition to being very absorbent. You will need at least 24 – which have to be folded in order to fit your baby properly – as well as plastic pants and special nappy pins with self-locking heads.

You might consider using the following:

Muslin squares are made of soft natural fibres and are useful as first nappies for tiny babies as they can be folded very small; they are not, however, very absorbent. They also make handy cloths.

Shaped terry nappies come ready shaped with a thicker absorbent layer in the middle; the rest of the nappy is made of a thinner type of towelling which may make it more comfortable for the baby to wear. These are more expensive and take longer to dry than folded squares.

One-way nappy liners are small oblongs of disposable material which can be used inside nappies, both terry and disposable. They are made of a special fabric which draws moisture away from the baby's body but not back the other way. The urine is thus absorbed into the nappy while the baby's skin is kept relatively dry; this can be helpful in preventing nappy rash, particularly at night if your baby sleeps for long periods.

Nappy liners are made of paper and are used inside fabric nappies. They catch most of the baby's faeces which can then be easily discarded.

Disposable nappies

There is a wide variety of plastic-backed, all-in-one disposable nappies to choose from, and these are generally the most practical. They come in different sizes to suit babies of all ages from birth onwards, and can usually be bought cheaply in bulk from discount stores. An alternative type consists of plastic pants with a pocket for a disposable pad. Disposables are more convenient than fabric nappies, and particularly helpful when you travel with your baby.

Changing your baby's nappy

You should always try to have everything you will need to change your baby close at hand before beginning. Nappies should be changed whenever you feel your baby is wet. If wet or soiled nappies are left on for long periods, the resulting ammonia will cause irritation and nappy rash (*see* p. 324).

When your baby feeds, the digestive tract is stimulated and inevitably he will wet or soil a nappy. For this reason, many breastfeeding mothers choose to change their babies' nappies midway during a feed, before changing breasts. This also helps to ensure that a sleepy baby is awake enough to empty both breasts before finally falling asleep.

Your baby can be changed on any clean, soft surface. It is best to do this while you kneel or sit on the floor, where there is no chance of your child rolling off and hurting himself. However, in the first week or two after the birth, when your ligaments are still soft, it is a good idea to do changing on a table, to protect your back.

The room should be warm (*see* pp. 213-4), and your baby will like having a colourful mobile to look at. It may take some time before he enjoys having his body exposed, but after a few weeks he is bound to look forward to this time of playful contact. If he is fretful at first, it is best to get it over with as quickly as possible, but if not, take your time to play with your baby and encourage him to enjoy the freedom of being without a nappy. This will allow the skin to dry properly and will help to prevent or heal nappy rash.

It is best to avoid the use of baby lotions, powders, creams and pre-packaged baby wipes. In particular, strong antiseptics and perfumed cleansing agents may disturb the baby's natural oil balance, and will make his skin more prone to irritation and rashes. You can make your own baby wipes by putting damp cotton wool pads into a plastic bag.

To clean your baby, remove the dirty nappy, cleaning away faeces with any unsoiled portion of the nappy. Use warm water and a few clean pieces of cotton wool to remove urine and any traces of faeces from the genitals, taking care to wash the creases thoroughly. With baby girls, it is not necessary to fold back the labia to clean inside, nor, with boys, to pull back or clean underneath the foreskin. Like the inside of the ears and nose, the labia and foreskin are self-cleaning in infants. Push back your baby's legs by pressing gently on his feet and clean his bottom, using a

Equipment for changing nappies

- A good supply of nappies
- Plastic pants and nappy pins (if using fabric nappies)
- Plenty of cotton wool and tissues
- Mild pure vegetable oil (optional)
- A small bowl containing warm water
- A clean, soft towel
- A change of clothing

Your child's first wardrobe

- 4–6 vests: the wide-necked envelope type are best as babies hate having tight things pulled over their heads.
- 4–6 all-in-one stretch suits (e.g. Babygro's): buy ones with poppers on the front (and along the legs) as you then will not need to turn over the baby to remove them.
- 2 shawls: pure cotton or woollen ones are lovely but flannelette squares are perfectly adequate.
- 2–4 cardigans or jackets.
- 4 pairs of socks/bootees: cotton in summer, wool in winter.
- 1 hat: the type will depend on the season.
- 2 pairs of mittens: to wear outdoors in winter. It will be more useful to have additional vests and stretch suits than elaborate clothes or nightdresses.

new piece of damp cotton wool whenever necessary. If you need a cleansing agent, use a natural oil on a piece of cotton wool. With girls, always wipe from front to back so that bacteria from the anus do not reach the urinary tract and the vagina. Dry the whole area thoroughly, especially in the creases.

The quick-dip method This is a very easy way to clean your baby. Fill the hand basin in your bathroom with some warm water. Expose the lower half of your baby's body – there is no need to undress him completely – and remove the nappy. Make sure you have a clean, dry towel close at hand.

Holding your baby, gently lower his feet, legs and buttocks into the water. With one hand supporting him under the arms and around the chest, use the free one to rinse and clean the genital area. Then gently lift up the baby and wrap him in the towel, ready for drying and a cuddle.

When you are away from home As well as the items listed above, you will need plastic bags for soiled nappies. You could also buy one of the very convenient portable changing mats which convert to a light bag; one of these will hold everything you need to change your baby.

Dressing your baby

You do not need many clothes for a newborn baby, but what you do have should be practical and easy to put on and launder. Pure cotton is best for items that will go next to your baby's skin, as is pure wool for jackets, cardigans and shawls.

The first wardrobe

It is generally not worth buying clothes in the newborn size as most babies outgrow them within a few weeks. Instead, start with clothes for a three-month-old – you will probably find that your baby can wear them from the start. Very young babies generally do not like being undressed, so buy simple clothes that open easily and are stretchy.

Undressing and dressing

When undressing your baby, make sure that the room is warm (*see* p. 213). If you smile, talk or sing it will help to make the process more enjoyable.

You can dress and undress your baby either when he is lying on his back on a flat surface or when he is sitting on your lap. Always have everything you need close at hand, and handle your baby firmly and gently. When passing clothing over his head, stretch the necks wide with your fingers. When putting on sleeves, place your hand through the opening in reverse and take hold of the baby's hand; then slip the sleeve over his hand and arm. When undressing him, pull the clothes rather than the baby!

Handling and carrying your baby

Human babies take longer than any other mammals to become physically independent of their mothers. It is almost as if the period of gestation lasts for 18 months – nine months in the womb and another nine in the arms or close to the body of the mother, until the child begins to crawl away towards independence.

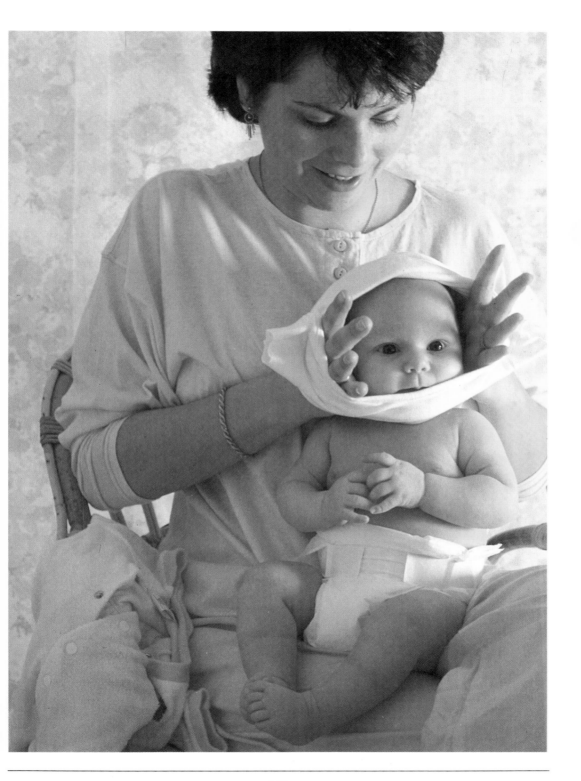

Buying a sling

When deciding which sling to buy, the following considerations are important:

- The sling should be soft and comfortable to wear, and made of an easily washable fabric.
- It should comfortably envelop the baby's curled body, supporting his head and neck adequately.
- The fastening method should be simple and secure, and ideally you should be able to put on the sling without assistance.
- You should be able to use the sling either in front or on your back.

It will also take a few weeks for your baby to gain proper control of his head, and you may be afraid to lift or handle him at first. However, provided you support him properly, there is no reason to be afraid. Babies are hardy and resilient creatures, and will soon let you know if they are uncomfortable. If possible handle your baby from the moment of birth.

The need for physical contact and body warmth is of prime importance in infancy and throughout childhood. Experience with premature babies in a special baby care unit in Bogotá, Colombia has shown that even the tiniest babies thrive better when held continually against the warmth and heartbeat of their mothers. Such holding and carrying is often of great especially important for premature babies, those who have had difficult births and those who have been born by Caesarean section.

Baby slings

In traditional societies throughout the world, babies are carried against their mothers' bodies while the women work. This continual and close body contact provides the babies with warmth and security, as well as stimulation from the sounds, smells and sights of all that is happening around them.

From the safety of their mother's breast or back, these children are part of their community from early infancy, as well as benefiting from the familiar sound of their mother's heartbeat and the sensations of her movements and of being carried, just as they were in the womb. They can easily communicate with their mother, who can breastfeed them whenever they are hungry or attend to any other needs at a moment's notice.

The importance of carrying babies has been underestimated in most industralized societies, where infants have been habitually placed for long periods in cots and prams and somehow distanced from their parents.

It is possible to carry a baby in a sling from birth, provided that there is adequate head and neck support. Babies tend to fall into a deep sleep when carried in this way, and it is an invaluable method of calming a fretful child. If you have problems with your spine or if you develop backache or shoulder or neck pain, you should not use a sling for prolonged periods.

Travelling with your baby

We live in a world where ease of mobility is almost a prerequisite and, luckily, small babies travel well. Although moving around with your baby – to the shops, to visit friends and relatives, to go on holiday or to move to another city or country – may seem daunting, the following tips make it easier and safer.

- Use a baby sling to carry your child (see above).
- Always be aware of safety aspects when buying a carry cot with transporter, pram or pushchair. Ensure that the brakes operate perfectly, that wheels are of good quality with plenty of tread, that fingers will not get caught in hinges, that pushchair straps are not worn or damaged.
- When travelling by car, always have your child safely strapped into a specially designed seat suitable for his age. You can now buy safety seats for infants which face backwards and fit on to passenger seats; they are held in place by car seat belts (the seats

themselves have straps to hold the baby in place). Carry cot restraints have now been proved to be unsafe: while the cot remains secured, in an accident the baby may be flung out.

- Always ventilate a car in hot weather and heat it in cold. *Never* leave a baby alone in a car.
- Drive carefully to minimize the risk of injury if you should have to stop suddenly.
- If you travel by air, feed the baby during take off and landing to avoid pressure changes in the baby's ears. Do not travel by air if the baby has a severe cold; the alterations in air pressure will be painful and could damage his ears.
- In areas of the world where you may be doubtful about hygiene, it is preferable to breastfeed to avoid infection. If you must bottle-feed, use bottled or doubled-boiled water to make up the feed, and be extra careful when sterilizing equipment.

Keeping your baby clean

Except for wet and/or soiled nappies, small babies do not get very dirty. As long as the genital area, hands, face, neck and skin creases are cleaned daily, they do not need a bath very frequently. You may find that your baby begins to enjoy being bathed only after the first few weeks, but if bathtime is enjoyable for both of you from the start, there is no reason why your baby should not be bathed every day.

Bathing

It is important to remember that bathing a baby is primarily for pleasure, cleanliness being only of secondary importance. Spending some time each day immersed in warm water is relaxing and refreshing, and a pleasant way to communicate with your child. Your partner may also enjoy this special time of the day. It is a good idea to bath your baby just before you expect him to be restless; this will relax him and he will probably sleep well after all the activity.

Bathing with your baby From the time of the birth onwards, many parents enjoy bathing with their babies. One partner can be in the bath with the baby while the other waits with a large, soft towel to take him when the bath is finished, but it is also quite easy to do this if you are on your own.

Ensure that the bathroom is warm enough, and that a non-skid rubber mat covers the bottom of the bath so that you will not slip. Before undressing yourself or the baby, run the water so that the bath is quite full and pleasantly warm (approximately 29°C, 84°F) – test the temperature with your elbow.

In the bathroom, undress yourself and then your baby. Place two large towels on the floor beside the bath. Slowly step into it, lower yourself into the water and then take the baby from your partner. Gently lower the baby into the water, holding him securely in your arms and talking reassuringly as you do so. Gradually allow his body to be fully immersed, while carefully supporting his neck and shoulders. As he becomes more confident, allow him to float freely, his head gently supported by your hand. If your partner or another helper is present, he or she can assist you. It will not harm your baby to nurse at the breast while in the water.

The best way to take the baby out of the bath is with your partner's help. Place the baby on a towel on your partner's lap; he or she can then wrap, cuddle and dry him while you dry and dress yourself.

If you are on your own, you should hold your baby securely while you step into the bath and gradually lower yourself into the water. When you have finished, kneel in the bath, holding your child securely against your body. Take one of the towels on the floor and wrap it around him, and place him on the floor beside the bath. Now drape a towel around yourself and get out of the bath. Dry the baby gently and thoroughly before drying yourself; then dress him.

Using a baby bath Baby baths do have a number of disadvantages:
- they may tip over and injure you or your baby.
- they may be heavy to lift when full, and you could strain your back.
- they are too small for the baby to experience swimming motions.

If you want to use a baby bath, make sure that the stand is 100 per cent

General hygiene

Skin To protect the natural oil and acidity balance of the skin, use soap infrequently and avoid special baby bath liquids. Clean, warm water is sufficient to clean your baby. If his skin is dry, you can add a drop or two of pure almond oil to the bath water, or massage it into the skin.

Scalp Use baby shampoo occasionally.

Eyes In the first week or two, clean the eyes with cotton wool moistened in water. Use a separate piece for each eye, wiping from the inside outwards.

Ears and nose Never attempt to clean inside any of the openings in your baby's body: they will clean themselves automatically. All you need to do is to clean gently around the outside of the nose and the openings to the ear canals with a damp face cloth or cotton wool.

Nails You should trim your baby's nails quite frequently as, otherwise, the baby may scratch his face. The best time to do this is when he is asleep. Use special blunt-edged scissors, available from chemists.

Navel *See* page 180 for instructions on the care of the cord stump.

Genitals *Girls:* do not try to clean inside the vulva; just wash the outside of the labia. *Boys:* do not attempt to pull back the foreskin to clean under it; this area is self-cleaning, and if you try to retract the foreskin by force you may cause damage.

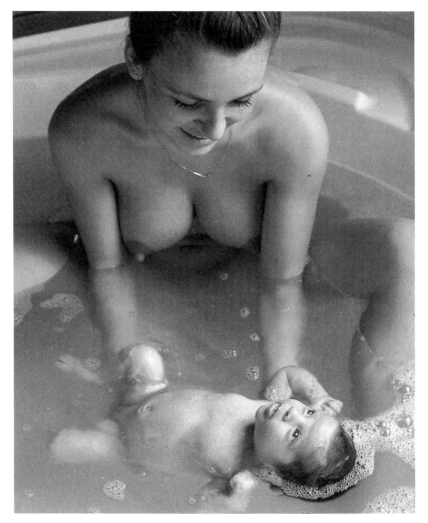

safe, or use a baby bath that fits securely over the bath. Use enough water so that it is deep enough for the baby to float, and test the temperature with your elbow beforehand.

Fear of bathing Some small infants dislike being bathed, and will yell loudly in protest no matter which way you try to do it. If this is the case, it is not necessary to bath your baby at all; cleaning the vital areas outlined above is all that is necessary. You can try giving him a bath again after a few weeks, when he may have forgotten the unpleasant experience.

Some babies fear the exposure of being naked rather than the bath itself. It can help to wrap the baby in a towelling nappy or small towel and then lower him, still wrapped, into the water, only removing the nappy or towel when he is accustomed to the feel of the water. Make sure that you have another, dry towel on your lap, ready to wrap around him as soon as he comes out of the bath.

Safety in the home

Although your baby will not be mobile for some months, it is best to make your home as safe as possible for him as soon as you can perhaps even before the baby is born. You can then look forward to his increasing development and exploration of the world without anxiety.

⚬ Never allow an infant to drink from a bottle which has been propped up, as this can cause choking.

⚬ Make sure that all carpeting on stairs is securely attached (and ban slippery rugs elsewhere) to avoid falls while you are carrying your child. Invest in a safety gate to go at the top of stairs.

⚬ Never leave your baby unattended in a bath or on any surface other than the floor.

⚬ Make sure that your infant is securely fastened into all baby seats, which should not be left on tables.

⚬ Always turn on the hot tap last when filling a bath, and turn it off first when the bath is full. Always check water temperature first (with your elbow or the inside of your wrist).

⚬ Use fireguards in front of an electric, gas and open fires; these should be securely attached to the wall.

⚬ Buy safety plugs to cover all unused electrical sockets; keep all electrical plugs and appliances out of the way of children.

⚬ Always put a cat net over the baby's carry cot, pram, etc: when outside; you may also need to do this indoors if you have a cat of your own.

⚬ Family pets may become jealous of what they consider to be a new rival. Keep them away from your baby while, at the same time, making a fuss of them. Then gradually introduce them to your child.

⚬ Keep all poisons and medicines out of the reach of children, locked in a special cabinet or box. Make sure that all alcoholic drinks, detergents and disinfectants are safely out of reach.

⚬ Keep all sharp kitchen utensils out of sight.

⚬ Never have a hot drink or smoke a cigarette while holding your baby.

⚬ Make sure that you do not leave such small objects as peanuts, marbles, raisins, seeds and dried peas within your child's reach. These may be inhaled and could obstruct his breathing.

⚬ Do not leave your baby on the kitchen floor where hot liquids could burn him if spilled.

⚬ Make sure that all toys your child is given are safe: make sure they will not come apart to be swallowed or to expose dangerous spikes, etc.

⚬ When you buy furniture or second-hand toys, make sure that all old paint is removed; this could contain lead which can cause brain damage if sucked.

Sleeping and waking

Newborn babies spend much of their time asleep – perhaps as much as 16–20 hours a day. They have similar sleep cycles to those of adults, which comprise patterns of REM (rapid eye movement) and NREM (non-rapid eye movement) sleep. REM sleep, which indicates dreaming, begins in the womb (see p. 60), and the sleep of a young infant may consist of 50 per cent REM sleep, compared to about 15 per cent in an elderly person. When babies appear to be dreaming, their bodies move reflexively or twitch, breathing can be irregular at times and facial expressions change. NREM sleep is more quiet and restful, with a slower heart rate and breathing and little movement of the body muscles or eyeballs.

When awake, some babies are quiet but alert, their brain patterns corresponding with those found in adults during deep meditation. These periods, usually lasting a few minutes, often occur during feeding, and the ability to learn is enhanced during them (see p. 185). Wakeful periods gradually increase until, at about three months, they usually have two fairly long periods during the day when they are wide awake, and attentive.

Coping with the erratic sleeping patterns of a baby can be one of the most difficult early adjustments to parenthood. This is particularly true if your baby has wakeful periods late at night or in the early hours of the morning. While this may be a wonderful learning time for your baby, who may seem to be getting quite enough sleep, you may become exhausted by the upheaval in your usual sleep pattern. Remember that, in the womb, your baby did not need to distinguish between day and night, and learning to associate darkness with sleep will take time. Until this happens, try to sleep whenever your baby does. You can encourage him to sleep at night by giving only essential, low-key attention in the evening, saving special stimulation and play for the day.

Falling asleep

A newborn baby can be placed either on his side or on his belly to sleep. If he brings up a little milk in either of these positions, it will run downwards and will not choke him, and if he sleeps on his belly, urine will drain downwards, lessening the likelihood of nappy rash.

If your baby sleeps on one side, you should place a rolled-up blanket behind his back to stop him rolling over. It is also advisable to alternate the side on which your baby lies, and to make sure that his ear is flat.

A baby will usually fall into a blissful sleep at the end of a satisfying feed, but if this does not happen, you can help him on his way by lulling him with motion. You can walk up and down rhythmically while holding or carrying him in a sling, or you can stand and sway or sit in a rocking chair. You could also try rocking him in a cradle or hammock. As a last resort, a short pram or car ride tends to put most babies to sleep.

Gentle music and – best of all – lullabies you sing to your baby can be a very pleasant part of the bedtime ritual. It does not matter if you invent the songs on the spur of the moment or sing the ones you learned as a child; your baby will love the soothing tones of your voice.

Waking in the night

After a few hours asleep, your baby may become hungry, cold, uncomfortable, or will simply not need any more sleep for the moment, and will wake spontaneously. He may also wake up for comfort.

Perhaps he will lie awake for a while before calling; a mobile or interesting patterns and textures to look at will provide quiet stimulation at this time. Very soon, however, he will make enough noise to attract your attention. It is best to pick him up as soon as you hear him, rather than wait for his cries to become urgent; if he is left to cry until he becomes overwrought, he will not feed or sleep well.

If you are lucky, your baby may soon sleep for periods of five or six hours at night, missing out a feed. However, most young babies wake up two or three times at roughly the same intervals as they are fed during the day, and it may be a year or more before your child sleeps through the night. His sleeping habits are bound to be somewhat erratic at first, but after a while he will develop a more or less reliable pattern, which may then be upset every few weeks when he undergoes a growth spurt and needs more milk.

You can minimize nappy changes by putting your baby in a double nappy with a one-way liner, or a nappy pad inside an all-in-one disposable nappy, before you go to bed. If the nappy is not soiled during the night, you will not need to change your baby before morning.

Where should my baby sleep?

When a baby wakes frequently at night for a feed, close proximity to his mother is important, and many parents therefore feel that the best place for their baby to sleep is in bed next to the mother, protected by the warmth of her body. In traditional cultures, it is customary for mothers to sleep in the same beds as their infants, but in Western society parents are often advised against this for fear they will crush the baby when they turn over in their sleep or because the baby might suffocate under the bedclothes. However, parents who do sleep with their young infant find that this never happens: even as they sleep they still retain an intuitive protective sense towards their child, and besides, the baby would soon let them know if he were uncomfortable.

Nevertheless babies can sleep anywhere, and some parents prefer having their infants sleep beside them in a carry cot or Moses basket. It is generally advisable to have your baby sleep in the same room as you until he is about six months old.

Your sleeping arrangements should suit your particular family. This is something to discuss with your partner before the birth, but you will probably not find out what is best for you until you experience your baby's sleeping pattern and individual needs.

The family bed If you wish to have your baby in bed with you from birth, this can have a number of advantages:

- If you are breastfeeding and your baby wakes up in the night, you only need to roll over to nurse him, without having to get up or even wake up properly. This will eliminate much of the fatigue caused by night feeds.
- If your partner is out working all day, these hours at night can form an important part of the relationship between father and child.
- Having the sweet and tender presence of a sleeping baby right beside you or between you and your partner is a delightful and rare privilege.

There may be another vital reason for having your baby in bed with you: it has been found that, in regions where babies traditionally sleep with their parents, the phenomenon of inexplicable cot death in infancy (see p. 306) is far less common. In addition, although not fully researched, it is now thought that sleeping with the mother may play an important part in the baby's development and future health.

A frequent concern is that the baby will roll off the edge of the bed, but this is unlikely as he will naturally snuggle up to your warmth. To avoid having to worry about this, some parents choose to sleep on a mattress on the floor during this time; others move the bed so that one side abuts the wall, and they then place the baby next to it.

For some couples, having their babies in bed with them creates anxiety, with one or both partners worrying that they will have no time to themselves and that it will be uncomfortable to make love in their baby's presence. There are a number of solutions. It is possible to make love in another room, and some couples put their baby to sleep on his own until the first night feed, and then bring him into the parents' bed for the rest of the night; in this way, the adults can have some time to themselves as well as having their baby sleep with them. Others make love when their baby is present but asleep.

You might be concerned that your baby will become so accustomed to the family bed that, later, he will not want to sleep alone. Actually, this is rarely the case. A child who benefits from the security of a family bed in early life eventually reaches a point – usually when he is about three years old – when he wants to sleep on his own, particularly if a new bed is introduced at the right moment and the child is free to start using it voluntarily. If a second baby is on the way, you can try to wean your child slowly into his own bed. Some family beds will include a toddler and a new

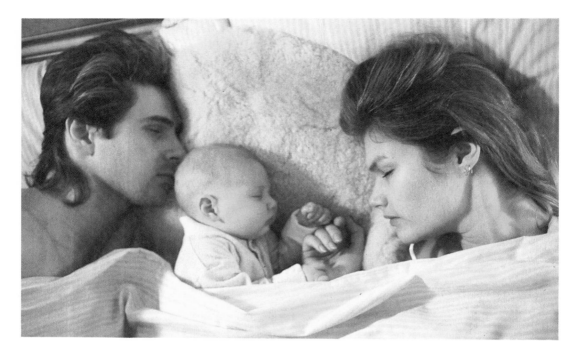

baby for a while, but this depends on your own personal preferences and the size of your bed!

Lined or quilted Moses baskets These light wicker baskets are easily portable, can be taken all over the house and placed (on a stand made for the purpose) right beside your bed at night. They are outgrown when babies are about four or five months old.

Carry cot These portable beds are very useful in the early months, and because they have hoods and windshields they can also be used outdoors. Most come with a transporter – a stand with wheels and a handle, which can be collapsed for storage – and so can be employed for outdoor walks or indoors to soothe a restless baby. If your baby is to sleep in a carry cot at night, make sure that the plastic inner surface is covered with a quilted or otherwise padded lining.

Cots These are too large for a young baby.

Baby fleece Specially treated sheepskins made for a baby to sleep on are now widely available, and will keep your baby cool in summer and warm in winter. They do not seem to absorb dirt easily and can be sponged; they are also machine washable, but do not require this very often. They can be placed in your bed, in a Moses basket or carry cot or on the floor. If your baby gets used to one of these, he will fall asleep in any corner quite happily.

C H A P T E R   1 7

EARLY PARENTHOOD

The first months of parenthood are usually very enjoyable, as the relationship between you and your baby unfolds and you settle into your new life together. This may also be a turbulent time, involving many physical and emotional changes. If this is your first baby, you will be learning to accept your new role as a parent and to accustom yourself to a relationship with the new person who is now central to your life.

Many people underestimate what is involved in caring for a new baby, and the challenge of parenthood can come as quite a shock. However, with planning and patience, caring for your baby is likely to prove a pleasurable and rewarding task. This chapter outlines some of the more common emotional aspects of life as new parents; you may find, too, that some of the topics discussed in Chapter 5 are also relevant now.

New motherhood

You will probably find that the many hours spent with your baby are delightful and deeply fulfilling. For many mothers, life with a new baby can be like falling in love, and everything may go smoothly and harmoniously from the start. However, the joys of new motherhood are usually balanced by the difficulties encountered during the first three months, and the psychological adjustment may be greater than you anticipate. With understanding and patience, problems can usually be overcome, and by the time your baby is about 12 weeks old, you will probably have settled into a comfortable way of life.

Coming to terms with the birth

Giving birth is a momentous experience, and in the days that follow, you will want to go over in your mind everything that has happened and perhaps discuss it with your partner, family, midwife or doctor. This re-experiencing is an important part of your recuperation, and many unexpected emotions may well up and need to be resolved. Some of these may be directly related to your experiences during the birth, and some may even stem from events earlier in your life.

The transition into motherhood involves letting go of the months of pregnancy as well as the events of the birth itself, and it is quite possible that your emotions may range from euphoria to depression, from a feeling of fulfilment to a sense of loss, from disappointment to profound gratitude. You may come to terms with all this very quickly or it may take time, but even if you need months, it is important eventually to accept all aspects of the experience, including the imperfections, and then put them behind you, so that you can feel at peace with yourself about the birth.

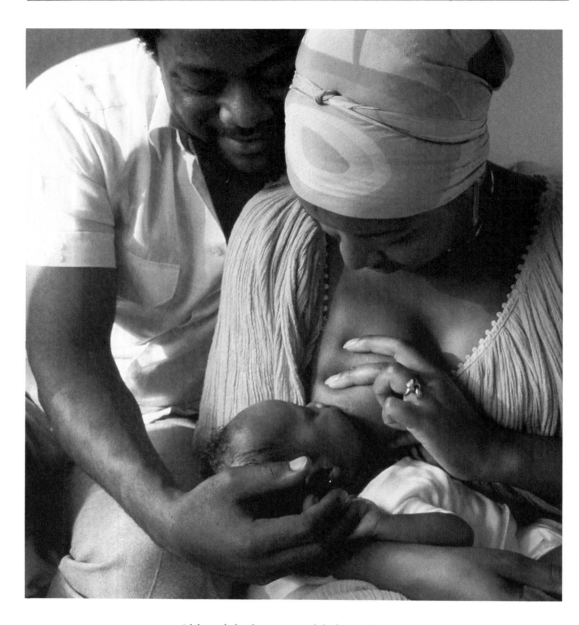

Although high spirits and feelings of satisfaction are common in the days and weeks after giving birth, it is also possible to experience disappointment, which may be related to the birth itself, if events such as an episiotomy, forceps delivery or Caesarean section leave you with feelings of invasion, anger or failure. Occasionally the disappointment can be focused on the baby, particularly if she is ill, premature or has an abnormality. In some families (particularly in certain cultures and societies), the sex of the baby is the prime consideration, and the parents may feel disappointed. These feelings usually soon disappear, but may continue and will then require counselling by experienced advisers (*see* page 347).

Your feelings about your body

Despite the radiant bloom of new motherhood which those around you may delight in and find very beautiful, it is not uncommon to feel uneasy about your body after childbirth. Your new maternal contours and still-flabby abdomen may make you think that pregnancy and childbirth have taken an irreversible toll on your body. If you have acquired stretch marks or a scar from a Caesarean, you are going to have to accept that they are unlikely to vanish completely, although once your body regains strength and a good muscle tone, they will fade.

In coming to terms with your body, it is helpful to accept that it is entirely natural and appropriate for you to be soft, cuddly and maternal at the moment. A positive attitude, setting aside time for rest and exercise, and care with clothes and appearance can transform the way you look and feel. However, lack of sleep and the new demands of motherhood may make this, for a while at least, easier said than done.

It is also natural to feel some anxiety about your attractiveness to your partner. Perhaps your altered form after the birth has come as a shock to him, or he may not have realized that it will take time before you are back to normal.

If you are breastfeeding, you may delight in nature's ingenuity and the way in which your breasts nourish your baby. However, it is also common to feel some ambivalence about the experience. At first, you may be shy about your body and find it difficult to breastfeed in front of others.

Your feelings about your body are also bound to be related to the sort of experience you had when you gave birth. If it was natural and spontaneous, you are likely to feel satisfied and fulfilled, and once any initial discomfort passes, you will probably be at peace with yourself quite soon. However, if the birth was difficult or medical intervention was needed, you may feel bruised or violated for a time, even if the procedures were carried out as gently as possible and were both necessary and helpful. In this case, gentle exercise and massage (see Part V) may prove beneficial.

Sleep and tiredness

The first major adjustment you are likely to face is learning how to cope with interrupted sleep at night, and you may find that you feel constantly tired or fatigued for the first few months. In traditional societies, the nursing mother has many people – usually her mother and other relatives – to attend to her needs and those of the rest of her family so that she can focus all her attention on her new baby. However, in most modern families, where the mother is alone much of the time, there is often a minimum of help available to deal with such basic necessities as shopping, cooking, washing and cleaning, and these routine tasks may seem insurmountable, especially if there are other children to care for.

Your social life

You may feel isolated after the birth of your child, especially if your partner goes out to work and you are alone at home most of the day, or if you are a single parent. You may become desperately lonely if you had an interesting job before the birth, or if you have moved to a new neighbourhood where you do not have friends or family. Being the primary carer of a baby can be quite a burden to shoulder without company or moral support.

A good solution is to get in touch with other mothers who live near you

Coping with tiredness

Tiredness will lessen in time, and your energy will return as your body acclimatizes to your baby's needs. The following suggestions may help:

- Try to stay in tune with your baby's rhythms, and rest when she sleeps or whenever you have an opportunity.
- Sleep with or beside your baby.
- Sort out your priorities, and only do housework that is really essential.
- Start exercising; this will increase your energy.
- Take care of yourself and eat regular, nutritious meals.
- If your partner's work is suffering because of tiredness brought on by interrupted sleep, it may be best for him, occasionally, to sleep in another room while you sleep with the baby.
- Accept all the help you can get, even if you feel strongly about managing on your own. If you have a partner, his help may be invaluable, and if friends or relatives come to call, perhaps they could help with household chores, rather than expect to be entertained.

by, say, visiting your local health clinic, birth centre or doctor's surgery and asking whether there are any parents' groups in your area, so that you can find out what activities are available for mothers and babies. You will discover that the company of other women, especially those with young children, is very valuable. See page 347 for organizations that may help.

You may, however, find that the dividing line between loneliness and being overwhelmed by too much company is a fine one. While you are bound to want to share your happiness with family and friends and will want their support, your relationship with your baby is a very intimate one, and having enough privacy and peace is important. Care should be taken to find a balanced solution – especially in the first few weeks.

Finding time for yourself

Another major change for a new parent is getting used to the lack of time to yourself, as most of your waking hours (and, perhaps, even much of the time when you should be asleep) must be devoted to your baby's needs. However much you delight in your baby, this can be frustrating as well as the cause of feelings of resentment and guilt. It helps to bear in mind that, although this period of imposed selflessness may seem interminable, it in fact passes all too quickly, and your child soon becomes independent.

While making the most of fulfilling your baby's needs, try to arrange to have at least an hour or two entirely to yourself each week, so that you can pursue a particular interest or treat yourself to a special outing, or just be alone and rest. Not only will these short separations do you the world of good, they will also provide a valuable learning experience for your baby.

It is important to make the most of the peaceful moments when your baby is fed and contented to spend some time alone with your partner, and to find a trusted person who can take care of your child so that you can go out together occasionally. Pamper yourself and each other sometimes.

If a second pregnancy follows closely upon the first, this can place even more strain on a couple's relationship, since two very young children require a lot of time and attention. It can seem that there is hardly a part of the day or night when both children sleep simultaneously, and keeping the household running can be a full time job for both parents. Sometimes the demands of daily life can be so intense that a couple become quite distanced from each other. It is important to keep the channels of communication open and try to find time to enjoy relaxing together.

Coping with your baby's needs

Mothering involves a great deal of unconditional giving, physical and emotional. While some women find it easy and enjoyable to fulfil their baby's needs, others find their baby's demands frightening and need to find ways of protecting themselves; most women experience both feelings.

Newborn babies usually have voracious appetites to ensure that they are adequately nourished for all the growing that is taking place. This can be source of delight, but it is not unusual to feel overwhelmed sometimes by the intensity of your baby's need for food. It is best not to feel pressured by other peoples' expectations. Realizing your own limitations is one of the first lessons of parenthood, and organizing your life to deal with this will ultimately benefit your baby. If you can, put aside non-essential things, and trust your own instincts and judgment.

New parents are often subjected to a barrage of advice which may be contradictory. There are fashions in childcare in every generation, and it may upset you to be given conflicting advice by 'experts', friends or family.

Life with a new baby is a process of exploration in which you learn together. When you have heard all the advice on a particular subject, it is then time to let your experience and your child's response guide you to the right solution to a problem.

The ideal meets reality

Most people idealize parenthood before a baby is born, and it is easy to deny the so-called 'negative' feelings which all parents experience at some time. You may be very surprised to find that, occasionally, you can actually feel angry with your tiny helpless baby whom you otherwise adore and who is so dependent on you for love and attention. It is common to become frustrated and resentful of the loss of freedom, the lack of sleep, the changes in your social and sexual life. Almost everyone feels like this at times, and there is no need to feel guilty about it – it is a normal part of loving someone very intensely.

Guilt is a familiar emotion to a new mother. You may feel guilty if you are unable to satisfy or understand your baby's needs, if you resent her domination of your life or if you have to compromise your standards in relation to housework, a job, personal appearance or in your relationship with your partner. You may also have feelings such as anger with a partner for not being sufficiently involved, or envy of friends who are not bound by the responsibility for a new baby.

In addition, you must face the fact that your influence as a parent will have a major effect on the life and personality of your child. Sometimes it can be difficult to deal with this new and seemingly awesome responsibility – you may simply not feel mature enough to make important decisions about the life of another person who is wholly dependent on you. How you handle this can be coloured by the experience of your own childhood. You may feel that your own parents were perfect and that you cannot equal their standards. On the other hand, you may feel that your upbringing was mismanaged and that you missed certain things, or that the trials and traumas of your childhood should not be repeated or projected on to your own child.

The issue of repeating patterns of behaviour is a complex and difficult one. Many men and women who were abused as children sometimes – and usually against their own conscious wishes – find themselves reacting in the same way as their parents did when they too were under stress. These reactions were learned during childhood, stored in the memory and re-emerge now. While child abuse is the extreme example, there are many other types of behavioural patterns, the reappearance of which can be distressing. If you find that this happens to you, you can develop a habit of self-observation to discover which situations trigger these patterns; then you can find ways to anticipate and avoid them or deal with them if they do occur.

Coping with any of the problems of parenthood is made much easier if you are in good physical shape. Making sure that you are eating and sleeping well and have sufficient exercise is more important than you may realize. Desperation can often be pre-empted by taking good care of yourself, and utilizing the skill of relaxation through deep breathing.

Open communication with a friend or your partner can be extremely

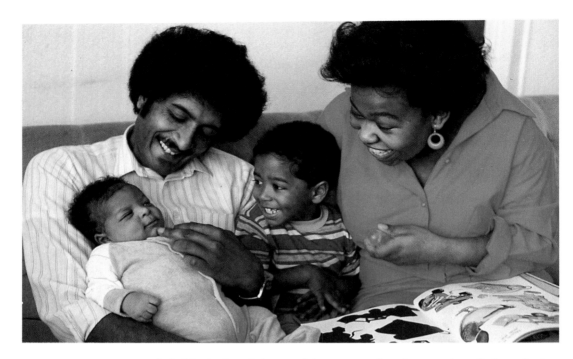

helpful – in fact, it is one of the most profound ways to benefit from sharing parenthood. Becoming a mother is a challenge to your own development, and affords you many opportunities to transform your weaknesses into strengths. It requires great courage to be open to change and self-realization, and even more to seek help. However, if your anger is intense or you find that your reactions to your baby are unacceptable and feel that this is affecting your relationship, the sooner you seek professional help, the better it will be for your long-term relationship.

New fatherhood

The new responsibilities of fatherhood can be a joy, despite the extra financial demands and the work involved in organizing the home. Coming home from work is an event which the new father may look forward to all day, and leaving in the morning may be difficult. Some men have a very strong paternal instinct which develops throughout the pregnancy. Occasionally such feelings towards a baby are more obvious in the father than in the mother, and in some cases, the man can become the major carer of the child and the home. Many men enjoy sharing all aspects of baby care, while others prefer to leave this to their partners and choose to carry on with their lives as usual.

Feeding and baby care
Many fathers derive great pleasure and satisfaction from the tender sight of their baby feeding at the breast. The mutual enjoyment and fulfilment of mother and baby and the calm, peaceful atmosphere can fill the home with a warmth which includes the whole family. The father's support can be a

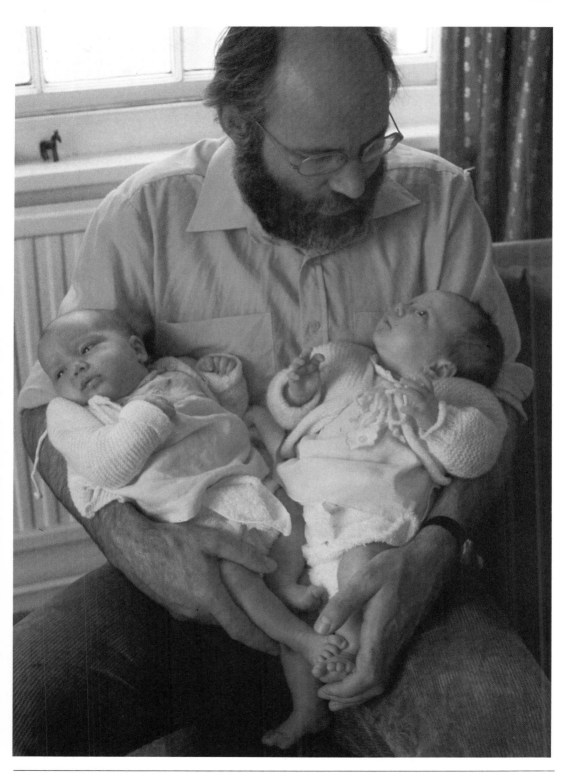

vital element in this, and especially so in the first two weeks of breastfeeding, as some women find that starting can be quite difficult. An encouraging, supportive partner who understands what she is going through can be invaluable. If your child is being bottle-fed, you too will be able to hold and feed her.

There are other activities which you can share with your partner. You may enjoy bathing with your baby, learning how to massage, change and dress her, talking and singing to her, playing with her, soothing her when she is fretful, comforting her when she cries and carrying her in a baby sling. You may find that you have a natural capacity to entertain and relax her, and this can be invaluable when your partner needs a rest as well as a source of pleasure for you.

Remember that your baby has been aware of your presence, the sound of your voice, the feeling of your hands, long before birth. You are already an important person in her life, and this relationship grows and flourishes whenever you spend time with her.

Coping with your emotions

There is another side to living with a baby which, to some degree, must play a part in every father's experience. There are bound to be times when you feel excluded from the love affair between mother and baby or even neglected by your partner. As a result, anger or jealousy of the baby is possible, despite the fact that these are irrational feelings to have towards such a tiny person.

If your partner is alone for many hours of the day with sole responsibility for the baby, and if her sleep is constantly interrupted, she may be under enormous strain and incapable of giving herself or your relationship the usual attention and care. Until your child becomes more independent, she may need to give almost all of herself, both physically and emotionally, to the baby. This can be difficult to cope with, especially if you are under stress yourself.

During the first three months, babies sometimes take a while to 'settle', and it is common for them to have a fretful time of day, usually between 5 and 10 p.m., when your partner may also be exhausted. If this coincides with your return from a tiring day at work, it may be trying to be presented with all these difficulties, which can be made even worse if the house is untidy, dinner is still uncooked and clothes unironed. This can result in friction between you and your partner.

Many of these problems can be alleviated with some forethought. Before going to work, you could possibly spend a bit of time helping out with household chores that may be fairly low on your partner's list of priorities. Life will be made more tolerable for her if you do your share of caring for the baby, giving her a break which can make all the difference.

Having angry feelings towards your baby and your partner occasionally is normal and very common. They can generally be dealt with by recognizing and allowing them in yourself, and perhaps talking about and sharing them with someone at an appropriate moment. If they seem overwhelming, some counselling may be helpful. The company of other fathers can be very useful: even though men may be reluctant to share intimate emotions, spending time with others going through a common experience is reassuring. Despite the normal ups and downs, a new baby is a source of immense pleasure and pride for the majority of fathers.

Making love after childbirth

For some couples, love-making resumes within two or three weeks after the birth, but it is very common – and perfectly normal – to find that months may pass before you begin to feel like making love again.

For some women, sexual desire returns soon after they have given birth, and there is no reason why they should not enjoy normal sexual activity. Of course, the timing of this will depend on how you feel, how the birth went and whether you need to recover from stitches or discomfort in the perineal area.

However, mothers tend to be fully absorbed in the great physical challenge of feeding and caring for their babies, and as a result, although she may have new and very deep feelings of love for her partner, this is often not a time when a woman is especially interested in genital sex. This may be heightened if she is afraid of becoming pregnant again too soon. In addition, as well as being nature's way of suppressing ovulation, the high levels of prolactin that occur during breastfeeding can reduce sex drive and may cause vaginal dryness, making penetration uncomfortable. A low sex drive in the months after giving birth is common in many women.

There is no need to worry or feel guilty if this happens to you, but you will need to understand that it can be especially trying for your partner. He may have great feelings of tenderness for you and a need for physical and sexual contact. If his needs are not understood, he may feel neglected or rejected. Remember that, before the birth, he had you all to himself, and is now having to learn to share you.

The solution to these difficulties can be found in open communication and sharing, with compassion and mutual compromise. There are many ways of being close that do not necessarily involve sexual activity. Bathing together, massaging each other, listening to music and enjoying a special meal together are some of the ways that you can encourage and discover new depths within your relationship, and of course there are many ways of making love without actual sexual intercourse. Both of you may need to feel cherished, protected, loved and understood in order to give your best to your child, and these are the aspects of love-making which take on added importance after the birth of a baby.

When you resume full sexual intercourse, this should be gradual. The tissues around the vagina may be sensitive, and you will probably need to use plenty of oil or other lubricant. Your partner should penetrate your labia quite slowly, taking particular care near the perineum and the entrance to the vagina. It is easier to control the rate of pentration if you are above your partner; the angle at which the penis enters the vagina will then also be altered so that pressure on the perineum is reduced. Any pain should recede in a few weeks, and intercourse itself will help to stretch the tissues.

If you are breastfeeding, you may discover that, when you become sexually aroused, your breasts leak abundantly due to the release of oxytocin. If this happens to you, it is a good idea to keep a small towel handy to wipe away the milk.

Making love after childbirth may be like starting your courtship again – beginning gently and gradually, and increasing in intensity with time. On the other hand, for some couples love-making can resume with intensity soon after the birth.

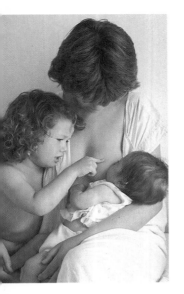

Other children

Once your baby is born, she is going to monopolize a lot of your time and energy, and despite all you may have done to prepare your older children (*see* p. 76), they are bound to experience a sense of loss as she takes their place in your arms. The way an older brother or sister copes with this will vary from family to family. At one extreme, sibling rivalry may lead to temper tantrums, regressive behaviour such as bedwetting and a variety of other signs that the child is angry or frightened of losing his special position within the family. On the other hand, the new baby may be accepted with love, interest and enthusiasm. The arrival of a new companion and friend is an event of major importance in your child's life, possibly the most significant since his own birth.

It is important to help your older child accept your new baby and to feel secure within the family and in his place within your affections. While you should make sure that you spend some time alone with him, giving him priority, you should also involve him with the baby. When you are feeding her, have him next to you for a cuddle, and explain why you are caring for the baby in a certain way, reminding him that you did just that for him when he was a baby. Try to be understanding if he is difficult for a while and cries a lot, and deal with any anger or aggression calmly and rationally. Remember that it is far better for these emotions to be released than repressed.

Looking ahead

Parenting is a learning adventure, which begins at or before conception and continues throughout life. All those involved will grow and learn from one another: parents are the central teachers of their child and, in return, your child will teach you to explore new realms of sharing, responsibility, love and care. Grandparents, too, should be included whenever possible in the joys and responsibilities of parenting your children.

You and your child have shared the nine months of pregnancy and the birth and, from her first breath, you will share her progress towards independence, as she masters the processes of feeding and digestion and learns to roll over, sit up, crawl, stand, walk and talk. This book takes you as far as the end of the first year of life, by which time your child will be three months old. Although you have already travelled far, the journey has just begun. Infancy is such a special time and passes so very quickly that it is important to make the most of it and to enjoy it with your baby.

Your child has her own destiny, her own life to live and difficulties to overcome. As a parent, you are able to be there to guide and help, but you will never be the sole determinant of your child's future. The great privilege of parenthood is to help another being through the early, most formative time of her life. At the same time, it provides a tremendous challenge for you to become more open, to mature and change.

Besides the responsibilities of parenthood, your children will provide you with a chance to find the child in you. You will remember how to play, be silly, laugh and cry. Once again, you will discover beauty in the simplicity of everyday things, and will become aware of the wonder of the natural world, as you accompany your children in the adventure of growing up.

Accepting a new brother or sister
Suggestions to help smooth the way towards your child's acceptance of the new baby:
* Help him to expand his horizons well before the baby is born – perhaps by starting him at a playgroup.
* Minimize any separation when the baby is born.
* Give him a special present when the new baby arrives.
* The father can help by making the older child his special concern.
* Devise special treats or activities that are only for 'big' boys and girls.
* Try to involve him in household activities such as tidying up, preparing meals, etc.
* Encourage him to hold and touch the baby freely. While you do need to supervise this carefully, try to relax – your baby is more resilient than you may realize.

PART V

SELF HELP

C H A P T E R   1 8

BREATHING

The breath is like a river of life, which ebbs and flows from the moment of birth until we die. As we inhale and exhale our very first breath of air, one of our fundamental body rhythms is set in motion, to continue throughout our lives. Our health and general well-being depend on the way we breathe, and this is particularly true during pregnancy, when a woman is breathing not only for herself but also for her baby.

What happens when you breathe

When you breathe, air containing oxygen passes through the windpipe (*trachea*) and bronchial passages until it reaches the *alveoli* in the lungs. There are billions of these tiny air sacs, covered with a fine network of blood vessels. Oxygen passes through the walls of these to enter your bloodstream, and it is then carried throughout your body by the haemoglobin in the red blood cells. Waste carbon dioxide passes the other way, to be expelled with the exhaled breath.

A similar exchange of gases occurs in the placenta. Oxygen from your blood passes through blood vessel walls in the placenta to enter the baby's bloodstream, and carbon dioxide from the baby passes out into your bloodstream, eventually to be eliminated with your exhaled breath.

Directly involved in breathing are the intercostal muscles between the ribs and, most importantly, the diaphragm, a strong muscular partition that lies just below the rib cage and separates the chest from the abdomen. As you breathe, the movements of your chest produced by these muscles cause your lungs to expand and contract as air is inhaled and exhaled.

During breathing, the up-and-down movements of your diaphragm massage all your internal organs and stimulate your circulation and digestion. The action of the diaphragm also affects your abdominal muscles, which contract and relax in a reciprocal action. If your breathing is out of balance, this will affect your abdominal muscles and, in turn, the whole abdominal and pelvic area and the deep-lying muscles located there. This is especially relevant during labour: when the diaphragm relaxes each time you exhale, the muscles of the pelvic floor relax as well; if the diaphragm is tense, tension in the pelvic floor will follow.

The diaphragm moves continuously in a rhythmic pattern of coordinated phases of contraction and relaxation. The relaxation phase (when you exhale) is longer than the contraction phase (when you inhale), and a slight pause follows each exhalation. Most of the time, breathing is involuntary and automatic, controlled by the autonomic nervous system in the brain.

The way in which we breathe is closely related to our posture and the way in which we use our bodies and live our lives. Many adults have forgotten how to breathe freely and may not be aware that the natural rhythm and flow of their breathing is disturbed. Poor breathing is usually combined with physical stiffness and postural imbalance: for example, tense shoulders, a stooped spine or a rigid pelvis will disturb the physiological balance of the body, restricting the circulation of blood to and from the lungs as well as the size and capacity of the chest cavity, and will thus affect breathing.

Our emotions also influence our breathing: stress and anxiety are common causes of restricted, shallow, rapid breathing. Over time, patterns of stress and tension can create a habit of this type of 'anxiety breathing'.

If you observe a baby or young child, you will notice that the abdomen moves in and out rhythmically with each breath, while the upper chest and shoulders remain relaxed and relatively still. Yet in many adults, it is mainly the chest that moves, while the abdomen remains still and sometimes rigid. We may also breathe too fast and emphasize inhaling rather than exhaling, inhaling the next breathe before we have fully emptied our lungs of stale air from the last. When this happens, about one-third of the stale air in the lungs is retained, which lowers the intake of oxygen and impedes the elimination of waste carbon dioxide. This reduces our vitality and effectiveness in everything we do.

Poor breathing affects all our bodily functions, our health, our state of mind and the quality of our lives. This is especially true during pregnancy and childbirth, when good breathing is vital to both mother and child.

Controlled breathing techniques

During the last few decades, many breathing methods or techniques have been taught to pregnant women to be used during labour – for example, psychoprophylaxis, the Erna Wright, Lamaze and Vellay methods, to name some of the most popular. All involve concentration on different 'levels' of breathing – from deep to shallow – and usually recommend that breathing should be lighter and more shallow as labour progresses.

These breathing methods were first introduced when women began to want more natural childbirth, and they were used in combination with a reclining or semi-reclining position in labour. By focusing her mind on her levels of breathing, it was hoped that the woman in labour would be able to dissociate from her body and thus gain control over painful contractions. Undoubtedly some women found this helpful. However, many others were disappointed by these techniques, finding that they proved difficult to remember in labour or were ineffectual.

In this book, we do not recommend any breathing techniques. Our main aim is to develop breathing awareness, so that you can learn to breathe in a full and relaxed way (correcting any poor breathing habits you may have acquired) for use not only during labour but throughout your life. By becoming more aware of your breathing, you will breathe more deeply and calmly, and during labour, you will be able to focus on your breathing to centre yourself and to surrender to the natural rhythms of the contractions.

Breathing awareness

Awareness of breathing can be cultivated during pregnancy, and will improve with practice. Daily repetition will deepen and improve your breathing, as well as providing both you and your baby with a few relaxing

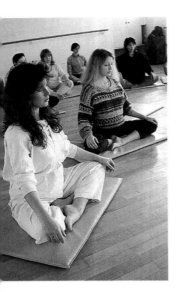

and peaceful moments each day. Although you may at first find it difficult to focus your attention on your breathing, after a few weeks it will become natural and spontaneous. Developing the habit of breathing deeply while you exercise or practise positions for labour and birth will extend naturally into the birth itself, and is the best possible way to prepare for breathing during contractions.

When we become tense or anxious, our breathing tends to become shallower and more rapid, and when we are afraid or in pain, we often hold our breath and restrict its normal rhythm. This sometimes happens during difficult or painful moments in labour and creates a vicious circle: stress causes tension and shallow breathing, which in turn causes the body to receive less oxygen, which produces more pain, which causes more stress and so on.

If you are able to focus your awareness on your breathing at such times – exhaling and inhaling calmly and deeply through each contraction while maintaining the normal rhythm of your respiration – you can reverse the process and reduce pain and stress. You will notice this happening when breathing through painful sensations while you exercise: often the pain dissipates and seems to melt away, bringing release and pleasure.

As your awareness of your breathing deepens, you will find that you have an invaluable tool for relaxing, calming and centring yourself. By spending some time quietly by yourself each day focusing on the natural rhythm and flow of your breath, you will begin to feel more in harmony with yourself and your baby and with the world around you. You will find a place deep within yourself to which you can return any time you need to, to relax and 'centre' yourself. With practice, this place will become so familiar that, when it comes to coping with the tidal waves of your labour contractions, you will know where to find your centre.

While developing greater awareness of your breathing, you could also be stretching and relaxing your body, releasing tension and stiffness and thus improving your posture and the mobility of your joints. By working simultaneously on your body and your breathing, you will make sure you keep yourself and your baby healthy during pregnancy, while preparing in the best possible way for the birth itself.

Daily deep-breathing practice

Choose a quiet place where you will not be disturbed, and make sure it is well ventilated. If weather permits, sit out of doors in the fresh air. You may wish to be alone, to include your partner or to practise in the company of other pregnant women. It is best not to eat for at least an hour beforehand.

Posture
You will need a blanket (folded into a square) and possibly a small, firm cushion or two; a wall can be used to help support your back if necessary. Sitting comfortably is most important, so try the following positions and choose the one that works best for you.

● *Kneeling.* Kneel on the blanket so that your buttocks are resting on your heels and your knees are slightly apart. If necessary, place a cushion or two under your calves so you feel comfortable and well supported.

- *Sitting on the floor.* Sit on the blanket. Draw one foot in towards your body; then draw in the other one and place it comfortably in front of the first, with both knees resting on the floor. Alternatively, if you can manage it easily, sit in a full lotus position (*see* exercise 5b, p. 250). If neither of these positions is comfortable, sit cross-legged against a wall and bring your lower back right up against it. If you like, you can stretch your legs out in front of you instead.
- *Sitting on a chair.* Sit in an upright position on a simple straight-backed chair, resting your feet comfortably so that the soles are flat on the floor.

Once you have found the most comfortable position, make sure that you are sitting with your back straight. You can do this by lifting up from your lower back and then opening your chest by relaxing and spreading your shoulders. Sway gently backwards and forwards from the hips until you find your body's central axis. Maintain this so that you do not have to strain to keep your back straight. Now relax the nape of your neck by bringing your chin down towards your chest.

Focusing

Place your hands gently and lightly on your lower abdomen and, without *doing* anything, become aware of the rhythm of each inhalation and exhalation, and the gentle movement of your abdomen. When you exhale, you will feel your belly moving away from your hands towards your spine as if it were emptying.

Exhale slowly through your mouth so that the breath is long and smooth and your lungs empty completely. After you exhale, pause, rest for a few moments and remain empty before you breathe again, this time through your nose. Wait for the inhalation to come spontaneously, and then, keeping your shoulders relaxed, breathe gently into your belly so that it feels as if your body is filling with air from the bottom up. Inhale towards your hands, allowing the belly to expand. Continue like this – breathing slowly, calmly and effortlessly so that one breath flows into the next, bringing a sense of stillness and peace.

Normally we breathe in and out through our noses. However, during labour most women instinctively breathe out through their mouths and inhale through their noses, and it may be helpful to practise this during pregnancy. If it is more comfortable for you to breathe in and out through your nose, continue to do so, but avoid inhaling through the mouth. Once your practice session is over, return to the way you normally breathe.

In the beginning, you may find that you are still breathing into your chest, and that your belly does not seem to move at all. If this is the case, make sure that your back is well supported and relax the nape of your neck. As you exhale, consciously draw in your abdominal muscles a little, away from your hands. At the end of the exhalation, rest a few seconds and then 'let go' as you inhale, breathing towards your hands. With a little practice, this will become more fluid, and soon you will be able to breathe more deeply quite naturally.

Working with a partner

Your partner can sit beside you and place one hand lightly and sensitively on your lower abdomen and the other on your lower back. Both of you should concentrate on your breathing. As you exhale, breathe *away* from the hand resting on your belly and *towards* the hand on your back. Then rest – be empty. When you are ready, breathe in *towards* the hand on your abdomen and *away* from the hand on your back.

Continue for a few minutes, and then swap places with your partner.

Breathing during labour

Having developed awareness during pregnancy, you will be able to breathe through your contractions in the first stage of labour in exactly the same way by simply relaxing in a comfortable position and focusing your attention on your breathing. As the contraction begins, concentrate on the exhalation and release tension with the breath. At the end of each exhalation, remain empty, rest and then allow the inhalation to begin, repeating the cycle through the wave of each contraction until it ebbs.

There is a lot of controversy about how women should breathe during the second stage of labour. Sometimes they are told to take a great big breath, hold it and push strenuously for as long as possible. Others may be encouraged not to push but to relax, breathe deeply and simply surrender to their bodily sensations. Deciding what to do in advance can be very confusing. You cannot really practise beforehand as you cannot anticipate what the expulsive reflex will feel like when your baby is being born. However, it will help to remember that the contractions of the second stage have a rhythm of their own, and that they are experienced as a very powerful urge to bear down, which is instinctive and involuntary.

It may be easier for you to surrender to these contractions at the time if, while breathing deeply, you practise positions for the second stage (*see* exercises 11a–e, p. 254) in the last few weeks of your pregnancy and visualize what is likely to happen. Try this: Squat down comfortably on your toes with your knees spread wide apart, and lean forward on to your hands. Imagine your baby deep inside your pelvic canal, the crown of his head resting on the pelvic floor, ready for birth. Focus your attention on your breathing, especially on the exhalation, and centre your awareness on your pelvic floor. Exhale slowly through your mouth, relaxing your lips and cheeks and 'blowing' the breath out gently until you feel completely empty.

While you are doing this, let go of all tension in your pelvic floor. Imagine your uterus contracting and pushing your baby downward, your pelvic floor expanding and opening, releasing and letting go as his head comes through the soft tissues of the vagina. Keep breathing deeply, concentrating on exhaling, and with each exhalation, imagine your vagina stretching and opening, releasing and letting go as your baby is born.

When you actually give birth, you may choose a different position, and you may perhaps release a lot of sound every time you exhale. Nevertheless, practising releasing the pelvic floor as you exhale will help you to be open and relaxed when the time comes.

After the birth

Knowing how to relax by breathing deeply will be useful throughout your life. When you are feeding your baby or if you are stressed or tired, trying to calm yourself or a crying baby or visiting the dentist, you will find it helpful to use your breathing to focus and centre yourself. A few minutes of attention to your posture combined with slow, deep breathing will quell anxiety, calm you and help you cope with any situation which life presents.

CHAPTER 19

BODY AWARENESS AND EXERCISE

Giving birth is, among other things, primarily a physical feat. The word *labour* implies that a woman needs all her strength to go up to and beyond the normal limits of her energy, and it makes sense to prepare to be at your best physically, in terms of both strength and suppleness, as you approach birth. In addition, exercise will help to ensure optimal health in pregnancy and to prepare you for the physical challenge of motherhood.

Developing body awareness

From an early age, our bodies express our feelings: when we are relaxed and happy, our bodies feel light, loose and comfortable; when we are under stress or anxious, they tighten. Tensions register on our musculature which, in time, will affect our posture, balance and the flow of energy.

The body stiffens to protect itself from both physical and emotional pain. For example, if you dislocate a joint, the surrounding muscles will stiffen as a defensive response; to ward off a blow to your belly, your abdominal muscles will tighten. Similarly, if you are emotionally hurt and cannot give vent to feelings such as anger or fear, you may suppress them by holding your breath, tensing your throat, tightening your abdominal muscles, lifting your shoulders and so on.

Due to the sedentary nature of modern life and inadequate physical education, we do not use our bodies to their full potential and rarely extend our joints to the limits for which they were designed. This means that our muscles are rarely fully stretched and so become stiff, losing some of their natural elasticity.

Such stiffness is caused partially by poor physical habits, such as sitting on chairs and driving cars rather than squatting, sitting on the floor and walking, all of which relax, exercise and use the body's potential for movement. Stiffness is also caused by emotional stress, which can arise at any time in our lives, including birth and infancy. Our bodies come to guard themselves against pain and fear by developing a kind of 'armour' in the musculature. This can be expressed as rounded shoulders, curvature of the neck and spine, distortion of the pelvis, tight hamstrings and inner thigh muscles, stiff knees and ankles and a host of other imbalances. The way to become more relaxed is, first, to recognize the stiffness in your body and then begin to work on gradually regaining elasticity by exercising in a very specific way.

When you begin to try the positions and movements in the exercises below, you will discover just how far you can go towards the complete movement. Very soon you will get to know the state of your body, and will be ready to begin work on regaining your suppleness and ability to relax.

Relaxation

Although the need for relaxation in childbirth is now widely recognized, many of the methods taught for its cultivation are ineffectual.

Relaxation is not merely a matter of lying down comfortably, letting go of your body and breathing deeply. This can be restful and invigorating, but will do nothing to release chronic stress patterns – when you get up, you will still be carrying around the same tensions. True relaxation comes from using your body, through exercise and breathing, to release stiffness and tension in the muscles, and learning to rid yourself of habitual body positions which limit your freedom.

Pregnancy provides you with a marvellous opportunity to begin to work on yourself. As your body changes, it has a natural tendency to soften and relax, and is predisposed towards health and healing. Becoming more in tune with your own body will also help you to focus on your baby and will enhance the depth of your communication with your unborn child.

Understanding exercise

There are many ways to exercise the body. The programme recommended in this book is made up of several different types of exercise.

Stretching exercises

These are derived from the basic principles of hatha yoga, and form the basis of most of the suggested exercises below. Typical ones are exercise 12, which lengthens and stretches the hamstrings at the back of the legs, and exercise 4, which stretches the inner thigh muscles.

Stretching is the most effective way of relaxing, and works on the principle of placing your body in positions in which the potential movement at the joints is maximal. Such positions have been carefully chosen so that gravity will assist the muscles to stretch passively without effort. In this way, they can gradually regain lost elasticity, and the movement of the joints will increase.

Fundamentally, these are not exercises but movements, which our bodies were intended to make with ease. Any small child can do them without difficulty, and by slowly regaining the ability to move in this way, you will enjoy a new suppleness, better posture and greater vitality.

As you begin to explore your body, you are bound to discover such phenomena as one knee being stiffer than the other, or the left shoulder being tighter than the right one. Although we are all born with a more or less symmetrical range of movement, the ways in which we habitually use our bodies give rise to imbalances, so that we stiffen up more on one side than the other. Stretching regularly restores balance and symmetry.

The exercises comprise a work-out for every part of the body, but concentrate particularly on the pelvic area to suit your needs during pregnancy. Many of the positions are, in fact, the most appropriate postures for labour and childbirth, so that regular practice will not only help you to have a healthy and comfortable pregnancy, but will also ensure that you are completely at ease when the time comes to give birth.

The effects and benefits of stretching

* Stretching is a passive, non-strenuous form of exercise which effectively releases chronic tension and stiffness.
* It lengthens and relaxes muscles and improves mobility of the joints by using gravity.
* It is ideal and safe exercise for pregnant women, but can be used to great effect by anyone.
* It makes the most of the natural increase in suppleness during pregnancy, due to the release of hormones which relax the ligaments that hold joints together.
* It will make it easier for you to adopt positions such as squatting and kneeling which are ideal for labour and childbirth.
* It helps you to 'make friends' with your pain, and to go beyond your normal limits. This is a most effective way to prepare for contractions during labour: by freeing yourself of unnecessary stiffness, tension and pain beforehand, you will be better able to cope with the powerful sensations that are experienced during childbirth.
* It improves blood circulation and breathing; regulates blood pressure and heart rate; improves and corrects posture to help prevent backache, cramps and headache; eliminates fatigue; and gives a sense of physical lightness and increased energy which is particularly helpful in late pregnancy.
* Most important of all, it will bring you more deeply in contact with your body, helping you to develop a new physical intimacy with yourself which will lead you to discover your own inner resources for giving birth.

Strengthening exercises

Some muscles require strengthening as well as suppleness. For example, the muscles of the buttocks, which support the lower back, should be firm and have good tone. If these are weak and flabby, the lumbar spine will be inadequately supported, resulting in back pain. It is also important for the pelvic-floor muscles to be strong as well as relaxed.

Strengthening exercises consist of the regular contraction of muscles. This is the sort of exercise used by weightlifters to develop muscular strength. Although to undertake this type of exercise exclusively would be unsuitable for pregnant women, it is important to include some during these months. Typical ones include exercise 10, which strengthens the buttock muscles, and exercise 9, which strengthens the pelvic floor. After the birth, gentle strengthening exercises can be used in combination with stretching to strengthen the back and pelvic floor to help the abdominal muscles recover their tone.

Aerobic exercise

This will get your breathing and heart going and will improve the performance of your circulation and lungs. Aerobic work-outs should be avoided in pregnancy, but some form of aerobic exercise is necessary.

Walking and swimming are the safest ways to ensure that you get enough aerobic exercise. You should walk, preferably outside, for an hour every day. Swimming is particularly beneficial.

Another way to exercise your heart and lungs is by dancing to music. In many cultures, dances are taught to pregnant women – in fact, belly dancing was first invented as preparation for childbirth. Many women find that circling their hips during labour dissipates pain and can help correct the position and rotation of the baby as it descends through the birth canal. Many women invent their own birth dance, seeming to discover intuitively the best way to ease their labour.

This is not a good time to take up strenuous sports such as cycling, jogging or tennis if you have never done them before. However, if you have enjoyed them regularly before pregnancy, there is no reason why you should not continue to do so, as long as you moderate your activity according to your comfort as your pregnancy progresses.

Centring exercises

Yoga-based exercises effectively increase a feeling of being centred on the inner self, a feeling that is deeply relaxing and calming. This sort of exercise is invaluable as a tool to reduce stress, and is also appropriate for labour and childbirth. Centring exercises will allow you to relax while your body is in action, and are a helpful way of focusing energy so that it can be put to the best possible use.

Resting

This form of exercise is what most people call 'relaxation', and involves the voluntary release of all the muscles of the body, combined with deep breathing. As well as resting your body, this is also a useful way of invigorating yourself and recovering energy, and it is a good way to become aware of your breathing rhythm and calm your mind. It is usually done in the 'corpse' position – flat on your back with arms, hands, legs and feet spread wide apart – but others are more appropriate in pregnancy, when your circulation may be affected if you lie flat. Of great benefit during pregnancy, it should be practised regularly at the end of each exercise session or whenever you feel fatigued.

Preparing yourself for exercise

The exercises below have been arranged as a work-out for the whole body, concentrating on the pelvic area and on the alleviation of postural imbalance and the minor discomforts of pregnancy. Some of them are intended as practice for labour and birth.

As you go through the whole sequence of exercises, you will begin to explore your body – noticing, perhaps for the first time, whether you are stiff or supple and which parts require exercise. After a while you will know which exercises are most beneficial, and you will then be able to create your own daily work-out to suit your own needs.

If you have a problem such as back pain, sciatica, varicose veins or piles, you will soon find out which movements and positions help to alleviate pain and improve the condition. Although some include cautionary notes, if you have a health problem it is advisable to check with your doctor that it is safe for you to practise these exercises.

Some of the exercises can be done with a partner. You may enjoy meeting other pregnant women to form an exercise group which can continue after the babies are born, and can then include post-natal exercise and baby massage.

Many couples greatly enjoy sharing a new awareness of their bodies, and can be a great help to each other. Including your partner in your programme of exercise and preparation will bring the two of you closer and establish a deeper communication between you, which will be invaluable during labour and birth and is the best foundation for the new challenges which lie ahead of you as parents.

Although men are usually physically stronger than women, they are often less supple. If your partner intends to help and support you during the birth, he may find that he too will need to spend some months beforehand loosening up, so that he can be at ease kneeling on the floor or positioning his body comfortably during your labour.

Getting started

Ideally, you should begin to exercise as soon as you know you are pregnant, or even earlier. However, it is never too late to start. Even if you begin towards the end of your pregnancy, you can still benefit greatly: your body naturally becomes more supple in the last weeks of pregnancy, and it will respond rapidly and instinctively to exercise.

The whole sequence of exercises, followed in order, should take about 60–90 minutes. If possible, the complete set should be practised daily, but if you are only able to spend 30 minutes every day doing the essential exercises listed on page 260 under 'Your daily work-out', with one or two sessions a week of the whole series in sequence, that should be adequate to ensure that you are at your physical best for pregnancy and labour. Obviously, the more time you are able to spend exercising, the more rapidly you will improve.

Choose any time of day, possibly dividing the exercises into a morning and an evening session. If you exercise first thing in the morning, you may find that your body is quite stiff and the movements are consequently more difficult. However, afterwards you should feel very invigorated and relaxed, with plenty of energy for the rest of the day. In the evening, after moving about all day, your body will be much looser and stretching will be easier. It is helpful to have a warm bath beforehand, and to empty your bladder and bowels before starting.

Try not to eat immediately before exercising – it is much better to do it on an empty stomach and then eat half an hour after the session. However, if you like, you can have a light meal an hour or so in advance.

Wear very loose, comfortable clothing, with bare feet. Find a clean, clear space where you can exercise undisturbed. There should be one empty wallspace available, as many of the exercises require a supporting wall. Make sure the room is warm and comfortably lit. If the room is not carpeted, place a few blankets on the floor, making sure that they will not slip out from under you. Peaceful music may be enjoyable and may enhance the process of relaxation.

Always begin a session with a few minutes of deep breathing. Then use it with each exercise, relaxing into the position and releasing tension with the exhalation. At first, you may find some of the positions a bit painful and difficult to hold for very long, but this initial stiffness and discomfort will soon disappear with practice, and each time you exercise, you will become more relaxed until, finally, you will be completely comfortable.

Start off cautiously, following the instructions for beginners. Hold each position for only a few seconds at first, gradually building up to a few minutes or longer as indicated. It is important to avoid strain, and to distinguish between pain that you need to go through and pain that is a warning signal that you are overdoing it. Read the instructions carefully, ensuring that you observe the cautionary notes and are feeling the stretch in the right places.

Your first aim should be to discover your limits in each exercise and to develop ease and comfort up to this point. When you have overcome your initial stiffness, you can extend yourself further. Proceed gradually, bearing in mind that, each time you practise, you will be freeing yourself of tension and will be more relaxed than you were before. Slowly your body will respond to your attention, and you will begin to notice a gradual but definite improvement after completing each exercise session.

The exercises

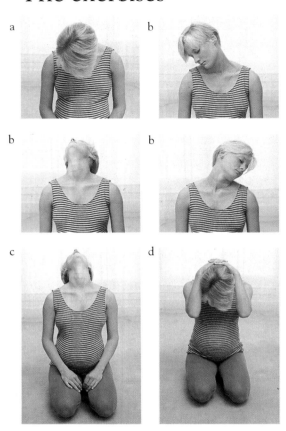

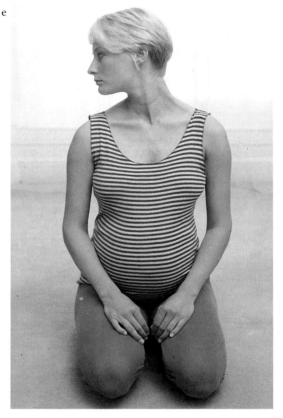

1 Head and neck exercises

a Sit comfortably cross-legged on the floor, or kneel. Let your head hang forward, relaxing the nape of the neck, the eyes, the shoulders and the face. Keep your back straight.

b Focus your attention on your breathing. Begin to rotate your head slowly while breathing deeply. Allow the weight of your head to carry it round in a wide circle. After you have done a few complete rotations, repeat in the opposite direction.

c Allow your head to drop backwards.

Open your mouth wide, releasing the tension in the jaws. Hold for a few seconds.

Close your mouth, bringing your teeth together to stretch the front of your neck. Hold for a few seconds.

d Drop your head forward.

Clasp your hands and place them on the back of your head so that your chin comes forward to rest on your chest. Drop your elbows.

Hold for a few seconds, keeping your shoulders relaxed and breathing deeply, concentrating on each exhalation. This will relax the back of your neck and your upper back muscles, and will relieve a headache.

Slowly lift your head, lowering your arms to your sides.

e With your shoulders facing forward, turn your neck and look round over your left shoulder.

Repeat to the right.

a

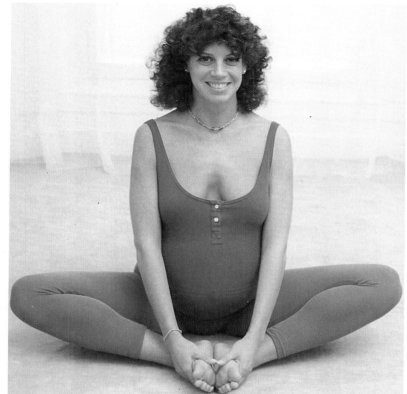

RIGHT

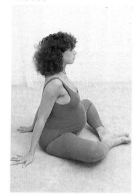

WRONG

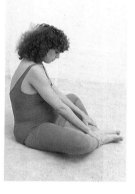

2 Cobbler's pose

This benefits the pelvic organs by improving circulation to this area. It relaxes the pelvic floor and widens the pelvis from side to side, increasing the flexibility of the joints and widening the front of the pelvic inlet. It also helps to correct the tilt and position of the pelvis. The key to this posture is to straighten your spine so that the hip joints can release. The cobbler's pose can be practised as often as you like and can be used as a sitting position.

How you feel In this position, you should feel the stretch on the inside of the thighs, in the groin and hip joints. You may also feel it in knees and ankles.

a Sit on the floor with your back straight and your legs stretched out in front of you. If necessary, use a wall to support your lower back.

 Bend your knees and bring your feet close to your groin.

 Bring the soles of your feet together, with the outer sides of both feet resting on the floor.

 Open out your thighs and lower your knees towards the floor.

 Now breathe deeply, concentrating on breathing down towards the floor and relaxing and releasing with the exhalation.

 Just before the inhalation, lift up from your buttock bones and stretch your spine from the sacrum upward.

b If you find it difficult to do the complete position at first, start with your feet about 30 cm (12in) away from your body and gradually bring them in towards your groin.

 Make sure that your lower back is straight and supported by sitting right up against a wall. Sitting on a folded blanket to raise your buttocks will help to straighten your back.

With a partner After loosening up on your own for a few minutes, you can increase the stretch by working with a partner.

 Sit in the position with your back straight.

 Your partner should sit behind you and place the soles of her feet on your lower back, applying some pressure to help you to straighten your spine.

 Breathe deeply and relax, lifting the spine from your partner's feet upward after each exhalation.

 Hold for a minute or so, and then change round.

a,b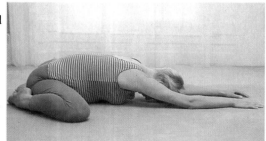

c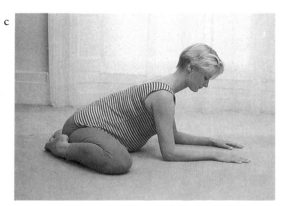

d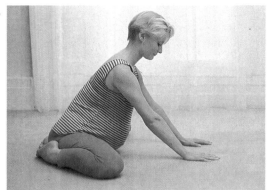

e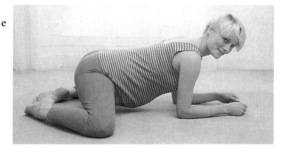

3 Kneeling with knees apart

This exercise releases tension in the groin and pelvic joints and, practised regularly, will help to restore their full range of movement and improve your posture. It will also greatly benefit your lower back, lessening or even eliminating pain in this area, including sciatica. It opens the pelvic outlet and lengthens and relaxes the muscles of your back, buttocks and pelvic floor, while at the same time taking the weight of your uterus and the baby off your back.

Start slowly with 3a, gradually stretching forward as your suppleness increases. Go only as far as you can without bending your back, and then stay there, breathing into it. Once you are at ease in this position, you may use it as often as you like.

How you feel You should be feeling the stretch mainly in the groin and possibly in your knees and ankles. This position also encourages a feeling of openness, which is good practice for labour.

a Kneel on the floor with your knees as wide apart as possible, your ankles turned out and your toes pointing inwards towards each other.

 If you can, sit between your feet with your buttocks on the floor. If this is too difficult, sit on your heels.

b Bring your shoulder blades down and towards each other at the back. Lift your spine up from your coccyx (tailbone) to the back of your head.

 Holding this position, move slowly forward from the hips, keeping your buttocks down as much as possible and your arms straight, until your hands reach the floor. You should begin to feel a stretch in the groin.

 Try making a gentle rocking movement, shifting your body weight from your arms to your legs.

 Breathe deeply in this position for a minute or longer, and then come up.

c If you can do the previous movements with ease, try resting on your forearms, keeping your back straight. Check in a mirror that your back is straight.

d If you can do 3c in comfort, try resting your head and chest on the floor.

 Stretch your arms out in front of you.

 Hold for a few minutes, breathing deeply, then come up.

e Come forward from the sitting position on to your elbows, lifting your buttocks and opening your knees as wide as possible.

 Rock backwards and forwards, shifting your weight between your elbows and your knees.

a: Resting position

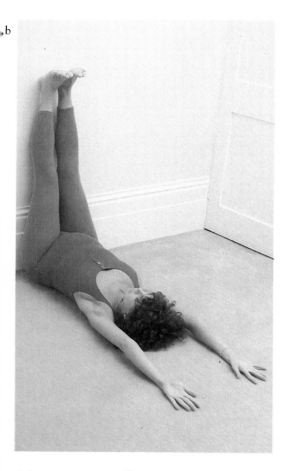

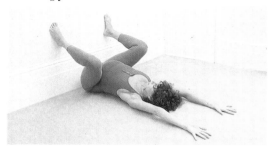

c

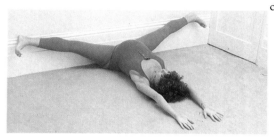

d

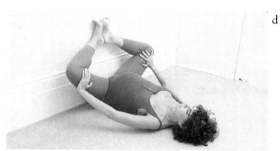

4 Legs apart on a wall

This exercise stretches the adductors – the large muscles that run along the inside of your thighs from the pubic bone to the knees.

Caution During pregnancy, particularly in the last weeks, some women find that they become dizzy if they lie flat on their backs. This is caused by the weight of the heavy uterus pressing down on major blood vessels and thus slowing down blood circulation. If this happens to you or if you are uncomfortable on your back, avoid all exercises involving this position.

If you feel uncomfortable while doing this exercise, eliminate it and concentrate on exercise 6.

How you feel You will feel this stretch in the inner thighs. Any initial discomfort is due to stiffness, but with a little practice it will disappear.

a Sit down sideways next to a wall, so that one hip is touching it. Swing round until your legs go up the wall and your upper body is lying flat on the floor with your buttocks close to or touching the wall.

  • Bend your knees as if squatting, place your feet flat against the wall and lift your arms up over your

head on to the floor. This is the resting position.

  • Breathe deeply into your belly, and relax your spine so there is no gap between your lower back and the floor.

b Straighten your legs up the wall.

  • Extend your heels so that the backs of your legs lie flat against the wall.

c Open your legs, allowing gravity to draw them down to the sides as far as they will go.

  • Bring the back of your knees towards the wall and extend your heels, bringing your toes towards your body.

  • Hold while breathing deeply. At first, you will probably be unable to hold this stretch for longer than a few seconds, but later, you may remain in it comfortably for 5–10 minutes.

d Bring the soles of your feet together, close to your body, and press your knees towards the wall with your hands.

  • To come out of this stretch, roll over slowly on to your side, wait a second and then come up on your hands and knees.

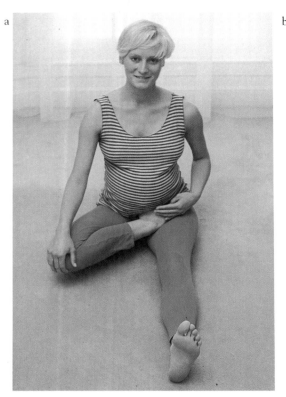

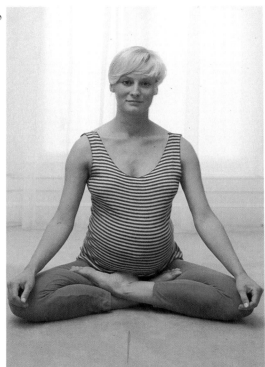

5 Knee stretch and lotus position

The knees are the largest joints in the body and tend to stiffen very easily. These exercises relax stiff knees and ankles as well as lubricating the hip joints.

The lotus position can be used for practising breathing and for meditation.

If you are not used to sitting on the floor or have never done this stretch before, you will probably experience pain around the knees and ankles. With practice, this will gradually subside, but it is wise to do the *half-lotus* 5a first, only attempting the *full lotus* position 5b when you can do 5a completely comfortably and your knee touches the ground.

Caution Knee joints are easily injured and should only be stretched very gradually, particularly if there has been a previous injury. Ensure your spine is straight.

How you feel This stretch extends the knees and is usually felt there and possibly in the ankles and hips. Take note of any pain in the knee. If there is, work into the stretch gently by supporting the knee on a folded blanket.

a Sit on the floor with your legs stretched out in front of you and your back straight.

  Bend one knee and, using your hands, bring the foot up to the opposite thigh as close to your groin as you can manage.

  Slowly and carefully, release your bent knee so that it moves down towards the floor, and then in towards your other knee. This is the half-lotus.

  After a few moments, change legs to exercise the other knee.

b Bending your right knee, hold your right foot with your hands and bring it up on to your left thigh so that the heel is near your navel.

  Now do the same with your left leg, bringing the foot up over the right one with the heel near your navel. The soles of both your feet should be turned up. This is the full lotus.

  Relax your arms so that your right hand rests on your right knee and your left hand on your left knee.

  Extend your spine from its base up to your neck after each exhalation.

  Hold this position for a few moments and then reverse so that the left foot comes up first. Hold for a few moments.

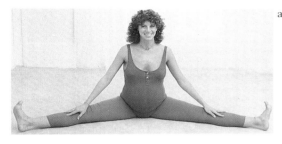

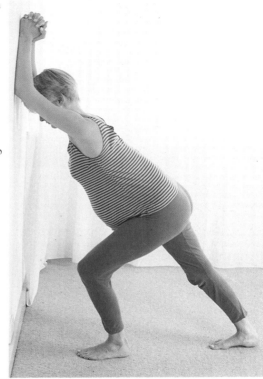

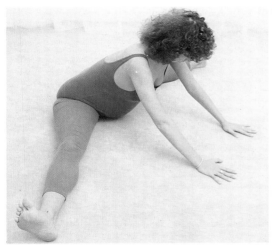

6 Sitting with legs wide

This is similar to exercise 4 as it also lengthens and releases the inner thigh muscles. It too encourages a feeling of openness, and can be used as a sitting position.

At first, you can try sitting on the very edge of a small, flat cushion or folded blanket and, once your legs are open, gradually slide off it. If you feel any discomfort, try massaging the painful spots while still maintaining this position. Do not go beyond 6a until you can do it with complete ease, which may take months of practice to achieve.

How you feel You will feel this stretch in the inner thigh muscles and at their insertion points in the groin and the knee.

a Sit on the floor with your legs wide apart and your back straight. You may support your back by placing your hands on the floor behind you.

● Move the backs of your knees towards the floor and extend your heels, bringing your toes up towards your body.

● Hold for a few minutes, breathing deeply, bringing the backs of your knees down towards the floor.

b If you can do 6a with ease, bend forward from the hips, keeping your spine extended and straight and lengthening your trunk.

7 Calf stretch

This relaxes and lengthens the calf muscles. As these govern the movement of your ankles, this will help to improve your ability to squat, and is beneficial when practised alternately with the squatting position (*see* p. 252). It will also improve the circulation to your legs, will prevent or ease cramps and swollen feet, will strengthen the ankles and make the calves more shapely.

How you feel You will feel the stretch in the calf muscles and Achilles tendons behind the heel.

● Stand facing a wall.

● With elbows bent in front of you, lean your upper body forward towards the wall and rest your weight on your forearms. Rest your head comfortably on your arms, keeping neck and shoulders relaxed.

● Place one foot about 30 cm (12 in) away from the wall and your other foot about 1 m (3 ft) behind and to one side of the first. Both feet should be pointing straight ahead, at right angles to the wall.

● Bend your front knee and straighten your back leg, pressing your back heel down so that all the weight of your body is on the back heel.

● Breathe deeply into the back heel. Hold for a few seconds, and then change legs.

● Repeat several times on each leg.

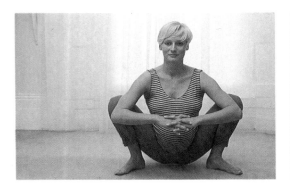 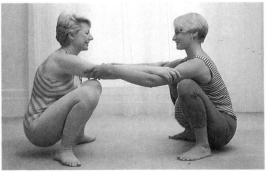

8 Squatting

This is the most important exercise to be practised during pregnancy. Squatting opens your pelvis, allowing your pelvic inlet, canal and outlet to be at their widest. In this position, the extensor muscles in the back and buttocks and the pelvic-floor muscles are lengthened and relaxed, and the tissues of the perineum are also at their most relaxed.

Squatting ensures good posture, improves blood circulation to the whole pelvic area and reduces constipation. It will also encourage the engagement of your baby's head in the pelvic brim. It is good practice to visualize your baby's head passing through your pelvic canal while you are in this position.

Even though squatting was instinctive and natural when you were a child, you may now find that full squatting – that is, with feet flat on the floor – is rather difficult. This is because you may not have used this position for a long time, resulting in stiffness in the ankle joints, Achilles tendons and calf muscles or in the knees and groin.

If this is the case, do not despair – with a little practice and perseverance, you can certainly become comfortable and flexible enough to use a supported squat during labour and delivery. Once it is easy, you should squat for a minimum of five to ten minutes daily – the more the better!

There are, in fact, two ways to squat:
1 Easy squatting on your toes
2 Full squatting on the heels
If you find it difficult to squat with your heels on the floor, start on your toes, spreading your knees wide apart. The following exercises, however, centre on the more difficult position with your feet flat on the floor.
How you feel You should feel the stretch mainly in the groin, but you may also experience it in your ankles, calves and knees.
Caution If you suffer from varicose veins in the legs or piles (haemorrhoids) or if you have had a stitch in your cervix (*see* Miscarriage, pp. 323–4), you should only do easy squatting or support your buttocks on a low stool or a pile of books (*see* below). If you have sciatica or pain in your lower back, squatting should

be done very gently and should not increase the pain. Care should be taken to keep your back straight by holding on to something for support.

   Stand with your feet 60–90 cm (2–3 ft) apart. Keep them parallel and pointing straight ahead so that they only turn out minimally as you squat down.

   Keeping your back straight and feet flat, squat down.

   Clasping your hands, spread and hold your knees apart with your elbows.

   Try to keep your spine straight with your weight on the outside of your feet, lifting the arches.

   Hold for a few minutes or for as long as you like if you are comfortable. Then come forward to kneel or stand up.

   If you find it difficult or impossible to squat with your feet flat, try holding on to a firm support such as a door handle or window ledge. You can also try placing a firm cushion or a book under your heels, or a few large books under your buttocks, removing them one by one as your squatting improves. For some women, it is easier to squat against a wall so that there is just a touch of support in the lower back.
With a partner Stand facing your partner, with your feet about 30 cm (12 in) apart and your toes pointing forward.

   Keeping your elbows straight, clasp each other's arms above the elbow.

   Holding on to each other for support and balance, squat down together slowly, turning your feet out slightly and finding the right distance from each other for a comfortable balance.

   Spread your knees as wide as you can, and keep the weight of your bodies on the outside of your feet, lifting the arches.

   Hold for a few seconds at first, then come up. Later, you can build up to three to five minutes.

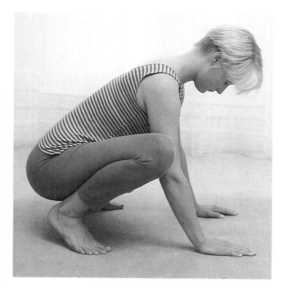

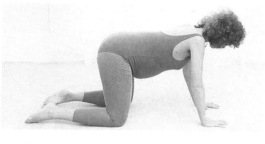

a

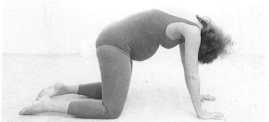

b

9 Pelvic floor exercise

By practising this exercise regularly, combined with deep breathing, you will be able to help your pelvic-floor muscles relax. This will be helpful in the second stage of labour, lessening the likelihood of a tear. In addition, it can help or prevent urinary incontinence, varicose veins and prolapse.

This exercise should be practised daily, particularly in late pregnancy.

Caution If you have vulval varicosities or piles, do this exercise while kneeling on all fours, with your head down and buttocks up.

- Stand with your feet about 60 cm (2 ft) apart.
- Squat down on your toes in the easy squatting position (*see* exercise 8). Lean forward on to your hands, keeping your arms and back straight, and spread your knees wide apart.
- Tighten your pelvic-floor muscles, drawing them upward as you would if you were trying to stop yourself from urinating in midstream.
- Hold for a few seconds and then slowly release them. Repeat several times.
- Make the same movement while breathing deeply. Tighten your pelvic-floor as you inhale, and then hold it tight as you exhale and inhale again. Then release slowly as you exhale. Repeat several times.
- Do the exercise again, this time releasing in four stages little by little, like a lift going down four floors and stopping momentarily at each one.
- Repeat the exercise, this time visualizing your baby's head passing through your pelvic canal during the second stage of labour. Each time you breathe out, imagine that you are breathing your baby out as you release your pelvic-floor muscles.

10 Pelvic tuck-in

During pregnancy, your lower back is subject to extra strain because of the extra weight you are carrying. Tightening and releasing your buttock muscles will strengthen them and improve their tone, increasing the support they give to your lower back and preventing or alleviating pain in the lumbar spine.

This exercise also helps your posture by correcting the angle of the pelvis so that it tilts forward as it should. It may also relieve sciatic pain. Additionally, it is a good practice for labour: a gentle pelvic rocking movement can lessen pain and help the baby descend through the birth canal.

a Go on to the floor on your hands and knees, with your knees about 30 cm (12 in) apart.

b Tighten your buttock muscles, tucking in your pelvis so that your back arches like a cat's.

- Hold for a few moments, then release, making sure you do not hollow your back. Repeat several times.
- Make the same movements in quick succession, rocking your pelvis gently up and down.

a
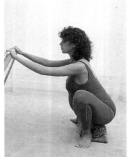
b c
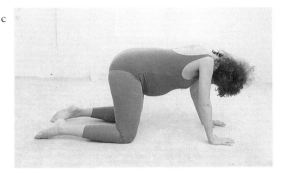

d
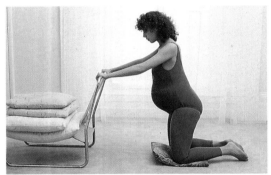
e
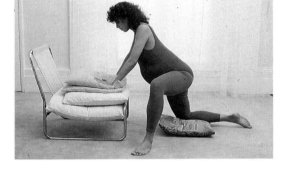

11 Movements for labour

These movements are used instinctively by women in labour, and it is helpful to practise them during pregnancy so that they become part of your body language.

Rotating your hips, rocking or walking will help you to cope with contractions, and will enhance the dilation of your cervix and the rotation of your baby. When practising these movements, try to imagine that you are in the midst of a strong contraction: breathe deeply, concentrating on the exhalation as if breathing through the contraction.

a *Squatting.* Squat down on to your toes and then stand up. Repeat this several times.

- Try squatting and then coming forward into the kneeling position, and finally back to a squat.
- If squatting is difficult, try placing a cushion under your heels and holding on to the back of a chair or lean forward over a pile of cushions.

b *Standing.* In this position, gravity will help your baby to descend and the labour to progress.

- Stand with your feet 30 cm (12 in) apart and gently rotate your hips in slow, sensuous circles.
- Tuck in your pelvis each time you move towards the front, and let go as you move towards the back.
- Repeat a few times, and then try in the opposite direction.

c *Kneeling on all fours.* Many women find this movement extremely useful in labour as it helps to reduce pain, and encourages the rotation of the baby.

- Kneel on the floor on all fours, with your knees about 30 cm (12 in) apart.
- Breathe deeply and rotate your hips in slow, sensuous circles.
- After a while, do the same in the opposite direction.

d *Kneeling upright.* Kneel upright with your knees slightly apart.

- Place your hands on your hips and make circular movements like a belly dancer. You can also do this while holding on to something firm for support.
- After a while, repeat in the opposite direction.

e *Half kneeling/half squatting.*

- From the upright kneeling position, lift up one knee and place your foot flat on the floor, so that you are in a half kneeling/half squatting position.
- After a while, change legs and repeat on the other side.

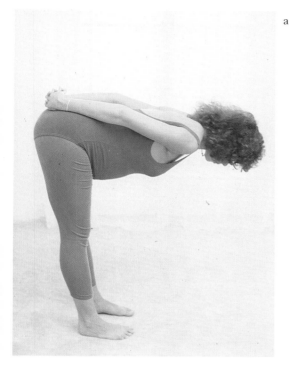
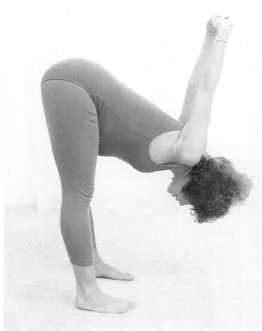

a

b

12 Forward bend

This lengthens and relaxes the hamstring muscles in the backs of your legs. This improves blood circulation and has an energizing effect, helping to prevent unnecessary fatigue.

Stiff hamstrings affect the curvature of the spine and thus distort posture. This exercise serves to correct the tilt of the pelvis, is excellent for developing good posture and also relaxes the pelvic-floor muscles.

Begin this movement slowly, not attempting exercise 12b until you can do 12a with ease. It is very important to keep your back straight, so check in a mirror if you are unsure. When you first begin, spend only a few seconds in the forward bend position, coming up slowly each time. Overbending in this exercise will place strain on your lower back.

How you feel You should feel the stretch in the hamstrings, at the back of the legs. No pain should be felt in the back.

a Stand with your feet about 30 cm (12 in) apart, parallel and facing straight forward.

● Spread your toes and lift your arches. Become aware of how your feet contact the floor. Breathe deeply, directing the exhalation to your feet.

● Keeping your back straight from its base to your head, drop your shoulders and open your chest by bringing your shoulder blades together at the back.

● Clasp your hands behind your back.

● As you exhale, and while keeping your back straight, bend forward slowly from the hips until you feel a stretch at the backs of your legs.

● Tighten your knees and breathe deeply, exhaling through your legs and feet down towards the floor.

● Stretch your spine by lifting your trunk forward from the pubic bone to your chin, keeping your back and the nape of your neck relaxed.

● Hold for a few minutes, breathing deeply. Come up as you exhale, whenever you feel like it.

b From the same position, lift your clasped hands and arms up as far over your head as you can, keeping your spine straight and your body extended in front.

If your hamstrings are supple, you probably did not feel much of a stretch in 12a and b. In this case, you might like to bend forward from the hips and rest your palms on the floor in front of you, keeping your spine straight. Hold for a minute or so, breathing deeply, and then come up.

13 Forward bend with legs apart

This stretch relaxes the hamstrings, improves blood circulation to the whole pelvic area as well as to the trunk and head, and relaxes the pelvic floor. It is similar to exercise 12 but the legs are positioned further apart. Follow the instructions for no. 12, but stand with your feet 1 m (3 ft) apart, and turn your toes slightly inwards.

a

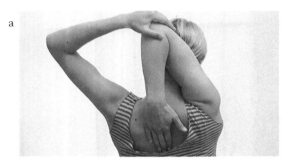

b

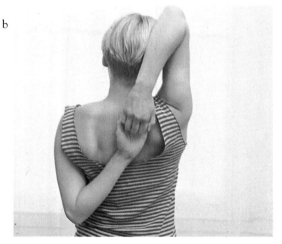

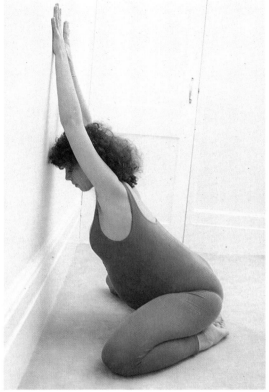

14 Standing shoulder stretches

These will release tension in the shoulders and open the chest. Regular practice will improve your breathing and blood circulation to the whole area, and thus to the whole body. Your lung capacity will increase, improving your respiration and your baby's.

These stretches can also help to relieve heartburn and pain in the ribs and will also tone up and exercise the breasts and the muscles which support them.

a Stand comfortably with your shoulders down and your pelvis tucked in.

● Raise your right arm over your head, bend the elbow and place your hand, palm down, on the middle of your upper back.

● Using your left hand, pull gently on your right elbow to bring it behind your head and increase the stretch.

Hold for a minute or so, and then repeat on the other side.

b If you found exercise 14a quite easy, complete the movement by bending your left elbow and bringing up your left hand to clasp your right.

● Hold for a minute or so, and then repeat on the other side.

15 Kneeling shoulder stretch

This will relax the shoulders, open the chest and stretch the muscles that support your breasts. It will also improve blood circulation and increase your lung capacity. It is helpful for relieving heartburn or pressure on the ribs.

How you feel You should feel the stretch in your shoulders and upper arms only. If you feel any discomfort in your back, you need to come a little closer to the wall.

● Kneel with your knees about 30 cm (12 in) in front of a wall, and spread apart.

● Drop your shoulders, and make sure your feet are turned inward, toes pointing towards each other.

● Lift your arms up over your head, and keeping your elbows straight, place your hands on the wall above your head about a shoulder's width apart.

● Reach up as high as you can without lifting your buttocks. Extend your fingers, and let your trunk relax forward so that the front of your body – your abdomen and chest – is extended.

● Breathe deeply, and hold this position for a few minutes. Concentrate on lowering your shoulder blades away from the back of your head and neck, while bringing your breastbone towards the wall.

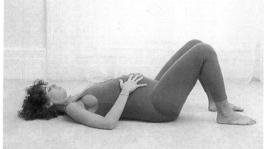

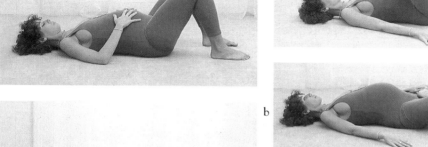

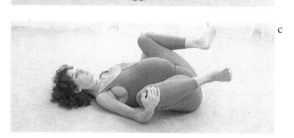

16 Pelvic lift

This exercise strengthens the buttock muscles while stretching the front thigh muscles. Regular practice will strengthen your lower back, and ease or prevent backache or sciatic pain. It is also a safe way to extend your spine and will help to correct the tilt of your pelvis and ensure good posture.

How you feel You will feel this stretch along the front of your thighs.

Caution If you feel uncomfortable when lying on your back, especially in late pregnancy, omit this exercise.

a Lie on your back on the floor with knees bent and arms by your sides. Breathe deeply into your belly, relaxing your spine.

● Bring your feet in close to your buttocks and parallel. Feel how your spine touches the floor.

● Tighten your buttock muscles and tuck in your pelvis, so that your lower back lies flat on the floor.

● Hold for a few seconds, and then relax. Repeat several times.

b Lying in the same position, inhale as you tighten your buttocks and lift up your pelvis by pressing down on your heels. Your spine should lift up off the ground as far as your shoulder blades.

● Hold this position for a second, keeping your buttocks tight and lifting your pelvis towards the ceiling.

● Come down slowly as you exhale, releasing the spine one vertebra at a time. Repeat several times.

17 Lower back release

Caution If these exercises make you uncomfortable, omit them.

a This is very soothing and relaxing, and relieves fatigue, particularly in the last part of pregnancy.

● Lie on your back on the floor, bending your knees and crossing your legs at the ankles.

● With your arms by your sides, rotate your legs gently, making a circular movement with your hips, thus massaging your lower back on the floor.

● Make two or three circles, and then repeat in the opposite direction.

b This can help to relieve the pain of sciatica.

● Lie on your back on the floor and stretch your legs out in front of you. Bend your right leg at the knee, clasping your right foot with your left hand, bring your foot up to the top of your left thigh.

● Lower your right knee towards the floor, and breathe deeply.

● Hold for a minute or so, and then repeat with the other leg.

c While lying on your back, draw your knees up to your shoulders as if squatting. This will relax your lower back and spine.

a

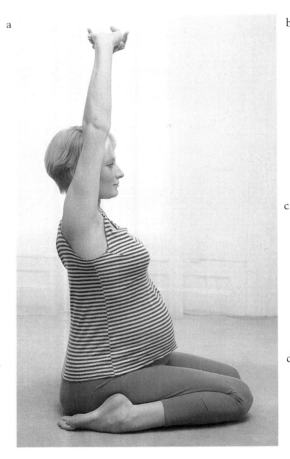

b

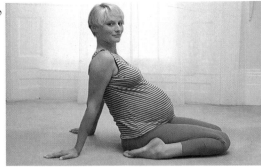

c

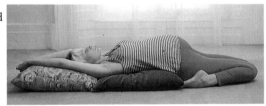

d

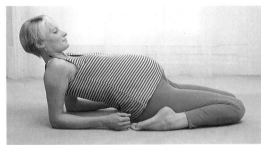

18 Sitting between your feet

This exercise will stretch the front of your body, relaxing the front thigh muscles. It will also relax the digestive tract, and may be useful for alleviating feelings of fullness and heartburn. It will also extend the ankle and knee joints, and will improve the circulation to the legs.

Proceed cautiously as you can very easily overdo it before you are ready. It is vital to be able to do exercise 18a with complete ease before progressing on to 18b and c. If you cannot sit between your feet, you will benefit more by practising just 18a until your ankles become more flexible.

How you feel You should feel this stretch in the thighs and perhaps in the knees and ankles. If you feel any discomfort or back pain, you are going beyond your limit and straining the lumbar spine.

a Kneel down and sit between your heels, with your toes pointing inwards towards each other and your buttocks touching the floor. Keep your spine erect from its base to your neck.

* Keeping your pelvis tucked in, gently raise your

arms over your head, palms reversed. Hold for a second or two, then relax.

b If you can do exercise 18a comfortably, try leaning back on to your hands, tightening your buttocks and keeping your arms straight and knees together. You should feel the stretch in your front thigh muscles.

c If exercise 18b was easy to do, lean back on to your elbows, keeping your buttocks firm, knees tightly together and pelvis tucked in.

* If you feel a good stretch in your thighs, do not attempt to go down any further, but relax and breathe deeply, concentrating on the exhalation.

d If you did not feel a stretch when you did exercise 18c, lie back completely, keeping your buttocks tight, lifting your pubic bone and stretching your arms up over your head. You can place one or two large cushions under your back so you can relax completely.

* Breathe deeply, concentrating on the exhalation. After a few minutes, come up slowly in stages.

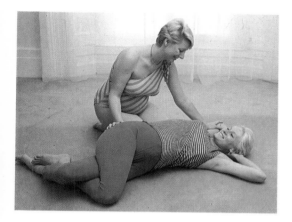

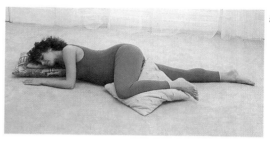

a

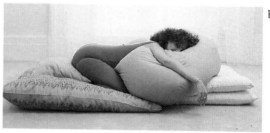

b

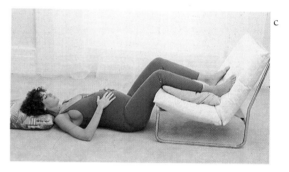

c

19 Spinal twist

Twisting the spine will stimulate the lubrication of the joints between the vertebrae. This exercise stretches all the oblique muscles along your sides as well as those that support your breasts and the intercostal muscles between your ribs; and it is very relaxing for the lower back, helping to relieve or prevent lower back pain and sciatica.

How you feel You should feel this stretch all along the sides of your body. When you do the exercise with a partner, you will feel a stretch above your armpit, in the muscles that support your breasts.

 This exercise is best done with a partner but it can also be done alone.

 Lie on your back and clasp your hands behind your head. Your partner should kneel beside you on your right side. Breathe deeply into your belly.

 Cross your right leg over your left, tucking the right foot under the left calf.

 Keeping your right elbow and shoulder flat on the floor, rotate your hips to the left so that your right knee moves towards the floor.

 Your partner should place one hand on your right elbow to hold it down, while applying gentle pressure behind your right hip bone to assist the rotation of your pelvis. If your shoulders are stiff, you may find it painful to keep your elbow down, and if the pain is intense, put your arm down alongside your body and ask your partner to hold down your shoulder instead. If you find it uncomfortable to cross your legs, simply bend them together to one side.

 Hold this position for a minute or two, breathing deeply, and then change to the other side.

 When rising from the reclining position, roll over on to your side and come up on to your hands and knees.

 If you spend five minutes in this position, breathing deeply, you will feel very rested and invigorated.

20 Resting

You should rest for at least five minutes after a stretch session. The most efficient position for complete relaxation, and the one most commonly used, is lying flat on your back on the floor. However, if you feel uncomfortable lying on your back, other positions may be more suitable.

a *Side lying.* Lie down on your side, placing a pillow under your head. Stretch out your bottom leg, and bend your top one, placing a pillow under the knee of that leg. This position is also suitable for sleeping.

b *Kneeling position.* Kneel comfortably on the floor or on your bed, with your knees apart and your upper body supported by a pile of cushions so that you can rest. This is a good resting position for pregnancy, and it is also useful during labour.

c *Resting on your back with your feet up.* Lie on your back on the floor, with a cushion under your head, and your feet and lower legs supported on a chair or bed. This position is useful if you have varicose veins or swollen ankles, but should not be used if you are uncomfortable lying on your back.

Your daily work-out

Ideally, all the above exercises should be done in this order at least once a week. In addition, there are some essential exercises which should be practised daily as well as any others which you find particularly helpful. The essential exercises are:

- Cobbler's pose (no. 2)
- Kneeling with knees apart (no. 3)
- Legs apart on a wall (no. 4)
- Calf stretch (no. 7)
- Squatting (no. 8)
- Pelvic-floor exercise (no. 9)

These can quite easily become part of your daily life – for example, you can sit in the cobbler's pose while watching television or kneel with knees apart while reading or playing with a child. In addition, you can exercise your body by making a point of sitting on the floor or squatting on a low stool rather than using a chiar.

Always begin your work-out with a few minutes of deep breathing, then start with the essential exercises and continue with the other movements as you feel inclined.

Everyday posture

Good posture during pregnancy is vitally important. As your baby grows and your uterus enlarges, your body has to accommodate and adjust to the dynamic changes that are necessary if you are to carry your pregnancy in a balanced and harmonious way. If your posture is incorrect, your body will be stressed, resulting in tension, discomfort and pain.

Regular exercising will help to correct and prevent postural imbalance, but it is important to combine this with a conscious awareness of the way you use your body. You may find that you have developed certain habits which misuse your body and will have to be corrected. To check your posture, make use of the following hints for body awareness.

Standing

Stand sideways in front of a full-length mirror. Without doing anything, become aware of your posture.

First of all, check your feet. They should be parallel to each other rather than turned out, and should grip the ground firmly, with your weight evenly distributed between toes, balls of your feet, heels and the outside edges. The inner arches should be slightly raised.

Next, check your knees. These should be just slightly bent, and relaxed rather than tight.

Now pass on to your pelvic area. Your pelvis should be tucked in slightly and should not dip too much in front. To get the right feeling, tighten your buttocks and tuck in your pelvis so that your lower back is almost flat, rather than arching. Over-arching, or hollowing, the back is one of the most common causes of back pain in pregnancy. If you have a tendency to hollow your back, make sure that you practise the pelvic exercises (nos. 10 and 16, on page 253 and page 257) daily.

Next, continue up the spine to the upper part of your torso. Keeping your pelvis tucked in, lift up the front part of your chest and spread your shoulders so that the shoulder blades come towards each other. While doing this, take care that you are not beginning to hollow your back.

Now check your shoulders. They should be loose and relaxed, and dropping down towards the floor rather than lifting towards your ears or bending forward.

Finally, your head should rest in a balanced position on top of your spine, with your chin tucked in just slightly. Check that you are not throwing your head forward or clenching your jaws. Your jaws and throat should be relaxed and loose.

Walking

Make sure that you keep your feet parallel to each other when you walk. Do not turn them out and 'waddle' – a common cause of pain in the sacro-iliac joints during pregnancy. Always wear flat shoes; high heels will throw your posture out of balance.

Keep your knees slightly bent, your pelvis tucked in and your spine and torso erect without hollowing your back. Relax your shoulders and swing your arms freely by your sides. Avoid habitually carrying a heavy bag over one shoulder as this will cause postural imbalance. Breathe deeply and evenly as you walk.

Bending and lifting

Never bend forward to lift an object or a small child. Stooping over and bending your back causes strain on the lumbar spine. Instead, squat down on your toes and lift the object or child while taking care to keep your back straight.

Sitting

Whenever possible, sit on the floor rather than on a chair or sofa. When sitting on a chair, avoid crossing your legs, make sure that you are sitting on your buttock bones and lift your spine and torso from the hips. Do not slump or allow your lumbar spine and pelvis or chest to collapse when sitting. To check that you are not doing the latter, lift your breastbone, drop your shoulders and bring your shoulder blades towards each other.

If you spend a lot of time at a desk writing or typing, make sure that your back is well supported and that you are not hunching forward over your work. Practise the shoulder stretches (exercises 14 and 15 on page 256), regularly to release tension in this area.

When relaxing at home or in company, avoid flopping into an armchair or on a sofa; rather, sit on the floor, your back comfortably supported by a wall, your legs crossed or in one of the sitting positions (exercises 2, 3, 5 and 18, on pages 247, 248, 250 and 258). It is also helpful to have a low stool or a pile of books on which to squat comfortably.

Lying down

Avoid lying and sleeping flat on your back. Instead, use extra pillows to make yourself comfortable on your side or front (*see* exercise 20a-c, page 259). It is best to sleep on a firm mattress; you may have to place a board under your mattress to achieve this.

Whenever you get up from lying down, roll over on to your side and come up on to your hands in a sitting or kneeling position, rather than tensing your abdominal muscles and lifting yourself straight up.

C H A P T E R 2 0

EXERCISING AFTER BIRTH

After you have given birth, you will probably spend the first week or two resting, getting to know your baby and becoming used to your new role as a mother. It is unlikely that you will have time for much exercise until your baby is a few weeks old. If the birth has been difficult or if you have had a tear, an episiotomy or a Caesarean section, you must allow the natural healing process to occur before you start exercising. It is advisable to wait about four to six weeks after a Caesarean before beginning, but make sure that you and your doctor have discussed this first.

The following exercises have been carefully chosen and arranged to stretch and strengthen your body safely. After childbirth, it is important to develop strength and good muscle tone before stretching and extending the body further, with vulnerable areas such as the lower back and abdomen being carefully introduced to new movements.

When you begin, follow the instructions carefully in sequence, exploring where your limits lie and then working gradually to go beyond those limits little by little, without strain. You are bound to find some exercises easier than others, corresponding to the degree of stiffness in different parts of your body. Concentrate on those you find most difficult, and work on them slowly until they become more pleasurable and easier to do.

One of the most difficult adjustments to make in the first few months of motherhood is getting used to broken nights and all the new demands on your energy, and you may find that you sometimes feel very tired. Exercising regularly can work wonders to restore your energy and lessen fatigue, even if you only manage one or two stretches at a time. While exercising your body, you will discover that it can be a wonderful way of relaxing with your baby, who will love to be included in the fun.

The pelvis Some of the exercises are intended to help you maintain the flexibility that you gained during your pregnancy. They will also improve the muscle tone of the uterus and will encourage it to return to more or less the same state as before.

The shoulders, neck and head Breastfeeding and looking after your baby involves hours of holding and carrying, which often causes tension to arise in these areas. In fact, the expression 'nursing shoulder' is often used to describe the stiffness in one shoulder which is so common in nursing mothers. You will find that the exercises which stretch and relax the muscles in your shoulders, neck and head are an invaluable way to release tension.

Areas of most concern are the following:

The pelvic-floor muscles To start with, you will need to strengthen and tone this area, and these exercises should be done as soon after the birth as you feel inclined. They will help to promote healing of the perineal tissues by improving the circulation of blood in this region, and will help you avoid problems such as urinary incontinence.

• *The abdominal muscles* It is essential to support and protect the spine while exercising the abdominal muscles, and to avoid strain in this area. The exercises suggested in this programme first gently stretch these muscles, then improve their tones and finally strengthen them without straining the back or the abdominal organs.

• *The lower back, buttocks and thighs* After a while, you can begin to strengthen the muscles in these parts, all of which have carried so much extra weight during pregnancy. Lower-back exercises are particularly important in the first few months.

The exercises that follow are arranged as a programme for the first 12 months after childbirth. You may add any of the exercises in the pregnancy section, and you should be ready to begin more extensive movements within 6–12 months. Hatha yoga is the ideal form of exercise with which to carry on at this stage.

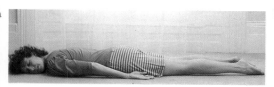
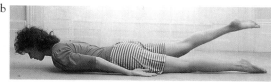
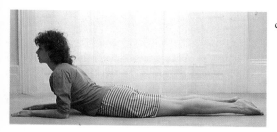
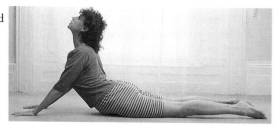

b

d

1 Strengthening the pelvic floor and lower back

This series of exercises does several things at once. It strengthens the pelvic-floor muscles, as well as improving circulation and muscle tone. It also begins to stretch the abdominal muscles. At the same time, the muscles in your lower back will contract, bringing strength to this area. Tightening and firming the buttock muscles will provide support to the lower back.

Note: If your breasts are very full and lying on your front is uncomfortable, try putting a pillow under your head or do exercises 1a and b on your back.

a Lie down on your belly with your arms by your sides, and your head resting comfortably to one side.

• Close your eyes and focus your attention on your pelvic floor.

• Breathe deeply, tightening your pelvic-floor muscles as you inhale, and releasing them slowly as you breathe out. Repeat several times.

• Now try tightening and relaxing your buttock muscles. Repeat several times.

b About a week or so after the birth, try lifting your head and one leg as you inhale, relaxing and returning to the resting position as you exhale. Repeat three or four times.

• Repeat with the other leg.

• Relax and breathe deeply.

c Two or three weeks later, come up on to your elbows, making sure that your shoulders are relaxed by pulling them down, away from your ears.

• Clench your buttock muscles firmly for seconds while maintaining this position.

• Relax as you exhale, and return to the resting position.

d After practising exercise 1c regularly for a few weeks, try coming up into the 'cobra' position – i.e. supporting your trunk with your arms and extending your neck. Push up with your hands and bend your elbows.

• Keep your shoulders down and relaxed and your buttocks firm, and breathe deeply into your belly.

• Hold for only a few seconds, and then, as you exhale, return to the resting position.

• Eventually, you can straighten your elbows.

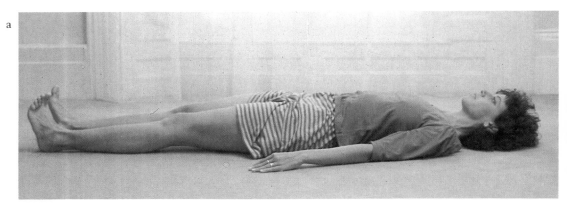

2 Toning the abdominal muscles

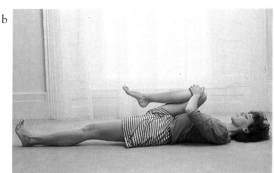

This sequence restores good tone to the abdominal muscles while avoiding strain. It also relaxes the lower back and tones the thighs, while gently stretching the hamstrings and calves at the back of the legs.

a Lie on your back, arms by your sides, with your body completely relaxed. Breathe deeply into your belly.
- As you exhale, tighten your abdominal muscles, drawing them down towards your spine.
- Hold for a few seconds, then release the muscles and breathe in at the same time, so that your belly relaxes with the inhalation.
- Repeat several times in harmony with your breathing rhythm.

b Bend your left knee, drawing it up towards your chest.
- Pull the knee firmly towards your body with your hands. Keep your right leg flat on the floor.
- Straighten the leg so that it is at right angles to the floor. Keep your knee tight, and point your toes towards the ceiling.
- Extend your heel, pointing your toes down towards your body. Slowly lower your leg to the floor as you exhale.
- Relax and breathe deeply. Then repeat the movement – knee to chest, toes to ceiling, heel to floor – five to six times.
- Relax and repeat with the other leg.
- Rest for a few minutes, breathing into your belly.

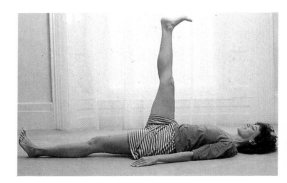

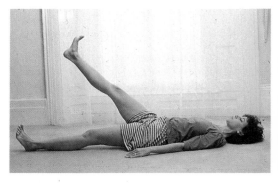

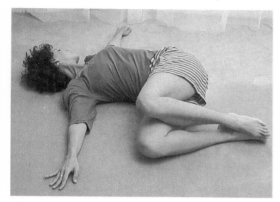

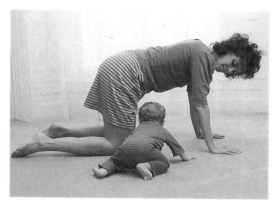

3 Spinal twist

This exercise rotates the whole spine, twisting each vertebra at the joints. This stimulates the secretion of lubricating fluids between the joints, and has an effect like 'oiling' the spine. It also opens muscles of the chest wall, releases tension in the shoulders and gently works the abdominal muscles while relaxing the lower back. Twisting in this way also stretches the oblique muscles along your sides and so helps to restore your waistline.

 Lie on your back on the floor. Spread out your arms at shoulder height on either side of your body.
 Place your hands palm down, and relax the whole of your body, breathing deeply into your belly.
 Keeping your shoulders, arms and hands flat on the floor, bend your knees and draw them, feet together, up towards your belly.
 Rotate your body so that the knees touch the floor on the left side of your body while you turn your head and neck to the right.
 Hold for a few seconds. Then reverse, bringing your knees to the right and your head to the left.
 Repeat several times in a fluid motion from left to right and back again, breathing evenly.
 Straighten your legs. Rest for a moment or two before getting up.

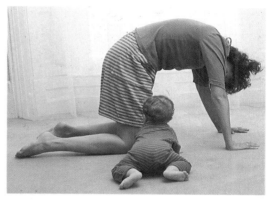

4 Pelvic tuck-in

See exercise 10, p. 253. This strengthens the buttock muscles which support the lower back, and also corrects the tilt of the pelvis, helping to relieve or prevent backache and poor posture. Your baby will enjoy lying underneath you and, later on, crawling through the 'tunnel' made by your body.

a
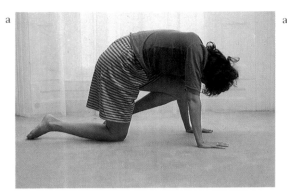

b
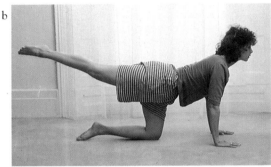

a
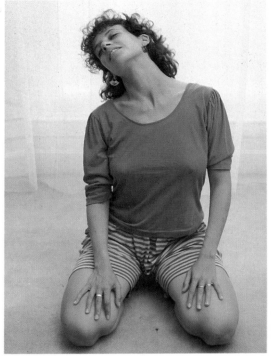

5 Leg lift

This alternately stretches and strengthens the front of
your body and your back, with the back, thigh and
abdominal muscles all working in a rhythmic flow of
extension and contraction. It is fun to do this one to
music.

a Kneel on all fours, with your knees slightly apart.
 As you inhale, tuck in your left knee, pulling it
towards your chest. Bend your neck to look down at
your knee. Hold for a second.
b As you exhale, extend your left leg, lifting it back
and up as high as you comfortably can. At the same
time, lift up your head and stretch your neck,
extending your chin.
  Hold for a few seconds, then relax.
  Repeat up to ten times in rhythm with your
breathing – i.e. breathe in and tuck in, breathe out
and lift up, then rest for a moment.
  Change legs and repeat on the other side.

6 Head and shoulder rolls

This exercise releases tension in the shoulders, and
will help to restore your energy and prevent or relieve
headaches. It is especially helpful after hours of
nursing and carrying your baby.
a Kneel on the floor, knees slightly apart, shoulders
relaxed and hands loosely resting on thighs.
  Become aware of your breathing.
  Relaxing your neck and shoulders, slowly rotate
your head and neck in a wide circle, allowing the
weight of your head to carry it around. Keep your
attention on your breathing, and your jaws loose and
relaxed.
b Draw up your shoulders towards your ears while
dropping your head forward. Allow your arms to
hang loosely at your sides.
  Slowly roll your shoulders backward and then
lower them, opening the chest, bringing the shoulder blades towards each other and lifting the head.
  In an even flow, raise the shoulders again and keep
circling them until they relax.
  Reverse: roll the shoulders forward, lowering your
head.

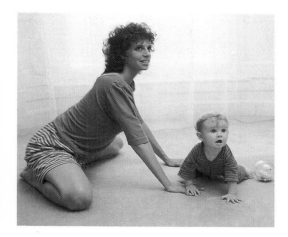

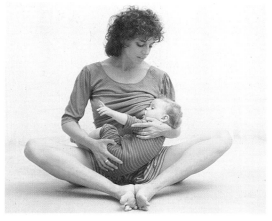

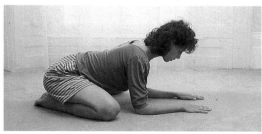

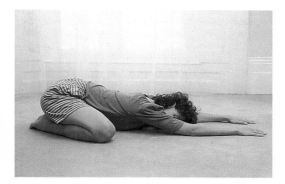

7 Kneeling with knees apart
See exercise 3, page 248. This will help to keep the pelvis supple and relax your lower back.

8 Cobbler's pose
See exercise 2, p. 247. This should have become familiar to you during pregnancy. Regular practice now will have the same beneficial effects, and will help to maintain or restore the flexibility you gained then. All the pelvic organs, especially the uterus, will be helped to recover their tone. In addition, the pose will strengthen and relax the pelvic ligaments and joints after childbirth.

When your baby is about four months old, try supporting him in the same position. This will help to strengthen his spine and maintain flexibility of the hip joints. From this position, your child will learn to support himself using his hands, and will then push up to start sitting on his own.

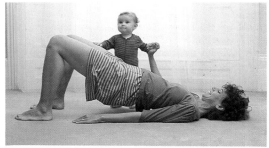

9 Pelvic lift
See exercise 16, p. 257. This strengthens and tones the buttocks and thighs, as well as strengthening the lower back and spine and relaxing the head and neck.

a

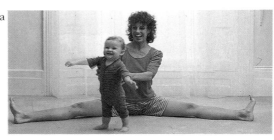

a

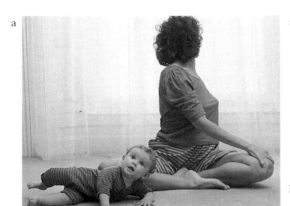

b

b

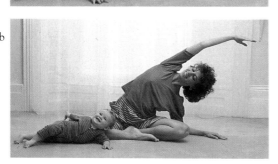

10 Sitting twist and side bends

Twisting will lubricate the spine, relax the pelvic area and help you recover your waistline; do not be surprised if you hear your spine click as you turn. Side bends will stretch the muscles along your sides – also helping the waistline – as well as the intercostal muscles in the chest. These exercises are also quick energy restorers.

a Sit with knees wide apart and feet tucked in towards the groin, while keeping your back straight and your shoulders relaxed.

● Become aware of your breathing and of both buttock bones in contact with the floor.

● Place your left hand on your right knee, and your right hand palm down on the floor behind you. Gently twist round, rotating your spine.

● Look round over your right shoulder and hold, breathing deeply into your belly for a moment.

● Relax and come forward again.

● Repeat the movement on the other side.

b While in the same position, bend over to the left. Place your left elbow and your left hand (palm down) on the floor.

● While keeping your right knee moving down towards the floor, stretch up your right arm and bring it up over your head.

● Hold for a few seconds, breathing deeply, and then repeat on the other side.

11 Sitting with legs wide apart and side bends

These exercises open the pelvis, maintain flexibility of the hip joints and stretch the hamstrings and inner thigh muscles. The movements will release tension in the inner thighs and groin, will condition and tone all the pelvic organs, and will correct the tilt of your pelvis, strengthening your spine and the sacral region. The side bends will also help restore your waistline and open your chest. Do each movement only once, and hold them for a minute or two – depending on how you feel.

a Sit with your legs as wide apart as possible, lifting your buttock muscles so that your weight rests on the buttock bones.

● Keeping your spine straight, extend your heels, bringing up your toes towards your body. If it is difficult to straighten your spine, try sitting on a folded blanket.

b Try lifting one arm over your head and bending sideways as far as you can manage without strain. It is essential to keep both hips down and avoid going beyond your limit. Repeat on the other side.

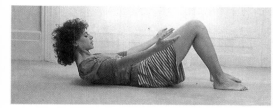

12 Abdominal toners

These movements work the abdominal muscles, helping to restore firm muscle tone without stressing the lower back or abdominal organs.
- Lie on your back with your knees bent and the soles of your feet flat on the floor.
- Breathe deeply. As you exhale, lift your head and arms, with your palms facing upward. At first, lift your head 5–8cm (2–3in) off the floor, gradually increasing with practice.
- Hold this position for a second or two, then exhale.
- Repeat about ten times, keeping your feet firmly on the ground.

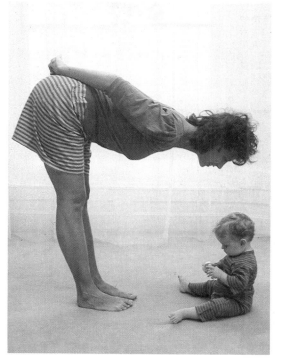

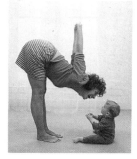
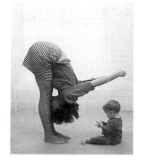

13 Forward bend

See exercise 12, page 255. This will stretch and relax both the pelvic floor and the hamstrings at the backs of your legs, which will increase your energy and lessen fatigue.

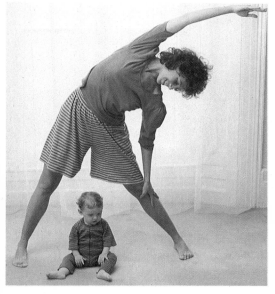

14 Side bends

These will stretch the muscles along your sides, and help restore your waistline. Repeat on both sides.
- Stand with your feet parallel to each other, 1m (3ft) apart.
- Bend over to the left, allowing your left arm to reach down your left leg.
- Lift your right arm up over your head, and breathe deeply into the stretch. Hold briefly, then come up as you exhale. Now bend to the right.

15 Sitting between your feet

See exercise 18, page 258. These movements will stretch the front of your body, especially the thigh and abdominal muscles, and will strengthen the lower back. They will also benefit all the abdominal and pelvic organs, and will enhance digestion.

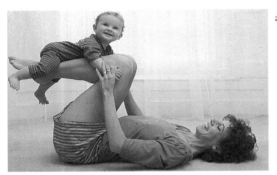

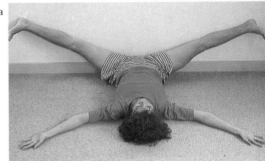

a

b

16 Baby bounce

This exercise, which is great fun for your baby, will relax your lower back while working your thighs.
- Lie on your back on the floor.
- Bend your knees, pulling them up to your chest.
- Put your baby on your shins and hold his hands.
- 'Bounce' your baby by moving your legs.

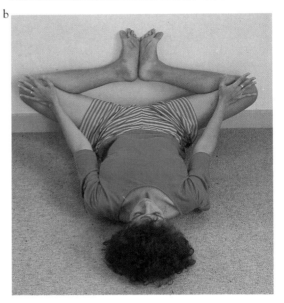

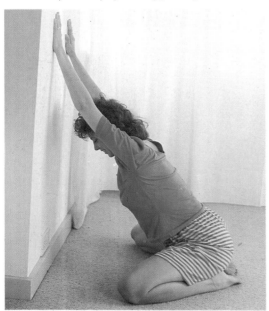

17 Kneeling shoulder stretch

See exercise 15, page 269. This will stretch the front of your body, releasing tension from the shoulders, chest and upper arms. It will also stretch the muscles that support your breasts, and will open the rib cage, improving general respiration and reducing any congestion. Practised regularly, this will loosen your shoulders, help tension headaches and provide relaxation and relief after hours of nursing and carrying your baby.

18 Legs apart on a wall

See exercise 4, page 249. This will lengthen and relax the inner thigh muscles, open the chest and release the shoulders. Because it promotes the return of blood from the legs to the upper body, it can help alleviate varicose veins and piles. Practised for five to ten minutes daily, it is deeply relaxing, and can be a great help if you are tired or lacking in energy. This exercise also has a beneficial, relaxing effect on the pelvic floor and uterus.

a Open your legs and allow gravity to draw them apart as far as they will go.

b Bend your knees and bring the soles of your feet together. Press your knees towards the wall with your hands.

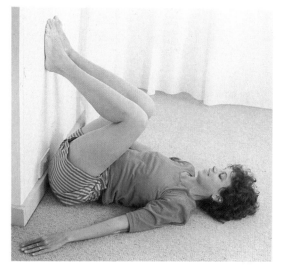

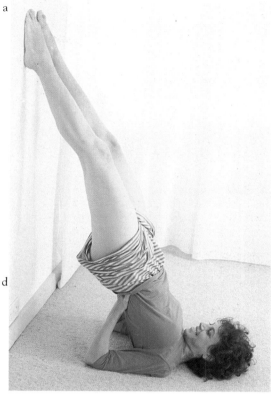

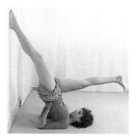

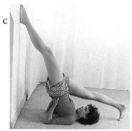

19 Shoulder stand

This will release tension in the shoulders, neck and hamstrings, and will strengthen the lower back and abdominal muscles. It will also stimulate the endocrine (i.e. hormonal) system, and will have a stimulating effect on the circulation. In addition, the pelvic floor and uterus will be toned, and a prolapsed uterus may be strengthened. Finally, it is deeply relaxing and calming. If you only have a little time to devote to exercising each day, try combining this with exercise 18 and doing them whenever you have 15 minutes to spare.

a Adopt the same position as in exercise 18, but bend your knees and keep them and your feet together, with your soles flat on the wall. Place your arms by your sides and tuck your elbows into your waist.

● Pressing with your feet, lift your trunk, raising your spine until your weight is resting on your shoulders and the back of your neck and head.

b Support your back with your hands as near to your head as possible. Breathe your elbows down.

● Straighten your legs, keeping the soles of your feet on the wall and your buttock muscles tight.

● Breathe deeply. As you inhale, tighten your pelvic-floor muscles, drawing them down towards your navel. Let go as you exhale. Repeat several times.

● As you exhale, return to the resting position, lowering your spine to the ground one vertebra at a time until the whole spine is in contact with the floor.

● Relax and breathe deeply, then roll on to your side and come up slowly.

c While in the shoulder stand, bring your left leg up over your head towards the floor, extending your heel.

● Hold for a moment or two, then bring your leg back up to the wall.

● Repeat with the right leg.

d If you can do exercise 18c easily, repeat the movements and touch the floor with your toe.

a

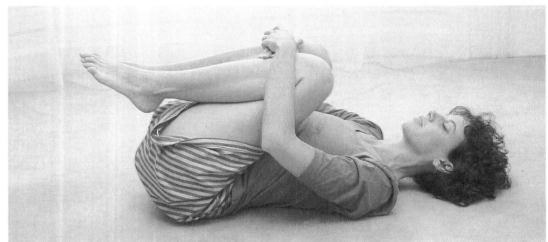

b

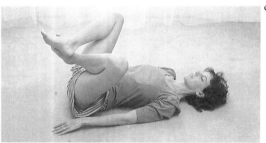

c

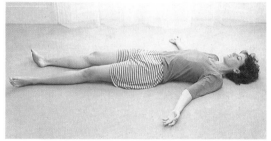

20 Resting

a Lie down on your back and bring your knees up to your chest, holding them there with your hands.

Breathe deeply into your belly, feeling your lower back relaxing every time you exhale.

Remain in this position for up to five minutes.

b Lie on your back with your hands by your sides, palms down, and your knees bent and ankles crossed. Rotate your hips, describing a large circle with your lower back.

Make five or six circles. Then reverse and rotate in the opposite direction.

c Lie on your back on the floor with your eyes closed. Extend your legs out in front of you and spread them comfortably apart.

Spread your arms out to either side, palms up.

Breathe deeply into your belly, relaxing and releasing tension in your body, starting with the toes, through the legs to the pelvis and genital area.

Breathe into your belly, chest, shoulders and down your arms to your fingertips.

Feel the way in which the back of your body is in contact with the floor, and imagine it is melting into the ground.

Relax the nape of your neck as well as all the little muscles of your face around the eyes, ears, nose and mouth, and release your jaws and throat.

Try to eliminate any thoughts that arise, focusing on the ebb and flow of your breathing for a while.

When you are ready, open your eyes and wriggle your fingers and toes. Stretch and get up in your own time.

C H A P T E R   2 1

MASSAGE

Through massage, we have the power to heal, comfort, soothe, stimulate and relax each other, and there is no more appropriate time to do this than during pregnancy. With most mammals, it is common for stimulation of the skin – for example, licking – to increase during this time, and many women find sensitive massage both pleasurable and necessary to enhance relaxation and to soothe away the minor aches and pains of pregnancy.

Massage is an intuitive and creative method of communication, helping both the person doing the massage (the *masseur*) and the person being massaged (the *subject*) to 'tune in' to each other, to discover a new way of being close and in harmony. It is a way of expressing tenderness and affection which is deeply sensuous and comforting without necessarily being directly sexual.

Our tactile sense is highly developed long before we are born, and throughout our lives, the touching and stimulation of our skin has a profound effect on us, enhancing both physical and psychological well-being. Learning to communicate with each other through touch during pregnancy can be invaluable in labour. The techniques described in this chapter were taught to the authors by Stephen Russell.

Learning to massage

Many methods of massage are practised throughout the world. Most of them originated in the East where, for centuries, massage has been a feature of daily life, particularly during pregnancy and after birth. The system described below is derived from a highly effective yet simple one used by the Taoists in China and based on the principles of acupuncture, which works at a profound level to stimulate the organs, release tension and help the person as a whole to achieve balance.

Rather than massaging the muscles directly, this type of massage follows subtle *meridians*, lines of energy which flow throughout the body. In the Chinese system there are 12 of these, and each organ is connected to a meridian at a number of points, known as *acupuncture points*. For example, there are 45 acupuncture points at which the specific energy of the stomach can be contacted and influenced. All the meridians are linked to each other so that, together, they form a continuous loop throughout the body.

With massage, we can affect the meridians to strengthen the flow of energy in the body and invigorate and purify it. This is done by stimulating individual acupuncture points – touching them for a fraction of a second as the hand passes by, making simple repetitive movements, and pausing before applying pressure. This will ensure the proper functioning of the organs, and will release pent-up energy or blockages caused by tension and stress. Although it can take years to learn all the individual acupuncture points, the movements themselves come naturally, and expertise is quickly gained as your intuitive sense of touch begins to surface.

Massage is particularly helpful in late pregnancy as a way to relieve the stress and discomfort that may arise as the spine adjusts to accommodate the extra weight of the uterus. As you approach the birth, this discomfort may increase, and massage may be given more frequently. Techniques which work on the back, buttocks, thighs and abdomen may be useful during labour, and a rapport built up during pregnancy will help you direct your partner to the ones which are of maximum benefit at the time. In addition, by massaging throughout pregnancy, your confidence will increase so that, by the time your baby is born, you will be ready to massage her effectively.

Practised regularly, massage will produce an immediate and obvious feeling of relaxation, and its deeper effects may last for weeks. It is completely safe, provided you follow the signals from your subject's body and only increase pressure if and when it is comfortable. The effects of massage will be optimal if both of you adopt, in turn, the roles of masseur and subject.

For many, massaging or being massaged may be an entirely new experience. However, it is not necessary to be an expert in anatomy or to learn any complicated techniques. What follows is intended as a guide to help you discover and enhance your own natural, intuitive skills.

Preparing for massage

Choose a time when you will not be disturbed, and arrange the room so that it is comfortable and warm, with soft lighting and perhaps some tranquil music. You will need a pile of cushions and a flat surface on which the subject will lie – a carpeted floor or a large bed are both suitable. Have a cover handy so that the parts of the body not being massaged can be kept warm. You will also need a vegetable oil – e.g. almond, olive or coconut.

It is essential that both the subject and the masseur are comfortable during the massage. The massage techniques outlined below involve positions that are likely to be the most comfortable for a woman during pregnancy and labour. If you are uncomfortable lying on your back, massage can easily be performed while you lie on your side. After the birth, massage using a reclining position, either on your back or on your front.

Pressure
The amount of pressure used can vary from a featherlight touch with the fingertips to a much firmer and deeper one, and both can be effective and powerful when used appropriately. It is best to employ a light touch to begin with, and then to increase the pressure gradually, 'listening' with your hands and never forcing your will on the subject. This is especially important when massaging a highly sensitive person such as a woman in labour or a young baby.

Massage should cease immediately if the subject indicates any discomfort. It is essential to bear this in mind when practising massage techniques that may be useful during labour. Remember that, although many women find massage in labour invaluable, some prefer not to be touched at all.

Hand movements

There are three basic hand movements:

  Stroking may be performed with all the fingers held together, or with one or two fingers only, or with the whole hand (fingers and palm).

  Holding involves using the fingertips or thumbs to exert an even pressure, with the hand(s) held in one place for a minute or so. If you encounter tension, reduce the pressure; it can subsequently be sensitively increased as the tension is released beneath your fingers.

  Percussion is difficult to describe but easy to perform. The shoulders, elbows and forearms are kept heavy but loose. The hands flop at the wrists as they beat rapidly up and down, as if you are drumming. The point of contact is the fingertips, or the outer edges of the little fingers as the hands are held in loose fists.

Warming up

Start by breathing together (*see* p. 239–40) to tune in to each other; relaxed deep abdominal breathing should continue throughout the massage. The masseur should look inward at his or her own body, relaxing and releasing any tension in the muscles of the jaws, shoulders, arms and abdomen and around the eyes. Meditate for a few seconds on your intention to heal, relax and soothe your partner. Rub your hands together vigorously to warm and energize them. After the massage, shake your hands loosely and vigorously from the wrists to release tension.

Massage for pregnancy

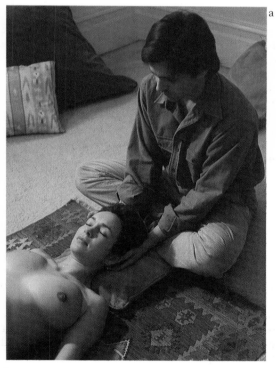
a

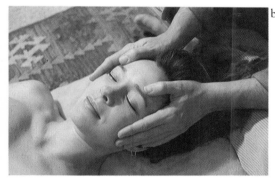
b

1 Face massage
The subject lies down flat, or with a few cushions under her back and head if lying flat is uncomfortable, and with a cushion under her knees to relax her back. The masseur then sits comfortably behind her head.
a Place your hands under the subject's head and slowly draw them backwards, gently stretching her neck, moving the head away from the feet.
b Place the fingers of both hands under her head with the heels of the hands held gently over the temporal bones above and slightly in front of each ear. Be aware of the rhythm of your breathing and that of the subject.

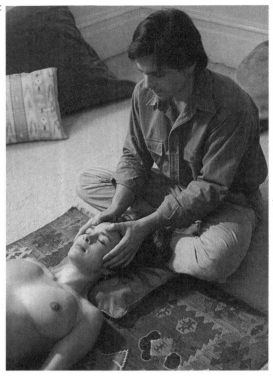

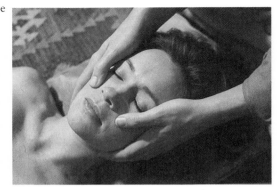

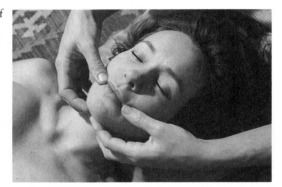

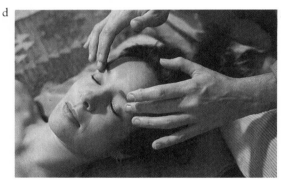

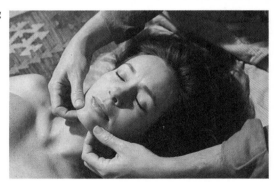

c Place your thumbs on the centre of her forehead about 1.5 cm (½ in) above the eyebrows, and lightly and slowly pull them away from each other towards the temples. Using a light, firm, even pressure, repeat the movement, smoothing away tension with your thumbs. This movement is very calming and reduces anxiety. Continue slowly for a minute or so.
d Rest your thumbs on the middle of her hairline, and place your middle fingers on the outside edge of each eye. Massage along the base under the eye towards the nose. Go round the inner corners of the eyes, and then along the eyebrows towards the ears. With featherlight pressure, continue circling the eyes slowly.

e Use your thumbs to massage across her cheekbones from midway down the nose to the bottom of the ears. Using a slightly firmer, even pressure, repeat the movement slowly for up to a minute.
f Massage her chin by placing your index fingers under the jawbone and your thumbs on the chin, one below each corner of the mouth. Circle your thumbs in the opposite directions, using a gentle yet firm pressure to move the flesh over the bone. Repeat for a minute.
g Work your way along her jawbone, starting with your fingers under the ears, and your thumbs moving outward from the centre of the chin towards the ears. Repeat slowly for up to a minute.

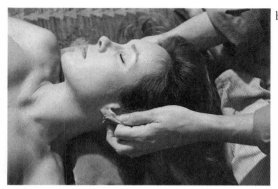

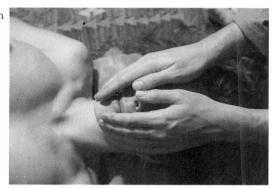

h Place your fingers behind her ears and your thumbs inside them. First, keep your fingers still to steady the ears while you massage every fold and crevice within the ears with your thumbs. Then keep your thumbs still while you massage behind the ears with your fingers. Cover every part, including the lobes. Continue for a few minutes, until the ears feel hot.

i Place one hand lightly over each cheek. Gently smooth your hands apart to reveal the features. Repeat slowly several times, at the end lifting your hands from the face very gently. Shake your hands loosely from the wrists.

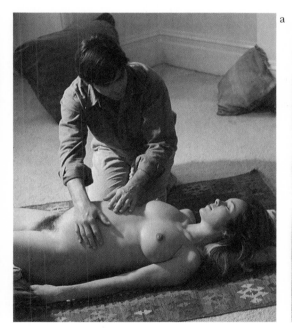

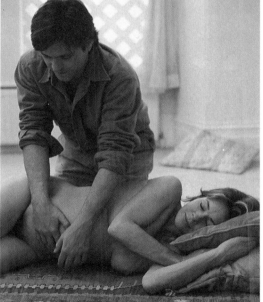

2 Belly massage

Position yourselves comfortably, with the masseur sitting or kneeling beside the subject. The latter should lie on her back with her head and knees supported by cushions, or on her side if this is more comfortable. Place your hands very lightly on her belly and become aware of the rhythm of your breathing and hers, and of the presence of the baby in her womb. Meditate on the baby's sensitivity to your touch.

a Using firm but gentle pressure, rub round and round the navel in a clockwise direction. Repeat gently.
b With the subject on her side, place both hands over and under her belly so that you feel as if you are supporting the baby. With firm and even pressure, draw your hands over the sides of the belly in an alternating rhythm. Continue for a few minutes.
c Now try techniques 1, 2, 3, 5, 6 and 7 in the baby massage section (pp. 284–5).

3

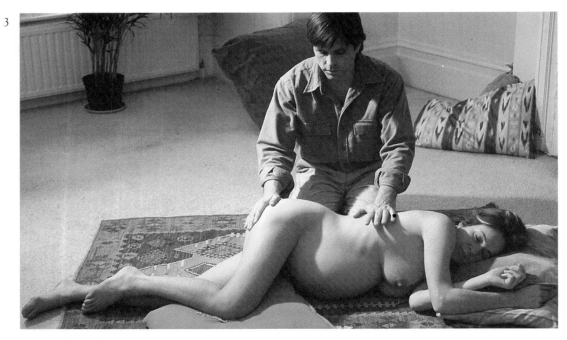

4

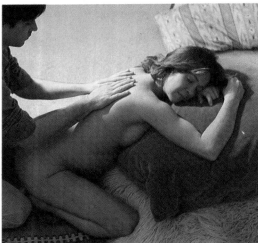

3 Hip massage

The masseur should sit or kneel comfortably beside the
subject, who should lie on one side with her head well
supported by cushions and an extra one placed under
the knee touching the floor.

Place one hand on the subject's hip and keep the
other in contact with her body. Using the whole
hand, rub from below and up and over the buttock,
over the base of the hip, around the top of the thigh
and back over the buttock again. The movement is a
circle covering the large mound made by the hip.
Using firm but gentle pressure, repeat the movement,
each circle taking about four seconds. Continue for
one or two minutes. Repeat on other hip.

4 Back massage

The masseur should kneel or sit comfortably behind the
subject, who will kneel forward over a pile of
cushions so that her trunk is completely supported. (A
non-pregnant subject can lie flat on his or her belly.)
a Using your middle fingers, massage down either side
of the spine from top to bottom with a firm but gentle
pressure. When you reach the sacrum at the base of
the spine, separate your hands, with one going over
each buttock. Draw them up the sides of the torso,
pulling upwards towards the armpits, then circle them
over the shoulder blades and back down the sides of
the spine. Repeat in a slow rhythm, continuing for
about three minutes.
b Try techniques 7, 9, 10 and 11 in the baby massage
section (pp. 285-6).

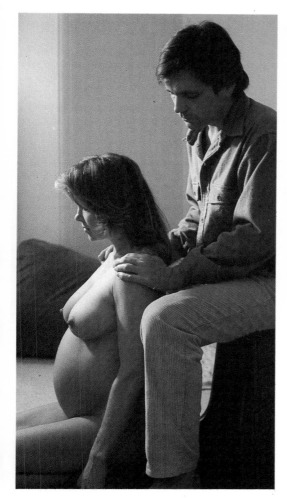

5

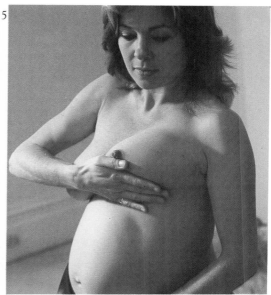

6

5 Shoulder massage

The subject should sit or kneel, and the masseur should stand, sit or kneel comfortably behind her. Using the whole of the palms or just the fingers, stroke with firm, even pressure from below each ear, down over the shoulder ridges and shoulder tips, over the deltoid muscles in the upper arms, and down the outside of the upper arms to the elbows. Each stroke should take about four seconds, and should be continued for up to 2–3 minutes.

6 Breast massage

This technique is useful for preparing the breasts for breastfeeding and for lubricating and softening the skin, and should be performed after bathing.

The ducts that carry breastmilk run from the outside of the breasts to the nipples, like the spokes of a wheel. With fingers held together, massage down from the circumference towards the nipples, stroking with the palms, then down the fingers. It is useful to regard the entire breast as a clock, and to work from '1 o'clock' to '2 o'clock' and so on, round the breast. The nipples can be gently massaged with almond oil.

Breast massage can continue after the birth; combined with the baby's sucking, it will help to ease engorgement or clear a blocked duct.

7 Perineal massage

During the last weeks of pregnancy, it is helpful to prepare the perineum for birth by increasing its elasticity and thus lessening the likelihood of a tear. This is easier to do if you are in a squatting position. Great sensitivity is needed when massaging this part of the body.

Oil is placed on the fingers which are then inserted into the vaginal opening; using a downward pressure, spread and flatten the perineum from side to side. Start with two fingers, and then, with practice, increase the pressure and the number of fingers, eventually using three or four. Alternatively, you may prefer to use your thumb. Gently stretching the perineum from side to side using the index fingers of both hands will also increase its elasticity, as will a kneading action using the forefinger and thumb of one hand.

Massage for labour

Massage can be performed during labour, using a light talcum powder or oil to reduce friction on the skin. In pre-labour, massage can be relaxing and calming. However, women vary tremendously in their need for or acceptance of massage.

It can be done in different ways, depending on the woman's preference. The time between contractions is for resting, relaxing and replenishing energy, so massage should be light and soothing, and it should take energy to the extremities by concentrating on the face, upper spine and limbs. The actual stroking is usually featherlight to calm and soothe, unless more pressure is appropriate. During a contraction, a different type of energy may be needed. Then, the pressure applied to the skin may be light or firm, and the massage often centres on the lower spine and the sacrum, from which the nerves supplying the uterus emerge.

However, any comforting massage can be used safely during labour. For some, merely having someone hold a hand on their sacrum or lower back is sufficient, while others may need a more vigorous massage. The latter can be done in any position except when the woman lies on her back. In a labour where back pain is a problem, massage can be an essential form of pain relief, and back massage is easy to perform if the woman in labour kneels and leans forward or stands.

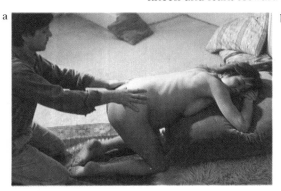

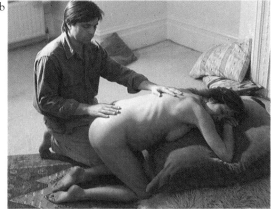

1 Lower back massage
a With the woman in a kneeling position, press your thumbs on the coccyx (the tailbone) at the base of the spine, moving up towards the sacro-iliac joints. The woman may like to direct her movements down towards your thumbs, thus creating just the right degree of pressure to ease pain in the lower back.
b Using your index fingers and palms make a gentle but firm circular movement over the lower back, harmonizing with the movements the woman may be making. At the same time, move your other hand softly over her back.
Alternatively, start in the middle of the sacrum and, using both hands, 'spread' the energy out over the buttocks towards and even down the thighs.
c Using the heel of your hand, apply firm, gentle pressure to the coccyx.

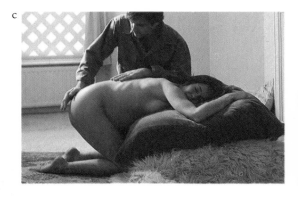

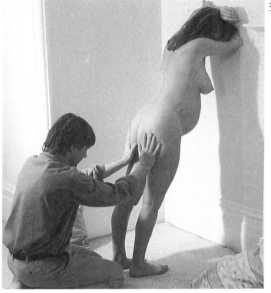

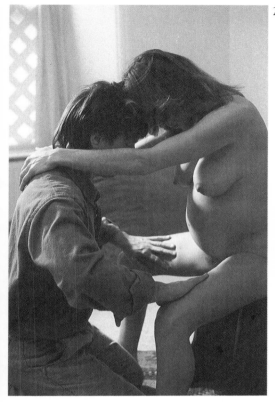

3 Leg massage

With the woman standing and leaning forward against a wall, and starting from the lower back, gently but firmly stroke down the centre line of the back of each leg towards the outer ankle. Repeat many times, each stroke taking about six seconds.

2 Inner thigh massage

With the woman sitting comfortably upright in a chair or on the floor or bed supported by cushions, place one hand on each of her knees, palms down and fingertips pointing towards each other. Slowly stroke up the inner sides of the thighs, over the fronts, then down over the outer sides and over the knees, starting again on the inner thighs. Continue in a slow, gentle rhythm for a minute or so, and then rest before starting again.

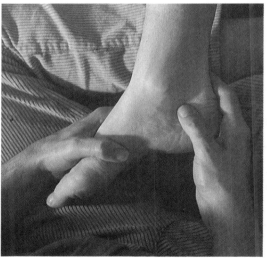

4 Foot massage

Massage the feet, concentrating on the fleshy parts of the heels behind the ankle bones, and making small, firm circles with your thumbs on the inner and outer sides of the feet.

Massage after the birth

In the East, massage is considered an essential to aid recovery from childbirth. It should be performed as regularly as possible, paying particular attention to the back and abdomen to help the spinal column settle back into its normal position and the uterus to regain its previous size. The pressure used should initially be very light, gradually increasing in intensity. Breast massage is also valuable at this time.

Baby massage

Babies enjoy being massaged from the first few days after birth, and practised daily, it can be a highly pleasurable and beneficial activity. Although it is a fairly new concept in the West, baby massage has been a common practice elsewhere for many centuries. It is particularly important in Eastern cultures.

Most mammals spend a great deal of time licking and fondling their young, and this skin contact and stimulation is necessary for healthy development. Through touch, a baby learns to experience pleasure; it enhances non-verbal communication between parent and child; and it is an invaluable way to give your baby a sense of well-being and relaxation. Another important benefit is that you will be able to help your baby release tension, which often arises as part of his adjustment to living outside the womb. Some babies adjust rapidly, but others may take several weeks to become comfortable and, for them, massage can be a way to smooth the transition. It can also be very useful if your baby is out of sorts or ill.

Many parents are concerned that, if they massage their babies, they might injure them, especially the very delicate, soft abdomen before the cord stump has dropped off. However, babies will soon tell you if you are intruding into a tense or painful area. In addition, the more tender areas in the abdomen can be relaxed indirectly by working on the baby's feet, ears, hands and back.

Preparation for baby massage

If you have practised massage during pregnancy, the techniques that follow will already be familiar to you. If not, try out one or two on an adult before starting on your baby. Abdominal and back massage are the most important techniques because many of the tensions experienced by a newborn are centred in the abdomen as the baby adjusts to drinking and digesting milk for the first time.

Newborns often have a relatively short attention span so the massage sequence should consist of only a few repetitions of each technique. It is best to perform a full sequence every day. How this is arranged obviously depends on both the masseur and the baby: some couples prefer to do the entire sequence once a day, whereas others split it up, doing only two or three techniques at varying times throughout the day. The advantage of doing the entire sequence is that your baby will become used to the feelings of well-being, confidence and buoyancy that this produces.

Each technique will have different beneficial effects on the body, and any that the baby does not enjoy should be sensitively explored to uncover any underlying tensions.

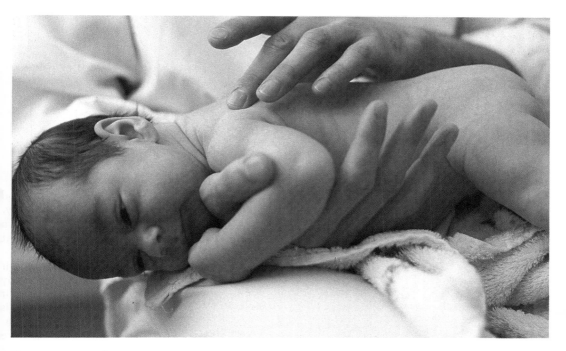

Getting started

Baby massage can be performed anywhere, but its benefits are optimal if a special setting is provided – i.e. a room that is warm with low lighting and tranquil music. Choose a time when he is not hungry and is likely to enjoy it. Ideally your baby should lie on a comfortable duvet or towel spread out on a carpeted floor. It is best to do massage when the baby is naked – especially after bathing – but it can be performed through the baby's clothing.

Massage may be performed without oil or powder, but a light dusting of talcum powder or a thin coating of a pure oil (e.g. almond or olive) will reduce friction and tone the baby's skin. It is important to keep your fingernails short, to avoid scratching him.

You can kneel on the carpet and sit upright, Japanese style, on the backs of your heels, keeping your spine straight. Alternatively, you may prefer to sit cross-legged, or with your back supported by a wall and the baby lying across your thighs. At other times, it may be more appropriate to put the baby on a bed or even hold him in the crook of your arm and use your free hand to do the massage

Before beginning, relax your jaw, eye, shoulder, arm and abdominal muscles. Your breathing should be rhythmic and flow evenly. When massaging, breathe deeply, allowing your abdomen to expand as your lungs fill with air, and continue to be aware of your breathing and the state of tension in your body.

Warm your hands before touching your baby, and if you are using it, place a little oil or powder in your palms. Begin with a very light touch and gradually increase the pressure as you become more confident and your baby gets used to being massaged. (*See* p. 274 for a description of the various kinds of pressure you can use.)

The techniques

1

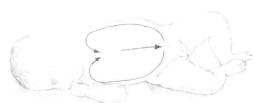

2

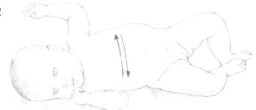

1 Chest and belly massage

With your baby lying face up, use the fingers of both hands to stroke down the midline of his torso from the chest to the pubic bone. Then separate your hands, move them to the sides of the torso and pull up into the armpits. Circle over each side of the chest and meet again on the midline.

Repeat the cycle with a slow and quite steady pressure, continuing for up to three minutes. Each cycle should last about ten seconds.

Benefits: calms; relaxes chest; balances heart and kidneys; strengthens digestive system.

2 Upper abdomen massage

With your baby lying face up, sit on his right side. You will be massaging across the upper abdomen in a band midway between the nipples and the navel, using a light touch of the fingertips or palms. Start by moving from left to right, with one hand deftly following the other to simulate a wave-like effect. After up to 180 strokes, the process is reversed, with you sitting on your baby's left and massaging from right to left. Rest for a second or two before changing direction.

Benefits: harmonizes liver and spleen; regulates digestive system; aids respiratory system and blood production; relaxes entire body.

3

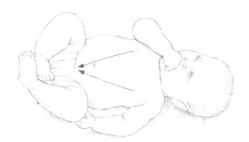

4

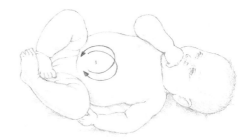

3 Diagonal abdomen massage

With your baby lying face up and using a featherlight pressure, run your fingertips diagonally down from, first, the left and then the right nipple to the centre of the pubic ridge at the base of the abdomen. Continue for a minute or so.

Benefits: regulates eating patterns; stimulates spleen, liver, kidneys, intestines and bladder.

4 Circling the navel

With your baby lying face up, use your fingertips to rub round and round the navel, first anti-clockwise and then clockwise, using gentle, steady pressure. Continue for a minute or so in each direction, but avoid the clockwise movement if your child has diarrhoea. This very natural movement can be performed without undressing your baby.

Benefits: eases constipation (clockwise) and diarrhoea (anti-clockwise); stimulates bladder, bowels, pancreas and stomach; strengthens liver.

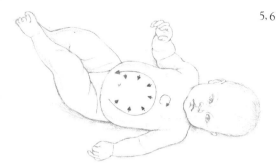

5, 6

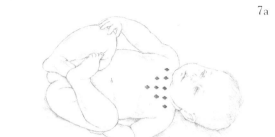

7a

5 Abdominal acupressure

Perhaps the most beneficial daily technique, this involves a few seconds of pressure on one spot, waiting for tension to release and then moving on to the next.

With your baby lying face up, visualize an inverted horseshoe shape on his abdomen, with the navel at the centre. Starting at the bottom right-hand corner, press lightly, with your fingertips pointing diagonally down towards the spine. Wait until your baby's body 'invites you in', and then allow your fingers to sink a little deeper. If you meet resistance at any point, never force your way in but let your fingers rest until the tension disappears. Slowly move around the horseshoe from right to left, releasing tight spots as you go. Each circuit of the horseshoe should last about three minutes.

This can also be used on a pregnant woman, when the horseshoe shape is wider and the points lie around the edge of the uterus.

Benefits: alleviates and prevents colic, constipation and indigestion; stimulates colon, stomach, liver, spleen and diaphragm; reduces sleeplessness and anxiety; deeply relaxes entire body.

6 Breastbone massage

With your baby face up or cradled in the crook of your arm, place two fingers on the chest at a point midway between the nipples. Use only enough pressure to move the skin in a small clockwise circle against the underlying breastbone. Continue for up to two or three minutes, each circle taking about ten seconds.
Benefits: stimulates heart and lung function; opens heart centre; regulates sleep patterns; calms and pacifies.

7b

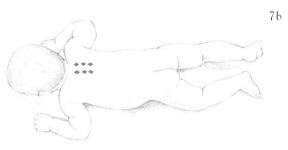

7 Percussion of the chest and upper back

Babies usually love this technique. Holding your hands in loose fists and keeping your wrists floppy, lightly and repeatedly tap the baby's body with the outer (little finger) side of your fists. Start slowly; with practice, the movements will speed up. Continue for up to three minutes.
a *Chest percussion:* With your baby face up, find a point midway between the nipples, and then one point on each of the collarbones which is directly in line with one of the nipples. Percuss in the centre of the triangle made by these three points.
b *Upper back percussion:* With your baby face down, visualize a band between the shoulder blades, and percuss in the area on either side of the spine.
Benefits: beneficial to respiratory system and heart; relaxes chest; induces relaxation and sleep.

8

9

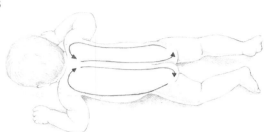

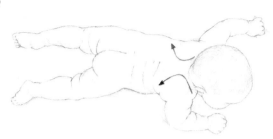

8 Full back massage

This technique is particularly beneficial and should be practised as frequently as possible. With your baby face down and using gentle pressure, massage down both sides of the spine from top to bottom with your middle fingers. When you reach the base of the spine, separate your hands, placing one over each buttock. Now draw your hands up the sides of the torso, lightly pulling up towards the armpits. Then circle your hands over the shoulder blades and on down both sides of the spine again. Continue for up to three minutes.

You can also try doing this with your baby lying across your thighs, or held upright, in which case use the index and middle fingers of one hand when massaging down the sides of the spine.

Benefits: invigorates lungs, heart, liver, spleen, kidneys and digestive system; strengthens back and spine; prevents sleeplessness.

9 Shoulder blade release

With your baby face down and using gentle pressure, massage down the back along the line of the shoulder blades with your middle fingers. Complete the triangle by massaging along their outer and upper edges. Repeat for up to two minutes, each stroke taking up to ten seconds.

Benefits: beneficial to lungs; releases tension from shoulders; stimulates acupuncture points which benefit intestines.

10

11

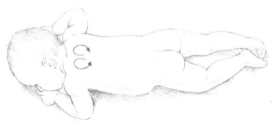

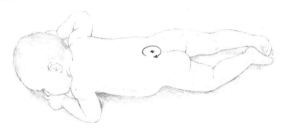

10 Upper back massage

With your baby face down and using a gentle, even pressure, place your fingers on the ridges of the shoulders, one hand on each side, and use your thumbs to circle around the fleshy parts above and between the shoulder blades. Continue for up to five minutes.

Benefits: relaxes neck and shoulders; releases tension from lungs; invigorates whole body.

11 Lower back massage

With your baby face down, use your palm to rub the lower back in a clockwise motion, taking a point on the second lumbar vertebra (directly behind the navel) as the centre. Use a firm enough pressure to create mild friction and heat, and move slowly, continuing for up to three minutes.

Benefits: strengthens lower back; stimulates energy flow in kidneys.

12

13

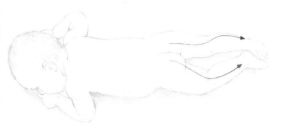

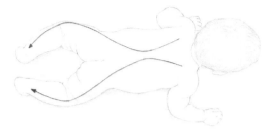

12 Back leg massage

With your baby face down, place a thumb on each buttock and gently stroke down the centre line of the back of each leg to the outer ankle. Use a gentle, even pressure, becoming slightly firmer as you get to the high point of the calf. Each stroke should take about six seconds, and the whole exercise can be continued for up to three minutes.
Benefits: releases tension; strengthens legs; indirectly benefits colon and bladder.

13 Brushing down

With your baby face down, place a hand on each shoulder blade. Lightly stroke your fingertips down to the kidney region, where the hands should meet and then separate out to the hips and down the outer sides of the legs – a light, sweeping gesture. Each stroke should take about ten seconds, and can be repeated for up to two minutes.
Benefits: clears energy; relaxes head, chest and abdomen; boosts kidneys.

15

14

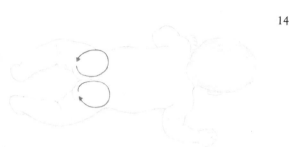

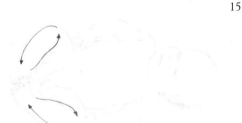

14 Hip massage

With your baby lying on one side, use your index finger to describe a circle, starting below the buttock, then going up and over the hip bone, around the top of the thigh and up over the buttock again, using firm, even pressure. Each circle should take about four seconds, and the movement can be repeated for up to three minutes. Repeat on the other side.
Benefits: relieves constipation; releases tension from hips and lower back; stimulates energy flow between head and feet; calms.

15 Lower leg massage

With your baby face up, use your thumbs to massage from the inside of each ankle to the inner side of each knee. Then circle your palms over the knees, and using your fingertips, massage down the edges of the shins, from the knees to the outer ankles. Each cycle should take about ten seconds.

Before or after doing this, try loosely jiggling the baby's legs from the hips, holding the ankles in your hands.
Benefits: stimulates energy; regulates digestive system and bowels.

16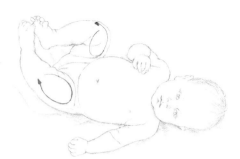

17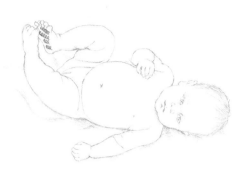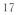

16 Thigh massage

With your baby face up, place one hand on each knee, palms down and fingers on the inside. Slowly stroke up the inner sides of the thighs and over the tops. Pull your hands down over the outer sides of the thighs and over the knees, and start again on the inner sides of the thighs. Start gently, increasing pressure gradually; the baby's legs will pull back and relax in time with the motion. Continue for up to three minutes, each cycle taking about ten seconds.

Benefits: releases tension from hips, thighs and genitals; strengthens circulation; increases vitality.

17 Foot massage

With your baby face up or sitting, use your thumb to make small circling movements across the sole of one foot, massaging from the outer edge of the sole under the toes to the inner edge in a horizontal line. Gradually move this line down towards the heel, massaging across for about three seconds before moving down. Massage at least once across every part of the sole, and then let your intuition take over as you massage the whole foot. Repeat on the other foot.

Turn your baby over and try percussing the sole of each foot with your fingerpads, as if you were tapping an hourglass to make the sand run faster. Continue for up to a minute.

Benefits: draws energy towards lower part of body; reduces tension in feet; stimulates whole body.

18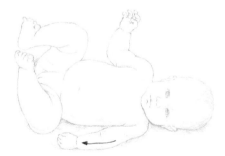

19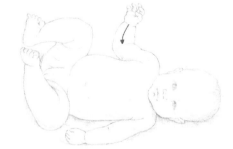

18 Outer forearm massage

With your baby face up, use your thumb or index finger to stroke down the centre line of the forearm from the elbow down the top side of the arm to the back of the wrist. Use a gentle, firm pressure. Each stroke should last three to four seconds, and can be repeated for up to two minutes on each forearm.

Benefits: draws energy away from ears (thus alleviating ear infections); releases tension indirectly from diaphragm; stimulates brain.

19 Inner forearm massage

With your baby facing you, hold one arm so that the palm is turned upward. With your index finger, run up the centre of the inner side of the forearm, from wrist crease to elbow crease. Use the lightest possible pressure, and repeat for up to two to three minutes on each forearm, each stroke taking two to three seconds.

Benefits: strengthens kidneys; brightens awareness; calms.

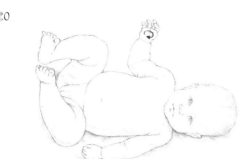

20 Palm massage

With your baby face up, use your thumb and index finger to make circles on one of the baby's palms. Repeat on other palm.
Benefits: stimulates reflex points to whole body; draws excess energy away from head.

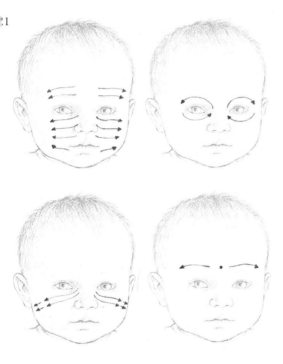

21 Face massage

Use technique no. 1 in the massage for pregnancy (see p. 275). Some babies are sensitive about having their faces touched, and it may not be possible to start this until your child is about six months old. At whatever age, begin with a very light pressure, and preferably practise on an adult first.

General movements

To prepare your baby for the development of mobility and to relax him, try these movements at the end of the massage sequence. Start gently and slowly, making sure that he is enjoying the experience. If he indicates discomfort, stop immediately and try another time.
Space flying Lift your baby, holding him firmly with one hand around either side of the chest. Move him in circles around an imaginary sphere with a diameter of about 60 cm (2ft). Make rhythmic circles in every possible plane – vertical, horizontal and diagonal – first anti-clockwise and then clockwise.
Back arching Sit with your back supported by a wall, and bend your knees. With your baby lying face up on your thighs, gradually allow his head to extend back over your knees so that he arches and gently extends his spine. He should enjoy this movement, which will strengthen the spine and promote head control.
Upside down Start this when your child is about six weeks old, and build up gradually to the full movement. Make sure that your hands are dry and also oil-free. Sit against a wall with your back supported and legs extended, and your baby lying face up on your thighs. Place your hands firmly on his hips, with your thumbs and index fingers nearest his feet. Gently and slowly lift him up, raising his legs, spine, neck and finally his head until his whole body is suspended. Hold this position as long as your baby enjoys it, and then gently lower his head, neck, spine and finally legs back on to your thighs.
Hip release Hold the baby upright, facing you, with one hand around either side of his chest. Using a slight, gentle, side-to-side motion, make his hips swing independently of his rib cage like a pendulum.
Leg shaking With your baby lying face up, hold his legs lightly by the ankles, one in each hand. Move them alternately back and forth, his knees bending in rhythm. Encourage but do not force the movement.
Baby dance Sit comfortably with the baby on your lap facing you. Placing your hands firmly around the sides of his rib cage, lift him up so that his feet rest on your lap. Allow him to adopt any position he wants.

Massage for illness

The Taoist massage system was devised as a form of body maintenance, to be used every day. It can also have therapeutic benefits if your baby is ill. If your baby shows signs of distress, has a fever or is in pain, you should consult your doctor immediately to investigate any underlying cause. Massage may then be used to release tension or alleviate the illness. Techniques appropriate to various ailments are:

* *Colic, indigestion, constipation, diarrhoea:* 1, 2, 3, 4, 5, 6, 8, 17
* *Respiratory problems:* 5, 6, 7, 8, 9, 10, 20
* *Sleeplessness, restlessness:* 1, 6, 7, 8, 17, 18, 20, 21
* *Teething:* 8, 9, 17, 21

PART VI

THE REFERENCE SECTION

All terms in SMALL CAPITALS refer to articles within this section.

Abdominal and pelvic pain in pregnancy *see* PAIN IN PREGNANCY AND AFTER CHILDBIRTH
Abortion *see* TERMINATION OF PREGNANCY
Abruptio placentae *see* PLACENTAL ABRUPTION
Abscesses, breast, *see* BREAST PROBLEMS AFTER CHILDBIRTH
Accidental haemorrhage *see* PLACENTAL ABRUPTION
Acne *see* SKIN CHANGES IN PREGNANCY
Age of mother *see* OLDER MOTHERS, YOUNG MOTHERS

AIDS

Acquired immune deficiency syndrome is caused by the human immunodeficiency virus (HIV) and is spread from person to person by contact with blood, semen or vaginal secretions. At present, it is known that over 50 per cent of those infected with the HIV go on to develop the full syndrome within three years, and the virus can be passed on before the infection has been detected. Most AIDS sufferers die within three years of the onset of symptoms.

The virus multiplies in the immune system and lowers the person's resistance to infection and can cause rare cancers. Drug addicts run a high risk of infection from shared contaminated needles; otherwise, women may acquire the virus via sexual intercourse with an infected man. Blood transfusions in Britain are probably safe: donors are now screened for the virus.

Women at risk from AIDS may elect to have a blood test to determine whether they carry the virus. The blood test is only positive three months after the woman acquires the infection from an infected partner. If a woman does discover that she is a carrier, she should not get pregnant. Quite apart from the risk to the unborn child, her own chances of developing full AIDS are doubled, the virus being stimulated by the changes of pregnancy. Two-thirds of mothers with AIDS give birth to infected babies, and the disease shows up within six months.

Alcohol

Drinking alcohol during pregnancy, and possibly also before conception, may affect the baby. The occasional glass of wine or spirits is probably safe, but many pregnant women choose to avoid alcohol completely.

The babies of women who drink heavily during their pregnancies may suffer from what is known as 'foetal alcohol syndrome'. At its worst, this may affect these children in four main ways: growth may be retarded or stunted; the brain may be small and there may be mental retardation; there may be heart, kidney and limb defects; and characteristic facial distortions may occur. Such distortions include low ears, a small jaw, droopy eyes and excess hair.

Although the full-blown picture is only seen in women who were alcoholics before the start of pregnancy, the higher the dose of alcohol in pregnancy, the greater are the likely effects on the baby. There is no hard-and-fast rule about this, however, because studies of affected twins have shown that one twin is sometimes more severely damaged than the other. The mother's nutrition may play an important role: a deficiency in zinc and other minerals, common in alcoholics, increases the effects.

Allergic rhinitis *see* COLDS, COUGHS AND RESPIRATORY INFECTIONS IN PREGNANCY

Allergies and hypersensitivity

During pregnancy, you may have a particular ailment for the first time, and it is worth examining your diet and your environment to see if it may be caused by an allergy. Possibly associated with allergy are asthma, sinusitis and recurrent COLDS, skin rashes and acne, migraine and headache, anxiety and DEPRESSION, TIREDNESS AND INSOMNIA, indigestion and HEARTBURN, CONSTIPATION, diarrhoea and recurrent cystitis.

If you suspect that a particular food is causing a reaction, you could try avoiding it, but during pregnancy be very cautious about making any major changes in your diet. If you give up one food, replace it with a near nutritional equivalent – for instance, substitute soya milk for cows' milk. You should also eat food that is as fresh and natural as possible, and avoid refined foods and those with added colourings as well as avoiding cooking in aluminium pots.

Babies in families with a history of allergies should be breastfed for as long as possible, to delay the first intake of foods commonly known to cause allergy. If these foods are avoided during infancy, the child will have greater tolerance to them later. You should avoid the same foods while breastfeeding, as they will reach the baby through the milk.

Common allergens

Allergen	Substitute
Dairy products (milk, cheese, butter, chocolate, cakes and biscuits)	Soya milk, vegetable oils, tofu
Refined and convenience foods with large amounts of sugar, food additives and/or colourings	Unprocessed wholefoods, fresh fruit, salads
Coffee (even decaffeinated), Indian and China teas, fizzy drinks and squashes	Herbal teas, spring or mineral water, fresh fruit and vegetable juices
Wheat, oats, barley	Rice flour or soya flour
Egg yolk, red meat, hormones in some meats	Vegetable proteins, bran, pulses, free-range meat

Grapes/raisins/wine, citrus
fruits, pears, apples
Insecticides and chemicals
used in preparing foods

Sprays, polishes, air
fresheners, washing powders,
soaps, etc.
Cosmetics, skin creams,
scent

Honey or molasses as
sweetener
Natural colourings
and organic
vegetables
Organic alternatives
from health food
shops
Hypo-allergenic
cosmetics and creams

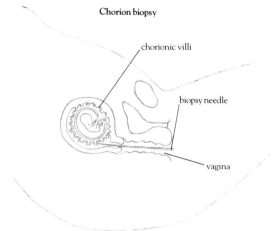

Chorion biopsy

chorionic villi

biopsy needle

vagina

Amniocentesis and chorion biopsy

These techniques are used to obtain small samples of cells
from the unborn baby, which are then used either to analyse
the chromosomes, to test for biochemical disorders of cell
function or to determine the sex of the baby in cases of
sex-linked disorders.

You may be offered one of these tests if your baby is at risk
of DOWN'S SYNDROME or, less commonly, if there is an
elevated level of alpha-foetoprotein (p. 86) in your blood.
You may also be offered a test if you have a family history of
an inherited disorder in which the risk of the disorder is
greater than that of the amniocentesis.

What happens

When amniocentesis is performed under local anaesthetic, a
needle is inserted through the abdominal and uterine walls,
and amniotic fluid is withdrawn from the uterus. The needle
is thinner than the one used to take blood, and the procedure
takes about twice as long as a routine blood test. About 20 ml
(less than 1 fl. oz) of fluid is taken, and this is replaced by the
placenta within 70 minutes. Babies usually seem to sense the
presence of a needle and move out of its way, and the
simultaneous use of ULTRASOUND ensures that the risk of
injuring baby or placenta during amniocentesis is minimal. If
the placenta covers the front wall of the uterus, the test is
delayed for a few weeks to allow the uterus to expand so that
the needle will not pierce the placenta. If the mother is
RHESUS negative and the baby is positive, the mother must be
given an anti-D injection at the time of the test.

Afterwards, the foetal cells are collected from the amniotic

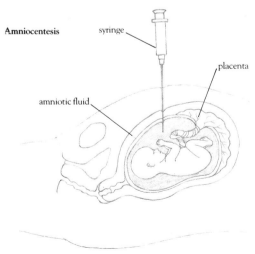

Amniocentesis   syringe

placenta

amniotic fluid

fluid and cultured for two to three weeks. As the cells grow,
the chromosomes contained in their nuclei can be examined
for abnormalities such as Down's syndrome, the enzymes in
the cells analysed for evidence of biochemical disorders, and
the fluid itself tested for its alpha-foetoprotein level.

In a chorion biopsy, a sample of chorion (placental tissue)
is taken, via a needle inserted through the cervix under
ultrasound control. This has the advantage that it can be
performed when the woman is only nine weeks pregnant,
whereas amniocentesis is not feasible before 16 weeks. It
takes two to three weeks for results to become available.

The risks of amniocentesis to the baby are well defined:
there is a 1 per cent risk of MISCARRIAGE following leakage of
amniotic fluid down the side of the membranes and out
through the vagina. The risks of chorion biopsy are probably
the same.

When the results of either test have been obtained, a
diagnosis is made. If the foetus is found to be abnormal, the
option of a TERMINATION is discussed. With chorion biopsy, a
vaginal termination is usually possible because the result is
available at 12 weeks; abortion after amniocentesis may
involve an induction of labour.

Counselling and support for the mother are important.
Although the doctor will be guiding the needle with a scan to
protect the baby and placenta, and neither procedure is very
painful, the insertion of a needle into the uterus is intrusive
and may be distressing for the mother.
See also CHROMOSOMAL AND GENETIC ABNORMALITIES, CON-
GENITAL ABNORMALITIES AND GENETIC COUNSELLING

Amniotic fluid

Polyhydramnios is an excess amount of amniotic fluid in the
uterus; a significant reduction is known as *oligohydramnios*.
Only rarely is a cause for either ever found: in most cases the
mechanism governing the production of fluid is merely out of
balance and the baby suffers no ill effect.

Polyhydramnios

Possible reasons for excess fluid include: DIABETES; TWINS,
where there is a normal amount of fluid for each twin,
producing an excess overall; and obstruction of the foetal
oesophagus or an abnormality of the nervous system, which
renders the baby incapable of swallowing the amniotic fluid,
which then accumulates. A large amount of amniotic fluid in
the uterus may be noticed during a routine ante-natal

checkup. An ULTRASOUND SCAN can measure the fluid and detect twins, and may also reveal a foetal abnormality. A glucose tolerance test (p. 85) will confirm DIABETES.

Excess amniotic fluid may cause no complications at all. However, if the uterus is greatly distended, there is a risk that premature labour may occur. The extra room in which the baby can move may mean that she does not settle into one position, and this can cause problems in labour such as TRANSVERSE LIE or a PROLAPSED UMBILICAL CORD. Excessive pressure on the mother's abdomen can cause BREATHLESSNESS, HEARTBURN and PAIN.

Once polyhydramnios has been diagnosed, bedrest will probably be recommended to reduce the risk of premature labour. If discomfort is severe, some amniotic fluid can be drained via a needle inserted through the abdominal wall. In labour, the baby should be carefully observed to detect cord prolapse or any awkward presentation.

Oligohydramnios
One reason for too little fluid is maldevelopment of the foetal kidneys or an obstruction preventing the flow of urine from the baby's bladder, with the result that the amniotic fluid contains no foetal urine. Obstruction of the baby's bladder may be relieved by inserting a plastic catheter to drain the fluid before birth. Severe placental insufficiency (see LOW BIRTH WEIGHT), may reduce foetal growth and amniotic fluid production, and the baby will need intensive ante-natal monitoring.

Oligohydramnios is usually noticed during a routine checkup. An ULTRASOUND SCAN offers more accurate assessment of amniotic fluid volume, foetal growth and foetal kidney and bladder function.

Anaemia
Red blood cells contain haemoglobin, which carries oxygen from your lungs to all your body tissues. During pregnancy, the overall number of red cells increases, but there is an even greater increase in the water in your body, resulting in a slight reduction in haemoglobin concentration. If the drop in the number of red blood cells (and, thus, haemoglobin) is excessive, you are anaemic.

Symptoms
You may feel tired, short of breath and lacking in energy. If the anaemia is severe, you will be unable to walk far or climb stairs. (These symptoms can also occur in unfit women who are not anaemic.) The baby is not usually affected. Anaemia can also contribute to tiredness after childbirth, and may reduce the flow of breastmilk.

A major aim of ante-natal care is to prevent anaemia, so that you have adequate reserves of red blood cells should bleeding occur during or after labour. The haemoglobin level in your blood should be checked twice during pregnancy, around 16 weeks and after 30 weeks. If the level is below 10 g per 100 g of blood, treatment is essential.

Causes
There are several reasons why some women become anaemic during pregnancy.

Mineral and vitamin deficiency Many women, especially if they have had heavy periods, begin pregnancy with low iron stores. The demands of the baby are then more than the body can meet, and the woman becomes anaemic. If reserves of zinc and cobalt and the vitamins B_1, B_6 and folic acid are also depleted, there is an even higher chance of anaemia.

Blood loss Excessive bleeding during childbirth may cause acute anaemia, in which case a blood transfusion will probably be needed. Less severe blood loss can lead to post-natal anaemia.

Sickle cell disease and thalassaemia These inherited abnormalities of haemoglobin structure (p. 34) are found in women whose families originated from the Mediterranean, the Near East, Africa, the West Indies, India and western Asia. If a woman is in one of the groups at risk, she will be tested in early pregnancy.

Treatment
Iron and folic acid supplements are often prescribed to pregnant women. In addition, the condition can be improved by eating foods rich in iron (p. 99). Avoid tea with or after a meal, as this reduces iron absorption. Women who cannot tolerate high doses of iron – which may cause HEARTBURN and CONSTIPATION – should experiment with organic iron tonics, which may be more easily assimilated. These are readily available from health food stores. Certain homoeopathic remedies may also improve the absorption of iron.

Anaemia caused by a lack of other nutients rather than iron deficiency often responds to a daily multivitamin tablet.
See also SICKLE CELL DISEASE AND THALASSAEMIA

Anaethesia *see* PAIN RELIEF IN LABOUR

Anal fissure
This is a crack in the mucous membrane lining the anal canal. Post-natal bruising can cause the underlying muscle to go into spasm, and this can be made worse by a vaginal tear or stitches. Hard stools create a superficial crack which then becomes infected, and a cycle of spasm and pain then continues. Anal pain that increases during bowel movements may be due to an anal fissure or prolapsed PILES.

Altering your diet to ease the constipation is the first step in treating this. Softening the stools and coating the lining of the anus by using a pure oil or suppositories with glycerine may also be helpful. If there is an infection, you will need antibiotics to clear it. As a last resort, surgery is sometimes performed to stretch the muscles surrounding the anus and reduce the spasm.

Anencephaly *see* NEURAL TUBE DEFECTS
Antepartum haemorrhage *see* BLEEDING
Arrhythmia *see* PALPITATIONS
Artificial rupture of the membranes *see* INDUCED LABOUR
Augmentation of labour *see* PROLONGED LABOUR: FIRST STAGE
Baby battering *see* INJURIES TO THE BABY
Baby blues *see* DEPRESSION AND STRESS
Back and pelvic pain *see* PAIN IN PREGNANCY AND AFTER CHILDBIRTH
Bicornuate uterus *see* CONGENITAL ABNORMALITIES OF THE UTERUS
Birth control *see* CONTRACEPTION

Birth injuries to the baby
Modern obstetric care is geared towards reducing the risk of birth injuries, and it is exceptionally rare for a baby to sustain severe trauma at birth. The best way to avoid injury to your baby altogether is to have good ante-natal care and to give birth actively using upright positions. Nevertheless, if after a premature or difficult labour a baby does sustain an injury, such is a baby's healing capacity that it is most likely to improve and disappear within a few days.

Bruising

Some babies are slightly bruised as they are born. Infants especially susceptible to this include premature babies, those delivered by forceps or vacuum extraction, breech babies and those whose blood-clotting systems have been affected because their mothers have taken large quantities of aspirin during pregnancy.

Pressure on the crown of the head may cause a swelling called a *caput*, which subsides within 48 hours. Occasionally the baby tilts her head during labour so that there is more pressure on it, and an egg-shaped lump appears on one side. This is known as a *cephalhaematoma*, and it consists of blood between the skull and the scalp. Although unsightly, this large bruise is best left untreated: it will gradually become flat over a period of weeks.

A forceps delivery may leave minor bruises around the ears, the angles of the jaw or the sides of the head. The use of vacuum extraction may cause swelling and a circular red line on the baby's head where the vacuum cap was applied. A breech birth may give rise to bruising on the buttocks and, in boys, the scrotum. These marks usually disappear within a few days.

The blood in any bruise is absorbed into the baby's bloodstream, and may cause mild JAUNDICE.

Head injury

Serious head injury in babies during birth is now very rare, due to the advances of modern obstetric care.

Rarely, the events of birth may damage the interior of the skull by tearing the meninges, the membranes that cover and protect the brain, and there may also be internal bleeding. Premature babies are the most likely sufferers, because their membranes may be exceptionally delicate and unable to withstand the normal pressures of birth. The birth needs to be made as easy as possible: the amniotic sac should not be artificially ruptured, and it is safest if the mother gives birth in an upright position. Minor tears in the meninges heal within a few days with no long-term effects, but major tears can cause internal scarring.

Shoulder and bone injury

Sometimes it is difficult to deliver the shoulders of a large baby, and damage may occur in the process of manoeuvring her to ease them out. The nerves running from the neck to the arm can be affected, causing weakness in the forearm and hand. Fracture of the collarbone occasionally occurs during delivery of the shoulders, but almost always heals very quickly and without scarring. Squatting or kneeling to give birth will prevent shoulder injury in most cases.

Birth injuries to the mother

Most women come through childbirth with only a bit of soreness and tenderness in the genital tissues for a few days.

Occasionally, more severe bruising or injury may occur, especially during difficult births needing FORCEPS DELIVERY or VACUUM EXTRACTION or during a CAESAREAN SECTION.

Injuries to the perineum and vagina

The most common perineal and vaginal injuries – tearing and episiotomy – are discussed on pages 336-7. Rarely, vaginal bruising (haematoma) occurs when blood from torn blood vessels clots under the skin. Haematomas are most common following a forceps delivery, but can also happen after a normal birth. Because its tissues are so stretchy, the vagina can swell without being painful, but if the swelling is large, the blood clot is removed under a general anaesthetic.

Injuries to the bladder

The base of the bladder and the urethra both lie beneath the pubic bone, which protects them. Rarely, the bladder may be bruised during childbirth (see URINARY TRACT AND KIDNEY PROBLEMS IN THE MOTHER).

Injuries to the uterus and cervix

The cervix occasionally tears slightly during labour, and may need stitching under a local anaesthetic.

Uterine tears are very rare. They may follow an exceptionally prolonged or neglected labour or – very rarely – during a labour following a previous Caesarean section. Rupture of the uterus is a major, life-threatening complication of labour, requiring immediate surgical treatment. The baby is delivered by Caesarean section, and the torn uterus is reconstituted by surgical stitching. In exceptionally rare cases suturing is impossible, and a hysterectomy (surgical removal of the uterus) performed.

Injuries to bones

The most common injuries involve the coccyx, the sacrum and the sacro-iliac joints. In a long labour when the baby fits tightly in the mother's pelvis, there may be pressure on the sacrum or coccyx, and the sacrum may twist on the sacro-iliac joints. In most women, this rotation corrects itself within a few days of the birth. The joint between the coccyx and the sacrum may be stretched. Both these injuries should be treated by bedrest initially. If there is pain, physiotherapy or gentle osteopathic manipulation may be needed. Post-natal yoga exercises may help (see Part V).

In very rare instances, an intervertebral disc in a woman's spine may prolapse or 'slip' (p. 327, Back and Pelvic Pain).

Birthmarks see SKIN PROBLEMS IN THE BABY
Bladder injury see URINARY TRACT AND KIDNEY PROBLEMS IN THE MOTHER

Bleeding

Vaginal bleeding during pregnancy and in the post-natal period should always be taken seriously. Heavy bleeding, especially if there is pain or if clots are passed, demands urgent medical attention.

Bleeding that occurs in the first half of the pregnancy is known medically as a *threatened miscarriage*; in the second half, it is called *antepartum haemorrhage*; after childbirth, it is *post-partum haemorrhage*.

Bleeding in early pregnancy

Slight spotting in early pregnancy usually originates from the uterine lining rather than the placenta and does not endanger the baby. It is commonly believed that bleeding is more likely at a time when a period would otherwise have occurred, but there is no statistical evidence for this.

Slight spotting can be caused by VAGINAL INFECTIONS or by CERVICAL EROSION. Both of these are diagnosed by a gentle examination of the vagina, and they are easy to treat and do not affect the baby.

More intense bleeding requires further examination and assessment. Particularly if there is pain, the cause may be a threatened or inevitable MISCARRIAGE. In very rare cases, it may be caused by an ECTOPIC PREGNANCY which also gives rise to intense pain on one side of the lower abdomen.

If the bleeding stops and the pregnancy continues, there is no increased likelihood that the baby will have been harmed. Bleeding in pregnancy is not a symptom of an underlying abnormality in the baby.

Bleeding in late pregnancy and labour

Vaginal bleeding may be a sign that labour is about to begin. If you pass mucus stained with blood, this is almost certainly the 'show' (p. 142), a normal event at the start of labour. Bleeding may also be caused by vaginal discharge or CERVICAL EROSION (see above). However, it should always be taken seriously, as it can originate from the placental site.

A low-lying placenta, called PLACENTA PRAEVIA, usually causes painless bleeding of bright red blood. At first, the amount may be slight, but it may become dangerously heavy later. Painful heavy bleeding may be the result of PLACENTAL ABRUPTION, when blood collects behind a correctly sited placenta and emerges through the cervix and out of the vagina. Emergency admission into hospital is essential for any bleeding.

Occasionally, excessive blood loss in labour indicates undiagnosed placenta praevia or placental abruption.

Bleeding after birth

There is always vaginal bleeding in the third stage of labour, during and after the birth of the placenta. Blood loss up to 500 ml (about a pint) is considered 'normal', although it is usually about half this. Giving birth in the upright position encourages placental separation and reduces blood loss.

Blood loss from the placental site As the placenta shears off the uterine wall, the site of attachment bleeds. If the placenta is very large, or after a multiple birth, the blood loss is correspondingly greater. Bleeding is stopped by further uterine contractions. Sometimes excessive bleeding means that the placenta has failed to come away completely from the uterine wall. The uterus is unable to contract to constrict the blood vessels at the placental site (see below). (See also PROLONGED LABOUR: THIRD STAGE.)

Blood loss from the uterus Occasionally, the uterus fails to contract, with the result that bleeding continues. Retained placental fragments may prevent adequate contraction of the uterus. Treatment is to massage the uterus manually through the abdomen, while giving the mother oxytocin to encourage contractions. Putting the baby to the breast will also help the uterus to contract by releasing maternal oxytocin. The retained placenta may be removed under epidural or general anaesthesia if the bleeding is severe.

Blood loss from the vagina or cervix Tearing of the cervix or vagina may cause excessive bleeding and need stitching (see TEARING AND EPISIOTOMY).

Blood-clotting abnormalities In very rare circumstances, particularly following placental abruption, the mother's clotting system may be affected.

Late post-partum haemorrhage This is defined as any heavy bleeding that occurs later than the fifth day after childbirth. The usual cause is the retention in the uterus of fragments of the placenta or membranes, but it occasionally results from an infection inside the uterus.

The initial treatment is to encourage frequent breastfeeding. This helps the uterus to contract and expel the remaining placental fragments. If this does not work, giving the mother ergometrine by mouth helps to stimulate contractions; it may also be necessary to give antibiotics for infection. In rare circumstances, a surgical dilation and curettage (D&C) under anaesthesia is needed to clear the uterine lining.

Blocked milk duct see BREAST PROBLEMS AFTER CHILDBIRTH

Blocked tear duct in the baby

Tears produced by the lachrymal glands lubricate the eyes and eyelids. Fluid drains out of the eye along a small duct, or canal, that runs from the inner corner of the eye into the back of the nose. Occasionally the tear ducts of newborn babies are blocked, causing their eyes to water.

In most cases, the ducts clear spontaneously by the time the baby is six months old. Occasionally it may be necessary for an opthalmologist to open the tear duct under anaesthetic.

See also CONJUNCTIVITIS IN THE BABY

Blood-clotting abnormalities in the baby see HAEMOPHILIA
Blood-clotting abnormalities in the mother see BLEEDING
Blood loss see BLEEDING
Blood pressure see HIGH BLOOD PRESSURE AND PRE-ECLAMPSIA, LOW BLOOD PRESSURE AND FAINTING
Blurred vision see HIGH BLOOD PRESSURE AND PRE-ECLAMPSIA, VISION IN PREGNANCY

Breast problems after childbirth

Common difficulties in establishing breastfeeding are discussed on pages 203-4. Here we are concerned with problems less frequently encountered.

Let-down failure

The let-down reflex is stimulated by the baby sucking the breast, which causes milk to be ejected from the nipple.

There are two common reasons for let-down failure: the baby may not be latching on to the nipple properly; or the mother is too unhappy or stressed to allow the hormones vital to milk production to be secreted. If the let-down reflex does not occur, the baby receives only the foremilk, which is less nutritious than the hindmilk. As a result, the baby is hungry, does not gain weight properly (see LOW WEIGHT GAIN AFTER BIRTH) and may even develop DIARRHOEA. Let-down failure is the most common reason for failure to establish breastfeeding in the early days after the birth.

Treatment Ensure that the baby is latching on and sucking properly, with the whole nipple and at least part of the areola in his mouth (pp. 200-1). Make sure that you and your baby are both comfortable and that the baby faces the breast. (See page 201 for alternative ways of holding him.)

Keep the baby close to you so that he can feed whenever he likes. Try massaging your nipples (p. 279), gently expressing some milk (pp. 204-5), bathing your breasts with warm water or applying warm compresses to encourage the let-down reflex. Once it starts, put the baby to the breast. As you begin to feed, breathe deeply, relaxing your shoulders and releasing tension. Try to be alone with the baby so that you can concentrate on relaxing, and take your time over feeds. Sometimes it takes a few minutes for the let-down reflex to occur once the baby starts sucking.

Insufficient milk

Sometimes a mother misinterprets her baby's frequent sucking as a sign that her milk is insufficient. However, he may be going through a growth spurt and is sucking more often to cause the breasts to make more milk – demand stimulating supply.

Women often think that they cannot produce enough milk for their babies, but unless your child is not putting on weight, this is unlikely to be true. A vicious circle may begin, in which anxiety affects the let-down reflex and the milk supply actually diminishes. If you keep calm, however, the only thing that will limit your milk supply is insufficient stimulation of the breasts.

Treatment Give yourself more time for your baby, and try to set aside a day wholly devoted to feeding him and making more milk. Feed him whenever he is hungry, even before he cries, both day and night. Eat nutritious food and drink plenty of fluids. Herbal teas such as fennel or dill will stimulate milk production. Try to deal with any anxiety or depression you may be experiencing. A talk with a good friend, relative, breastfeeding counsellor, midwife or health visitor may be all you need.

In the unlikely event that your milk really is insufficient, you may have to add supplementary formula to the baby's diet.

Cracked nipples

Occasionally a crack may develop in the skin of a sore nipple (pp 203-4), causing a sudden, sharp, piercing pain in the nipple.

Treatment If pain is extreme, you may have to rest the breast for a feed or two, feeding the baby from the other breast and manually expressing milk from the painful one. You can feed your baby using a teaspoon or bottle.

After a feed, allow the nipples to dry thoroughly and then apply a little calendula cream or tincture very sparingly to the nipples: too much will make the skin soggy. Before feeding, try dusting cornflour on your nipples using a piece of cotton wool; this will help seal the cracks and will protect them when the baby starts to feed. Do not wear a bra; instead, wear a light, loose-fitting top so that your breasts can breathe, and expose the skin to the air as much as possible. Wearing nipple shields for a day or two while feeding can be helpful. Make sure the baby latches on to the nipple properly. Seek help from a breastfeeding counsellor.

Thrush

If the soreness of your nipples persists, or you find that, after weeks or months of breastfeeding, they suddenly become red, you may well have thrush. This is uncomfortable but not serious, and it is quite easy to treat (p. 343).

Blocked milk duct

Sometimes the outlet to one of the milk ducts can become blocked. This may be caused by a tight, badly fitting bra pressing on and constricting a milk gland, or by thick milk preventing a duct from emptying properly. If you have a blocked duct, you will notice a lump in one of your breasts, usually on the lower side. If it is infected, it becomes painful, the skin reddens and you may become feverish.

Treatment Feed your baby frequently; the sucking will help clear the duct. Alter his position regularly to stimulate all parts of the nipple. Heating the breast gently with a warm compress before feeding may loosen any dry milk that is blocking the outlet of the duct. Get plenty of rest and eat well, drinking plenty of fluids to increase the volume of the milk.

Massage the breast after each feed (p. 279). Stroke from the lump towards the nipple, in the direction of the milk duct; this is easier if oil is applied to the skin. It is a good idea to start doing this as soon as possible as it will prevent infection developing in the blocked duct (see below).

Mastitis

If your temperature rises to about 37.5°C (99.5°F) and you have an inflamed patch and/or pain in one of your breasts, you have developed the breast infection known as mastitis. This involves inflammation of the tissues around the lobes within the breast, and is often caused by a staphylococcus infection within an untreated blocked milk duct or entering through a cracked nipple. You may feel as if you are coming

down with flu. Mastitis may develop into a breast abscess (see below) if it is not treated.

Treatment Try to continue feeding your baby, keeping the breasts empty and the milk flowing. The antibodies in the milk will protect your baby from the infection. Offer the sore breast first, to ensure that it is emptied regularly, massage the breast to enlarge the ducts, and change your feeding position from time to time to prevent cracked nipples.

Get plenty of rest. If possible, put yourself to bed with the baby until you have recovered. Eat well and drink plenty of fluids. Wear very loose-fitting, comfortable clothing, and go without a bra.

If the infection lasts more than 24 hours, visit your doctor, who may prescribe an antibiotic. It is important to take the complete course of tablets to prevent recurrence. Mastitis can also be treated homoeopathically, but antibiotics may be needed.

Breast abscesses

Inappropriately treated mastitis may lead to the formation of an abscess – a hot, painful, pus-filled swelling that usually causes a high fever.

Treatment An abscess can sometimes be prevented if a course of antibiotics is taken in the early stages. However, if it is not treated soon enough or proves to be stubborn to clear, your doctor may need to open it surgically to drain out the bacteria-filled pus. This is usually done in an operating theatre under general anaesthetic.

It may be necessary to stop feeding for a while if the abscess needs surgical draining, unless the drainage site is away from the nipple and does not prevent the baby from latching on. A full course of antibiotics is essential, even after drainage. You may have to stop feeding from that breast altogether if the abscess recurs or does not subside after drainage, because your milk will be providing food on which the bacteria thrive.

Breathing problems in the baby

Before birth, the baby obtains oxygen via the placenta. The change at birth involves dramatic physiological adjustments (p. 164), and a few babies may have initial breathing difficulties.

Birth asphyxia

Breathing is usually established within one minute of birth, during which time the baby is still receiving oxygen via the umbilical cord. Babies have the ability to survive on low amounts of oxygen for longer than adults.

Certain groups are more vulnerable to breathing delays, including premature babies, babies whose mothers have had pethidine, those whose mothers have undergone general anaesthesia, and babies with severe FOETAL DISTRESS.

If there is a delay in breathing, suction using a fine tube will clear the baby's airways of amniotic fluid; oxygen can then be given via a mask. If this is not enough, intubation – a soft tube inserted through the baby's mouth into the larynx to deliver oxygen to her lungs – is carried out. This artificial respiration is continued until the baby breathes spontaneously, usually within a few minutes. If necessary, an antidote to pethidine is also administered.

Respiratory distress syndrome (hyaline membrane disease)

In a few newborn babies, the lungs do not produce surfactant, the substance which lowers surface tension and allows the lungs to expand freely when filled with air. Very premature infants and those with diabetic mothers are particularly susceptible. Lack of surfactant means that some air sacs in the lungs do not expand when the baby inhales. As a result, her breathing may be very laboured and rapid, she may make a grunting noise when exhaling, her ribs and breastbone may move inward when she inhales and she may even become blue from lack of oxygen.

A baby with these symptoms will be kept in a special-care baby unit in a warm incubator with piped oxygen (see ILLNESS IN BABIES). If the effort of breathing exhausts the baby, oxygen is blown under pressure from a mechanical ventilator through a tube put in her mouth and down her windpipe. She will be given fluids, glucose, and proteins by drip, and will be constantly monitored to ensure her vital signs are all normal. This support system is usually only necessary for a few hours, but may continue for days depending on the severity of the lung problem. Once the baby's lungs are mature enough to start producing surfactant, recovery is usually rapid and complete. Although parents may find the technology alienating and frightening at first, long-term results have improved dramatically in recent years.

Fast breathing
This occurs in full-term infants when amniotic fluid in the lungs is not quickly absorbed into the body – i.e. 'delayed absorption'. The baby has to work hard, grunting and breathing rapidly, but does not usually go blue. With the help of some extra oxygen, the breathing generally slows down within a day, there are rarely any lasting after-effects and mother and baby do not need to be separated.

Meconium aspiration
Meconium is present in the amniotic fluid of about ten per cent of all babies (see MECONIUM STAINING), but meconium aspiration (when a baby inhales amniotic fluid containing thick meconium) is extremely rare. The fluid has to be thick and viscous to cause lung damage.

Giving birth in an upright position ensures that the baby's lungs drain as the chest is squeezed at delivery. If thick meconium is present, the baby's windpipe is cleared of all fluid as soon as she is born, and the mouth and larynx are suctioned. If meconium is inhaled, the baby may suffer from respiratory distress and is treated accordingly (see above). Recovery usually occurs within 48 hours; occasionally inflammation of the lungs may lead to breathing difficulties.

Breathlessness
Most women in late pregnancy feel breathless after exercising or walking upstairs, and this is no cause for concern. However, if you become breathless while at rest or after minimal exercise, you may be unfit to begin with, so that pregnancy is an extra strain on your system. Alternatively, you may be suffering from ANAEMIA or from a dietary deficiency. You may be expecting TWINS or a very LARGE BABY. You may find that you become breathless when lying on your back because blood flow to your heart is diminished. Whatever reason you suspect, a full medical examination is recommended. If no reason for your breathlessness is discovered, it is a good plan to take iron and mineral supplements and to become physically fit, gently and according to your doctor's advice.
See also HEART DISEASE IN THE MOTHER

Breech birth
In a few pregnancies a baby's *breech* (another word for 'buttocks') engages in the pelvis instead of her head. There are various types of breech. If a foot is born first, the baby is known as a 'footling', but if it is a knee, she is a 'kneeling'. Some babies squat, so that their feet and buttocks are born at the same time (complete breech).

Why some babies are breech
Many babies are breech in early pregnancy, but most turn as pregnancy progresses (many during the last few weeks). In most cases there is no obvious reason: the baby is breech because she is more comfortable that way.

A few contributory factors have been found. There are more breech births than the average with premature babies and TWINS, when there is an excess of AMNIOTIC fluid and with PLACENTA PRAEVIA. Occasionally, an abnormal shape of the uterus (see CONGENITAL ABNORMALITIES OF THE UTERUS) encourages breech presentation and, very rarely, an abnormality of the baby such as a NEURAL TUBE DEFECT gives rise to it.

If your baby is still breech after 35 weeks, you will probably be given a clinical examination, and an ULTRASOUND SCAN may be suggested to exclude the above possibilities.

Turning the baby during pregnancy
Your doctor may want to try and turn your baby, using a technique known as *external version*, in which gentle massage of your abdomen encourages her to do a somersault. The pressure of the massage is very gentle, as excess force could put strain on a short umbilical cord or the placenta.

The head is the heaviest part of the baby's body and tends to be pulled down by gravity. Specific exercises in the last weeks of pregnancy may encourage the baby to turn, starting at 36 weeks.

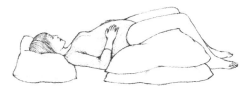

Adopt this position several times a day to encourage your baby to turn. At the same time, gently massage your belly in the direction in which you want her to move, after your midwife has told you which way she is lying. Once the baby has turned, discontinue this exercise and squat to encourage the head to engage.

Acupuncturists recommend the application of pressure, heat or acupuncture needles to a point on the outer edge of the little toe to encourage a breech baby to turn. This can be done in combination with the above exercise.

Problems with breech birth
If the buttocks are not engaged in the pelvis, the umbilical cord may prolapse (see PROLAPSED UMBILICAL CORD). The major problem otherwise is delay or difficulty in delivering the baby's head, which is the largest part of her body.

Giving birth to a breech baby
In some hospitals, all breech babies are automatically scheduled to be delivered by CAESAREAN SECTION. The theory behind this is that, when the body is born, the cord is compressed and the baby receives less oxygen, and for safety's sake the head must be born within five minutes. However, the need for routine Caesarean section for breech babies of normal size and weight in women with a normal pelvic capacity is questionable. Where the birth is active, the

potential for a normal vaginal delivery is greatly increased and the risks of complication are reduced considerably. If the following criteria can be met, you can opt for a vaginal breech birth:

- The baby must not be estimated to be larger than 4 kg (8 lb 13 oz) nor smaller than 2 kg (4 lb 6½ oz).
- It must not be a premature labour: the head of a premature baby is especially delicate.
- Your pelvic capacity must be assessed as adequate.
- The pregnancy must have been normal, with proper growth and development of the baby.
- The first stage of labour must progress well.

The first stage of labour The baby's heartbeat should be regularly monitored, and a vaginal examination should be done to exclude the possibility of a foot slipping through a partly dilated cervix (giving the mother the urge to bear down before the cervix is fully dilated), or of the umbilical cord prolapsing. If the breech is easily engaged in the pelvis, you can anticipate a normal second stage.

The second stage of labour The mother should not bear down before the cervix is fully dilated. A supported squatting position is safest for the vaginal delivery of a breech baby because it opens the pelvis fully, allows the best use of gravity, and encourages the baby's head to engage. This is preferable to the lithotomy position – i.e. feet up in stirrups – which is used in some hospitals.

Once the cord has emerged, the pressure of the baby's chest against the pelvic cavity will compress it and reduce the supply of placental blood. Gravity and gentle traction on the baby will assist the birth.

After the shoulders have emerged, the attendant carefully controls the speed at which the head is born. This usually occurs with ease, especially if the birth is active and the mother uses a supported squatting position (in which an episiotomy may be done if necessary). If epidural anaesthesia is used, the obstetrician may have to apply forceps to the head because gravity is no longer being used and the pelvis is not at its widest.

If a spontaneous birth is not possible with a breech baby, a Caesarean section may be necessary. This decision is made before or during the first stage of labour.

A breech baby's head will not have the same sort of moulding as one born head first, and the final head shape may not be obvious until several weeks after the birth.

Bronchitis *see* COLDS, COUGHS AND OTHER RESPIRATORY INFECTIONS
Bruising *see* BIRTH INJURIES

Caesarean section

When a Caesarean section operation is performed, the baby is delivered through a surgical incision made in the mother's abdomen and uterus. Then the placenta and the membranes are delivered, and the incisions are closed with stitches.

Why a Caesarean may be needed

Caesarean sections are performed either for the health of the mother or, more often, for the safety of the baby. Possible reasons include: a baby too large to pass through the mother's pelvis; a baby in an awkward position for normal delivery; a baby suffering from foetal distress; prolonged labour; and failed induction of labour.

Maternal reasons for Caesareans are less common. The mother's life may be in danger, perhaps from severe pre-eclampsia (*see* HIGH BLOOD PRESSURE AND PRE-ECLAMPSIA) or even eclampsia (*see* FITS IN PREGNANCY). There may be

severe bleeding caused by PLACENTA PRAEVIA or PLACENTAL ABRUPTION. The mother may be having an active attack of genital herpes (*see* VAGINAL INFECTIONS).

In Britain in the mid-1970s, Caesareans accounted for less than 5 per cent of all births. Today, however, about 15 per cent of babies in Britain and 30 per cent in the United States are delivered by Caesarean section, and in some hospitals the Caesarean rate exceeds 60 per cent. If this trend continues in Britain, in the near future one mother in five will give birth this way, and the Caesarean will then be one of the most common operations performed on women.

This rising rate is mainly due to the increasingly techno-logical environment for childbirth. The fear of litigation prompts many a Caesarean – the so-called 'safe option' in an era of defensive medicine. By contrast, when birth is active, and in countries where midwives manage the majority of births, the Caesarean rate falls to its lowest level.

While unnecessary Caesareans can be avoided, it is reassuring that modern skill and expertise generally ensure a positive outcome for mother and baby if a Caesarean does prove essential.

Types of Caesarean

It may be that, when you discuss the future birth of your child with your doctor and midwife, you all agree that a Caesarean is the most appropriate option in the circumstances, and a date is set for you to be admitted to hospital before labour begins. This is known as an elective Caesarean. In contrast, a Caesarean may be carried out as an emergency procedure once labour has begun. Modern obstetric units are equipped to deal with such an emergency at any time.

Caesareans also differ in terms of which form of anaesthe-sia is used. Until 20 years ago, all Caesareans were performed under a general anaesthetic, which meant that the woman was unconscious throughout the birth and could not see her baby until she recovered some time afterwards. Today, epidural anaesthesia provides an alternative which allows you to remain conscious throughout the operation, and to watch your baby being lifted out. You can then hold the baby immediately. Post-natal recovery is usually quicker, and an epidural is usually safer for the baby.

An epidural Caesarean cannot be done quickly, so a general anaesthetic is always used in an emergency. Some woman find the prospect of being conscious during the operation unappealing and prefer a general anaesthetic.

Hospitals vary in allowing partners to be present; most encourage this during epidurals, but may not if a general anaesthetic is needed.

Possible complications

When a Caesarean is needed in an emergency, the mother has usually gone into labour and the baby is ready to be born. On the other hand, babies delivered by elective Caesarean are sometimes found to be premature, even though the operation was scheduled for what was apparently the right time.

A Caesarean delivery remains more hazardous for the woman than natural childbirth, despite improved techniques in surgery and anaesthetics. Major risks include those of any major abdominal operation, especially if a general anaesthe-tic is involved – for example, excessive loss of blood and the possibility of injury to nearby organs such as the bladder or bowel. Post-operative problems also occasionally occur, such as infection, a blood clot in a leg vein or a pulmonary embolus – a blood clot that travels through the circulation to lodge in the lungs (*see* VENOUS THROMBOSIS AND PULMONARY EMBOLISM).

In a modern maternity unit, these risks are very small, but a Caesarean should be undertaken only when the benefits outweigh the risks.

The operation

Before a Caesarean section, your abdomen is shaved and prepared for surgery. After anaesthesia is administered, a catheter (a narrow tube) is inserted up the urethra to the bladder to drain urine, and an intravenous drip is inserted into your arm. The skin of the abdomen is disinfected and the surgeon cuts through the tissues to reach the membranes of the amniotic sac and the baby.

The skin incision is usually a horizontal 'bikini' cut along the hair line at the bottom of the abdomen. This has the advantage of running along natural lines in the tissues, which means less bleeding, less pain and faster healing. In some emergencies, a vertical skin cut is still occasionally used: this runs from below the navel to the hair line. A little less awkward for the obstetrician, it results in a more disfiguring scar. The incision in the uterus itself is usually horizontal and made in its lower segment (resulting in a *lower-segment Caesarean*); this reduces bleeding and minimizes any subsequent risk of scar rupture.

The baby is then lifted out, occasionally with the help of FORCEPS. The time that elapses from the first incision to the birth is about five minutes. The umbilical cord is clamped and cut, and the baby is handed to an assistant. If you are having an epidural Caesarean, you will then be given the baby to hold or, if he is present, the father could take her.

The placenta is delivered and checked, and then the layers of the uterus and abdominal wall are stitched one by one, with dissolving stitches. The skin will either be stitched or closed with small metal clips. It is common practice to leave a thin tube in the wound for a day or two so that excess blood and fluids can seep away. This causes little discomfort.

After the operation

Immediately after the operation, you will be put to bed, usually in the post-natal ward. After a general anaesthetic, many women feel groggy and will find it difficult to focus on the baby for some time. You may be in pain, needing an injection of pethidine until you are able to take ordinary pain-killing tablets. However, if you have had an epidural, pain relief can be achieved by simply leaving in the epidural cannula for 24 hours.

You can expect to feel more comfortable within a few days of having a Caesarean. Movement may be restricted for at least 24 hours by the intravenous drip providing fluids and nourishment, but you may be surprised by how soon you will be encouraged to move about. Early mobility eases breathing, improves healing and prevents blood clots developing in the leg veins.

Mother and baby usually stay in hospital between five and ten days. The stitches or clips are removed after a week or less, and there is a post-natal checkup at six weeks. While some women recover quite quickly, it can take others between six weeks and six months before full energy returns. Plenty of rest is essential, and gentle stretching exercises (*see* Part V) started six weeks after the birth will help.

Breastfeeding your baby Most women who have Caesareans manage to breastfeed their babies. Any problems are sometimes connected with the Caesarean itself – for instance, a general anaesthetic may have reached the baby and made her sleepy for a day or two – but more often they are linked to the reason why the Caesarean was done in the first place (e.g. LOW BIRTH WEIGHT AND PREMATURITY).

Much will depend on your own optimism and determination to succeed, and on the support of those around you. It is a good idea to begin as soon as possible after the birth (*see* Chapter 15). The ward staff will usually encourage you, and their support will be especially important if the baby is in a special-care unit and you are immobile for the first day or two. You will need help lifting and handling her, and your scar will need to be protected during feeds: to do this, you can either prop the baby up on pillows or lie on your side to feed her (p. 201).

Emotional reactions Many mothers feel a great mixture of emotions after a Caesarean. At the time, the joy and relief felt at having a normal baby are usually paramount. If the birth was difficult or complications arose, the Caesarean is usually welcomed as the only way to a safe delivery.

However, after any major operation, involving a general anaesthetic, depression is common, often on the third or fourth day. After a Caesarean, this may be compounded by painful breasts, indigestion, wind and after-pains. These discomforts, added to the difficulties of being physically restricted, can make the first days especially trying. You will need to rest and recuperate as well as get to know, feed and care for your baby.

A few women feel deprived of the experience of vaginal birth, angry at having 'failed' to give birth naturally and envious of others who have given birth normally. These feelings are entirely natural, and may surface weeks or even months later. Some mothers question whether there was a real need for the operation, especially if they felt pressured into having it at the time, or feel that the Caesarean resulted from unnecessary intervention. Such issues are usually resolved by discussion with your attendants as soon as possible after the birth and again in the weeks that follow. The obstetrician will explain why a Caesarean was the best course of action in the circumstances.

Many psychologists believe that a Caesarean birth may affect a baby emotionally, especially the minority who are separated from their mothers in special-care units (*see* ILLNESS IN BABIES) and who will need extra love and attention. It will not matter if 'bonding' (p. 169) is a little delayed as long as you are able to appreciate this special time in quiet and privacy when you are finally united with your baby. Most hospitals try to keep the separation of mothers and babies to a minimum, some allowing incubators to be placed next to the mothers' beds.

Repeat Caesarean sections

Medical policy concerning subsequent births differs widely. In many parts of the United States, once a woman has had one Caesarean, all her future babies will automatically be delivered in the same way, while in most other countries, this would happen if a woman has had two Caesareans.

The main concern in subsequent labours is strain on the scar in the uterus, which may tear or rupture. However, this is now very rare, and in most of Britain and Europe, each pregnancy is assessed on its own merits. Obviously if you had a Caesarean because your pelvis was abnormally small, any subsequent delivery would also be by Caesarean but, providing the reason for the initial operation does not recur, subsequent deliveries can usually be vaginal. You would go into labour spontaneously but with full surgical facilities on standby, and the obstetrician would observe your condition, the labour, and the scar closely; this is called 'trial of scar'.

Using upright positions in such a labour is not only safe but preferable. An active birth will usually shorten labour, help the uterus work better and relieve pressure on the scar. In the second stage, an upright supported squat is ideal. If there are any difficulties, the obstetrician may advise a FORCEPS or vacuum delivery to reduce the strain. After the birth, the scar is usually checked by internal examination, which takes just a few seconds.

Carpal tunnel syndrome *see* NUMB AND PAINFUL FINGERS IN PREGNANCY
Caudal anaesthesia *see* PAIN RELIEF IN LABOUR
Cephalhaematoma *see* BIRTH INJURIES TO THE BABY

Cerebral palsy

Cerebral palsy is not itself a disease: it is the name given to a number of chronic disorders of the brain in young children which impair movement of the body. A significant proportion of children with cerebral palsy – commonly (and wrongly) referred to as 'spastics' – are also mentally retarded. The incidence is constantly dropping because of improved obstetric and paediatric care. Cerebral palsy is most common in babies who were very small (*see* LOW BIRTH WEIGHT AND PREMATURITY), suffered from foetal distress, were very ill post-natally, or had a major congenital abnormality.

The child is usually ill at birth, and intensive care may be needed. Then a latent period of a few months usually follows, during which the baby's behaviour is only minimally abnormal. Developmental milestones are delayed, and gradually the full extent of the defect becomes obvious.

If cerebral palsy is suspected, a full examination and a neurological assessment are essential. During a series of family counselling sessions, the cause, the outlook for the infant and the degree of the burden for parents and family will be discussed. It is a highly specialized field, so most of the first three months of life will be taken up with planning the baby's treatment and care.

Cervical cancer *see* CERVICAL PRE-CANCER AND CANCER

Cervical erosion

The cervix has an inner lining consisting of delicate, red, mucus-producing cells, and an outer covering of thick, pink vaginal skin. Pregnancy stimulates the cervix to enlarge so that the cervical opening often 'pouts' and reveals the red inner lining. If the cervix tears during childbirth, even more of the red lining is revealed post-natally. This is known as *cervical erosion*, but the lining is not, in fact, 'eroded': it has simply appeared on the outer part of the cervix.

An erosion is a benign condition, which affects most women at some time in their lives. Most erosions produce no symptoms. Occasionally they cause a clear vaginal discharge or bright red bleeding, especially after sexual intercourse. The cells of the erosion are checked via a CERVICAL SMEAR to exclude abnormalities.

Although a cervical erosion usually does not require treatment, any bleeding during pregnancy calls for a thorough check by a doctor. If treatment is needed post-natally, because of a discharge or bleeding, heat is applied to the cervix for a few minutes to destroy the displaced inner lining. Over a few weeks, this is replaced by the thicker skin of the outer cervix. There may be a discharge or even bleeding during the healing phase, as new tissue grows to cover the affected skin.

Cervical incompetence

The criss-cross muscle tissue in the cervix (the 'neck of the womb') acts like a valve: it opens during childbirth but stays closed during pregnancy. In some women the valve is weak or opens prematurely, causing miscarriage or premature labour. This is known as *cervical incompetence*.

Incompetence is rare. Causes range from uncommon CONGENITAL ABNORMALITIES OF THE UTERUS to repeated dilation of the cervix during D&Cs (dilation and curettage) or TERMINATIONS. Following two or more miscarriages after 12 weeks of pregnancy, incompetence will be suspected. An obstetrician can confirm the diagnosis by a gentle vaginal examination or ULTRASOUND SCAN in early pregnancy; in between pregnancies, an X-ray can be taken.

When cervical incompetence has been diagnosed, a stitch (known as a *Shirodkar suture*) can be inserted into the cervix under general anaesthetic when the pregnancy reaches 12 weeks. This will hold the cervix closed throughout the pregnancy. It may cause a vaginal discharge until its removal and, very rarely, its insertion may stimulate the cervix and cause a miscarriage.

Cervical incompetence

membranes

cervix

suture

vagina

Although the stitch itself is hidden beneath the surface of the cervix, the knot is left visible so that the stitch can be easily cut, with minimal discomfort and without anaesthetic, at about 36 weeks. Many women expect to go into labour as soon as the stitch is removed, whereas in fact it usually takes a few weeks.

Cervical pre-cancer and cancer

Sometimes changes occur in the cells of the cervix. Early, pre-cancerous changes may develop over a period up to 20 years; they are symptomless, but if undiagnosed, they may, in some women, progress to become an invasive cancer. Doctors refer to pre-cancerous cervical change as CIN (cervical intraepithelial neoplasia), and grade it according to its seriousness: I (mild), II (moderate) and III (severe).

The cause of cervical cancer remains a mystery. It has, however, been related to sexual activity and to infection with the papilloma (wart) virus: the recent increase in the incidence of this infection has been matched by an increase in the number of women between the ages of 20 and 40 with pre-cancer of the cervix. Invasive cancer mainly affects women over 45, and thus occurs rarely during pregnancy.

Because pre-cancer is symptomless, it is wise to have regular CERVICAL SMEARS, or 'Pap' tests, to diagnose cell changes years before they become dangerous. If any abnormal cells are revealed, a *colposcopy* is recommended. This sophisticated test involves the doctor examining the cervix through a lens which greatly magnifies it, and taking a biopsy (small tissue sample) for microscopic examination.

Colposcopy during pregnancy is possible but treatment for pre-cancer can usually be delayed until after the birth. If colposcopy is essential, there is no risk to the baby because the cervix is merely inspected and not tampered with.

Some six to 12 weeks after the birth, small areas of pre-cancerous cells can be destroyed by laser or heat treatment (*diathermy*) under local anaesthetic. Very rarely, extensive areas of abnormal cells have to be removed surgically in an operation called a *cone biopsy* performed under a general anaesthetic. In this, a cone-shaped section of the internal lining of the cervix is removed and sent for examination. Cone biopsy may reduce fertility or cause CERVICAL INCOMPETENCE. This is not the case with laser treatment and diathermy.

The treatment of pre-cancer has a cure rate of more than 95 per cent. After treatment, there is an initial colposcopy checkup after six months, followed by annual cervical smears for the rest of the person's life.

In the extremely unlikely event of invasive cervical cancer being discovered during pregnancy, treatment depends on the degree of invasion and the stage of the pregnancy. The baby may need to be delivered early to make surgery or radiotherapy possible.

Cervical smear

The cervical smear – also called a Papanicolau or 'Pap' test, after the doctor who invented it – is a basic screening test designed to detect CERVICAL PRE-CANCER AND CANCER. It will also diagnose some VAGINAL INFECTIONS.

The test is performed by inserting a speculum into the vagina to expose the cervix which is lightly rubbed to remove some of the surface cells, which are then examined under a microscope. Ten per cent of those with abnormal cells may not be shedding them at the time of examination, so a repeat test is recommended. If the smear suggests anything suspicious, a colposcopy is recommended.

Pregnancy is an ideal time to begin having regular smear tests if you have not done so already. A cervical smear may be part of your first ante-natal visit, or you may not have one until your six-week post-natal checkup. The current DHSS recommendation in Britain is to have a smear every three to five years and to begin at the age of 35. However, many gynaecologists now feel that routine testing should begin when a woman becomes sexually active with intervals of one to two years.

Chilling *see* HYPOTHERMIA IN THE BABY
Chlamydia trachomatis *see* VAGINAL INFECTIONS
Chloasma *see* SKIN CHANGES IN PREGNANCY
Chorion biopsy *see* AMNIOCENTESIS AND CHORION BIOPSY

Chromosomal and genetic abnormalities

There are 46 chromosomes in human cells – 23 identical pairs – which contain thousands of genes made from spirals of DNA which store hereditary information. Every gene performs a unique function in the cell.

Chromosomal abnormalities

Inherited abnormalities may consist of an alteration of an entire chromosome, the presence of an extra one or the total absence of one. This will be visible when cells are cultured and the chromosomes examined under a microscope. The best-known chromosomal abnormality, DOWN'S SYNDROME, is the commonest cause of mental retardation in Britain.

These are a variety of other abnormalities that can affect a baby, some very serious, others barely noticeable. In cases where there is a family history of chromosomal abnormalities, individual genetic counselling is essential.

Single-gene defects

If an individual gene is abnormal, it cannot be seen under a microscope, but it can be identified by analysing the DNA or by examining the products of the gene and deciding whether or not they are normal. The technology of gene probing is a new and exciting advance which will be used increasingly in the future.

X-linked genes (sex-chromosome abnormality) All women have two X chromosomes, and all men one X and one Y. Certain diseases are carried by some women on one of their X chromosomes but, because the healthy one is dominant, the affected women are completely normal. However, they have one chance in two of passing on a defective X chromosome because, at conception, the women provides one X and the male an X or a Y. Consequently, female children have a 50 per cent chance of *carrying* the abnormal gene, while half of all male children will *suffer* from the abnormal gene (i.e. they will not have a healthy X chromosome to mask its effects). The most well-known diseases caused by an X-linked abnormality are HAEMOPHILIA and DUCHENNE MUSCULAR DYSTROPHY.

Recessive genes In this, affected children carry two defective genes of the same type, which cause part of the body's metabolism to malfunction. There are over 200 known defects and, with advances in molecular biology, the list increases every year. Specific enzyme tests are available for about 60 of these defects, enabling ante-natal diagnosis. In most cases a first child is not diagnosed ante-natally because the disease is not suspected.

The inheritance is recessive – that is, both mother and father must contribute one abnormal gene. One in four of their children is affected (by having two abnormal genes), two are carriers (with one normal and one abnormal gene) and one is unaffected (with two normal genes).

You are more likely to be a carrier if you have a family history of a disease (e.g. CYSTIC FIBROSIS) or if you are a member of a particularly ethnic group. For instance, Afro-Caribbean people and those originating around the Mediterranean may be subject to, respectively, SICKLE CELL DISEASE AND THALASSAEMIA; and TAY SACHS DISEASE is more common in Ashkenazi Jews.

The majority of chromosomal and genetic anomalies appear without warning in a first baby because it is impossible to screen all pregnancies for every possible defect. Once there has been an affected baby or if there is a family history, ante-natal diagnosis can be considered.

See also CONGENITAL ABNORMALITIES AND GENETIC COUNSELLING, PHENYLKETONURIA, THYROID DISORDERS IN MOTHER AND BABY

Cigarettes *see* SMOKING IN PREGNANCY

Circumcision

Male circumcision – the removal of the foreskin from the penis – began as a religious custom among Jews and Muslims, whose nomadic desert life meant that there was a high risk of infection from grains of sand under the foreskin, and today it is a social custom in many parts of Europe and America. It is not more hygienic to be circumcised and there are few medical grounds for removal of the foreskin – such as if the urinary opening in the foreskin is too small. In some hospitals, circumcision is performed shortly after birth, after the umbilical cord has been clamped; according to tradition the Jewish circumcision ritual takes place on the eighth day after the child has been born.

In a ritual circumcision, no anaesthesia is used. The foreskin is cut and the penis wrapped in a tight dressing to prevent bleeding. Dressings are changed every 24 hours, but in the first few hours need to be checked frequently because of the risk of bleeding. Bleeding can be stopped by gently squeezing the penis until medical help arrives. A more modern technique involves inserting a plastic shell and ring around the foreskin, which, deprived of blood, drops off in a day or two.

If the wound becomes infected, the baby will be in pain every time urine touches the sensitive skin. This is eased by leaving the nappy off, but antibiotics may also be needed. Babies may be irritable for days or weeks afterwards; massage (pp. 282-9) may help to release tension in the back, abdomen and thighs.

Many parents are opposed to circumcision because of the pain and trauma experienced by the baby, which may have long-term psychological effects. While female circumcision (removal of the clitoris) is generally accepted as barbaric, religious tradition and the widespread use of male circumcision have, perhaps wrongly, prevented people from viewing the two as comparable.

Cleft palate and hare lip

The palate, or roof of the mouth, develops from three bones: one in the centre front and two at the back and sides. If these bones fail to fuse, the result may be a hare lip (a vertical split in the upper lip, usually on one side) with or without a cleft in the palate at the back.

Cleft palate and hare lip affect one in 600 babies. Ante-natal diagnosis is not generally available, so the condition is usually first noticed at birth. The cause is unknown in most cases.

Breastfeeding is usually possible. If milk flows into the nose, a special teat can be used on a bottle; the mother may choose to express breastmilk (pp. 204-5) into this.

Although the initial reaction of parents towards the malformation may be one of shock, modern plastic surgery can achieve amazing results. Several operations are usually necessary, but the outlook, even for children with severe degrees of cleft palate, is generally excellent.

Clubfoot

About one in 1000 babies is born with a deformed foot that turns downwards and inwards. This is known as 'clubfoot' or *talipes*. Most cases are mild, and virtually all respond to manipulation and massage two or three times a day, performed by the parents under the supervision of a physiotherapist. Splints and boots may need to be worn at night. In severe cases, the tense, shortened ligaments holding the foot in position need to be released surgically. With modern surgery and physiotherapy, most babies with clubfoot will be able to walk normally and wear ordinary footwear.

Colds, coughs and other respiratory infections in the baby

A baby with a cold may also develop a cough as a result of mucus trickling down the back of the throat, or because the windpipe (trachea) is also infected. The cough is designed to get rid of excess mucus, and so should not be suppressed. It is also quite common for infants to develop a FEVER, with some VOMITING or DIARRHOEA. The vomiting and diarrhoea may be caused by the baby swallowing mucus, but may be due to some infection of her digestive system (*see also* DIARRHOEA AND GASTRO-ENTERITIS IN THE BABY).

Treatment

Most babies develop a cold at some time or another, and this can cause the parents anxiety, especially the first time it occurs. Babies are resilient, however, and generally deal very efficiently with common ailments. You can speed the healing process by breastfeeding more frequently: the extra fluid will keep the nasal discharge clear, watery and flowing easily. Carrying the baby around a lot will also be beneficial, although this may be tiring for you.

If central heating is making the air very dry, use a cold-steam vaporizer to humidify the environment. Encourage the baby to cough and bring up mucus by massaging her chest and back.

Young babies often become distressed because they cannot breathe and feed at the same time. If the baby's nose seems very blocked, moisten some cotton wool in water or breastmilk, and gently wipe the mucus from the nose to relieve the blockage.

Complications

Viruses are responsible for straightforward colds. Complications arise when bacterial infections are superimposed on a viral one. If your baby suddenly seems ill (as opposed to simply bad-tempered), if she runs a very high fever, has a thick green nasal discharge, a wheezy cough and/or severe diarrhoea, or goes off her feeds, you should seek urgent medical advice. The baby may have croup, bronchitis or pneumonia.
See also EAR INFECTION IN THE BABY

Colds, coughs and other respiratory infections in pregnancy

Colds and infections of the upper respiratory tract such as bronchitis are common and may be a great problem during pregnancy, when hormonal changes often cause the linings of the nasal passages and sinuses to swell. Any infection will be very difficult to clear.

Coughs may be infective or even allergic in origin. Care should be taken not to strain any muscles in the abdomen and back during coughing bouts. Humidify the atmosphere around you, especially if you have central heating, inhale steam two or three times a day, have postural physiotherapy to drain the sinuses, remove any obvious allergens from your surroundings or diet and avoid smoky rooms. Decongestants may occasionally be appropriate while certain homoeopathic remedies may be very helpful. If nothing else works, your doctor may prescribe antibiotics.

Symptoms such as sudden excessive pain, breathlessness or coughed up blood should be reported to your doctor.

Congenital abnormalities and genetic counselling

A congenital abnormality is defined as any defect present at birth. Although many parents worry about having an affected baby, only a very small percentage of babies are born with a significant abnormality. The majority of abnormal foetuses are miscarried. The effects of congenital abnormality range from minor to major disability.

Causes and prevention

Faulty nutrition (*see* Chapter 7), ALCOHOL, DRUGS AND CHEMICALS, RADIATION, being a member of certain families or ethnic groups more susceptible to particular CHROMOSOMAL AND GENETIC ABNORMALITIES, maternal age (*see* OLDER

MOTHERS) and contracting RUBELLA or certain other infections during pregnancy have all been implicated as the causes of particular disorders. However, no cause is ever found in most cases.

All parents try to ensure the well-being of their children, but only some abnormalities are preventable. For example, improved nutrition before conception can reduce the risk of NEURAL TUBE DEFECTS, and immunization can prevent RUBELLA IN PREGNANCY. (See also p. 11.) Nevertheless, most congenital abnormalities are unavoidable.

Diagnosis and genetic counselling

Routine ante-natal care detects certain congenital abnormalities, and couples with a family history of any such abnormality and those who have lost a baby or already have an affected child will receive special ante-natal attention. In high-risk pregnancies, diagnosis may be obtained by AMNIOCENTESIS AND CHORION BIOPSY or by FOETOSCOPY.

Genetic counselling is designed to give individuals advice about genetic disorders, the possibility of having an affected child and the options for prevention and treatment. Family doctors, midwives, obstetricians and specialist geneticists may all become involved in this. Counselling is divided into three phases: pre-conceptual, which relies on an exact family history; diagnosis during pregnancy; and post-natal diagnosis, when the problem already exists in the baby.

An accurate assessment of the possible risks involved in subsequent pregnancies depends on an accurate diagnosis. The parents are then given the odds: for instance, a 41-year-old woman has a two per cent chance of producing a baby with a chromosome abnormality.

Those whose babies are at significant risk may decide to attempt a pregnancy and opt for TERMINATION if amniocentesis or chorion biopsy reveals that the baby is affected. Another solution may be artificial insemination or in vitro fertilization.

General counselling

The need for counselling may arise at different stages of the process of having a baby.

Before and during pregnancy A couple who know that there is a significant chance of a congenital abnormality in their baby are faced with some very difficult decisions. There is the possibility of making up of tests to check whether the baby is affected. This can be very valuable if the results reveal that the baby is unaffected and all anxiety can be laid to rest. However, if the test is positive, parents are faced with the choice of terminating the pregnancy or proceeding with it and thereby accepting the responsibility and reality of parenting an abnormal child.

Your doctor will be able to advise you on the practical outlook for the future and help you make this very difficult decision. Opting for termination may involve disappointment, sadness and grief (see LOSS OF A BABY). Alternatively, accepting nature's course carries with it difficulties that are almost impossible to predict. You will need time to weigh up the situation, listen to advice and finally discover the right solution.

After the birth If it has not been predicted beforehand, discovering that a newborn baby has a major defect comes as a great shock, and parents may be faced with the possibility that their new baby may have to have corrective surgery very soon. This is bound to be a very stressful time, especially if decisions have to be made in the first few days, when the mother is still recovering from the birth. Parents will need special care and counselling, with time afterwards to integrate their feelings and recover.

The long-term outlook A disabled baby requires extra care and attention. Most mothers love their disabled child intensely, and the rewards of caring for such a baby may be profound. Some disabilities are easier to live with than others, and the additional strain on the whole family should be realistically assessed.

Care can be very costly, possibly including re-organization of the home, hiring extra help and loss of parents' earnings. This can mean major sacrifices on many levels: reduced career prospects, fewer holidays, less time to devote to each other and to the rest of the family. There is a higher divorce rate among parents of disabled children and more adjustment difficulties with siblings.

It is inevitable that, in coming to terms with a congenital abnormality, parents will search themselves for possible causes. They may have a deep-seated feeling of responsibility or guilt, or they may blame each other. These feelings are common and often unconscious; they need to be resolved, perhaps with the help of counselling, so that a realistic perspective may be regained. If there has been a termination or the child has died, support may be necessary to help them cope with death and bereavement. Parents are also likely to feel considerable anxiety about a subsequent pregnancy, even if the abnormality is of a type unlikely to recur.

It should be realized at an early stage that the affected child may also have to deal with the stigma of a major abnormality. In minor or correctable abnormalities, the effects are minimal, but when a major abnormality is present, they can be very difficult to cope with – at a physical, intellectual and psychological level.

All in all, the presence of a child with a major abnormality will challenge the whole family at the deepest level, but like many difficult situations, the challenge can bring out the best in everyone. Parents need to be counselled and reassured, to overcome their guilt and come to terms with reality, and there are specialist geneticists and counselling groups for all the major disorders, giving advice and support. However, despite the many problems it entails, parenting a disabled child can be a wonderful experience.

See also individual abnormalities and conditions

Congenital abnormalities of the uterus

Sometimes there are variations in the normal development of the female genital organs. The most common is a bicornuate uterus, when the two 'halves' of the uterus which normally join together remain separate, resulting in a heart-shaped organ.

Most women born with a bicornuate uterus have no problems during menstruation, pregnancy and childbirth, the abnormality often being discovered by chance. However, the condition may cause CERVICAL INCOMPETENCE. Occasionally, a bicornuate uterus leads to a BREECH presentation or a TRANSVERSE LIE. After the birth, there may be a retained placenta (see PROLONGED LABOUR: THIRD STAGE).

It is usually not necessary to treat the bicornuate uterus itself; instead, treatment consists of dealing with any problems that it may cause.

Other malformations are much less frequent.

See also RETROVERTED UTERUS

Congenital heart disease

This is the most common serious congenital abnormality, affecting six babies in 1000, four of whom will have major abnormalities. Despite advances in medicine, the underlying causes of most heart defects are unknown. A minority may be related to DRUGS taken during pregnancy or RUBELLA infection. The first eight weeks of pregnancy are the time of most risk for the developing foetal heart.

Diagnosis and treatment
Not many affected babies are diagnosed before birth, but some hospitals have advanced ULTRASOUND equipment for women at high risk. Most congenital heart disease is diagnosed by cardiac examination after birth. Abnormalities may cause a heart murmur (turbulence possibly caused by the abnormality), but murmurs may be present in babies with perfectly normal hearts.

The most common abnormalities are a 'hole in the heart', where there is an opening between the left and right sides of the heart, and narrowing of one of the major arteries carrying blood away from the heart. Often correctable by surgery, these defects may not show up for years.

Severely affected newborns have obvious breathing problems and their skin may be blue from lack of oxygen. These babies need emergency treatment in a specialized unit. Advances in cardiac surgery mean that a corrective operation is possible for an increasing proportion of babies.
See also CONGENITAL ABNORMALITIES AND GENETIC COUNSELLING, ILLNESS IN BABIES

Conjunctivitis in the baby

Often known as 'sticky eye', this infection, common in the first week of life, causes the mucous membrane (the *conjunctiva*) that lines the front of the eye and the eyelids to become inflamed. The affected eye looks red and pus may cause the eyelids to stick together, especially after the baby has been asleep for a few hours.

If a newborn develops a pus-filled discharge from the eye, your doctor will probably take a swab, to ensure that the conjunctivitis has not been caused by such rare but serious infectious agents as gonorrhoea (which shows up on the first or second day after birth) and chlamydia (on the third to fifth days), which can be contracted by a baby during his passage though the mother's vagina. Conjunctivitis can also be caused by other bacteria, a BLOCKED TEAR DUCT or irritants such as dust.

Bacterial conjunctivitis will need careful treatment with antibiotic drops to prevent scarring; gonorrhoea may need additional antibiotic injections. Treatment otherwise is to bathe the eyes with warm saline solution every few hours or more often if the eyelids become stuck together. Use separate pieces of cotton wool for each eye, wiping from the nose outwards.

Constipation in the baby

If a baby is constipated, passing a stool causes obvious discomfort, and the stool itself is hard. Lack of frequency is usually unimportant.

For the first few days after birth, babies pass greeny-black meconium (p. 182). If no meconium has been passed by the time the baby is 72 hours old, a doctor should check that nothing is blocking the rectum.

Once all the meconium has been passed, the newborn's stools go on to develop their typical appearance. This will vary according to whether the baby is breast-fed or bottle-fed.
The breastfed baby Constipation in a breastfed baby is virtually unknown. As long as the stools are liquid and yellowish she is not constipated, even if she has a bowel movement only once a week. The baby is simply absorbing most of her food. If constipation does occur, it can usually be alleviated by giving the baby extra fluid, especially in hot weather. Otherwise, some adjustments to your diet may be the answer.
The bottle-fed baby There are several likely reasons why a bottle-fed baby may become constipated. Occasionally a baby may show an intolerance to protein in cows' milk by becoming constipated. In this case, a change to a different type of milk, perhaps a soya-based one, may solve the problem. More often, the cause of constipation in a bottle-fed baby is the parents' misguided belief that increasing the strength of the formula by adding more powder to a feed will boost growth. In fact, it does no such thing. What it does do is to cause constipation.

If adding extra fluids does not soften the stools, a daily teaspoon of fresh orange juice slightly sweetened with honey may do the trick. Certain areas of Britain have such hard water that, when used to make up feeds, it contributes to constipation: use bottled spring water for a while and see if there is any difference.

Enemas should never be given to a baby. If she seems to be continually constipated, take medical advice. Massage (pp. 282-9) may succeed where all else has failed.

Other causes of constipation
Very rarely, constipation is the result of a deficient nerve supply to the large intestine (colon) preventing contraction of the lower part. This exceptional condition, known as *megacolon,* is diagnosed by X-rays and a biopsy, and then the affected area of the intestine is removed surgically and the healthy intestine is attached to the anus.

Even more rarely, constipation may be caused by the genetically inherited disease CYSTIC FIBROSIS.

Constipation in pregnancy

During pregnancy, food moves at a slower rate through the intestines, and constipation may result. The major cause is a diet deficient in fibre. The bulk that this provides acts as the vital stimulus to the lower bowel to contract and expel its contents. Food fads in pregnancy (p. 97) often lead to high-calorie, low-roughage diets. Iron tablets may also cause constipation.

Treatment
Altering your diet will almost certainly ease constipation. Eat more whole grains, fresh fruit (unpeeled), vegetables (steamed and raw) and salads. Drink plenty of fluids, taking mineral water between meals. If you find that iron supplements cause constipation, try a different brand or see page 99 for a list of foods rich in iron that you can eat instead.

If you suspect that your constipation is a reaction to something you eat, experiment with omitting various foods. At different times, try eliminating dairy products, coffee and wheat products for a week or two, and see if there is any difference.

Avoid straining when using the lavatory; instead, try deep breathing. Massage, yoga and/or HOMOEOPATHY may also help. Laxatives are almost never necessary, but if you do use one, bulk laxatives are preferable to the stimulant varieties. If you suffer from severe chronic constipation, take medical advice.

Contraception *see* chart on pages 304-5
Controlled cord traction *see* PROLONGED LABOUR: THIRD STAGE
Convulsions in the baby *see* FEVER IN THE BABY
Convulsions in pregnancy *see* FITS IN PREGNANCY

Contraception

If you want to plan your family, the best thing to do is to discover an effective contraceptive method that suits both you and your partner. Virtually all family planning services and prescribed supplies are free on the National Health Service. They can be obtained from hospitals and clinics and from most family doctors (the latter, however, cannot supply free sheaths). Your nearest family planning clinic to you will be listed in the Yellow Pages under 'Family planning'.

The following is a brief summary of the types of contraception available. The rates of effectiveness given for each method depend on that method being used correctly on a consistent basis.

Method	How it works	Effectiveness
Natural methods		
Breastfeeding	Ovulation is suppressed by increased amounts of prolactin in the blood.	Unpredictable. Decreases after a few months, and drops when feeds are reduced.
'Rhythm method' and fertility awareness (see pp. 20–2)	Avoidance of sexual intercourse when woman is fertile, established by taking temperature every morning, examining consistency of cervical mucus, doing calculations with a calendar or using all 3 methods.	85–93% (those using all 3 methods to determine 'safe' period)
Barrier methods		
Diaphragm and cap	Soft rubber dome (diaphragm) or smaller device (cap) covers the cervix and prevents entry of sperm. Left in for 6 hours after last sexual intercourse, and used with spermicide.	96–98%. Can be put in any time up to 3 hours before love-making.
Contraceptive sponge	Polyurethane sponge containing spermicide is inserted into the vagina any time before intercourse. Must be left in place for at least 6 hours after intercourse.	Unknown
Sheath (condom)	Thin rubber sheath rolled on to erect penis will prevent sperm entering womb. A new condom must be used for each intercourse.	97% (more if used with spermicide)
Contraceptive pills		
Combined pill	2 synthetic hormones (oestrogen and progestogen) suppress ovulation, affect lining of uterus and cervical mucus. Pill is usually taken for 21 days, then stopped for 7 days to allow withdrawal bleeding. Dosage as low as possible.	99%. Should be used only under strict medical supervision. Takes 2 weeks to become effective.
Mini pill	Progestogen-only pill taken at same time each day. Will thicken cervical mucus to make it difficult for sperm to enter uterus and for uterus to accept fertilized egg.	96–98%. Takes 2 weeks to become effective.
Injectable contraceptive (e.g. Depo-Provera)	Progestogen is injected into a muscle, from which it is slowly released into the bloodstream for about 3 months. Acts like the mini pill and also suppresses ovulation.	98%
Coil (IUD, intra-uterine device)	Small plastic and copper device inserted into uterus renders uterus unsuitable for implantation of fertilized egg. Must be checked by doctor annually, and woman must check strings (attached to coil) at least monthly.	96–98%. Coil changed every 3-4 years if it contains copper. May be expelled by uterus.
Sterilization		
Female sterilization	Fallopian tubes are blocked or cut to prevent eggs from being fertilized. Procedure is done under anaesthetic, and a hospital stay of 24 hours is needed.	99.9%
Vasectomy	Man's vasa deferentia (tubes through which sperm travel from the testicles) are cut so sperm cannot be ejaculated. It is a 10–15 minute procedure, carried out under local anaesthetic.	99.9%. Only very rare failures

Advantages	Disadvantages	Comments
No periods. Does not interfere with love-making.	You never know when you will ovulate.	Must be used with another method (e.g. barrier method).
May be only acceptable method because of religious or personal beliefs.	Cannot be used if woman's periods are irregular or if she has just had a baby. Needs full cooperation of both partners.	Methods must be taught by someone with specialist training. Can be used in combination with a barrier method.
Can be used as and when necessary and involves less health risk than other methods.	Need to plan ahead before love-making. Can be messy to insert and remove. Allergy to spermicide possible.	Fit checked after birth and annually thereafter.
After insertion, no need to think about it. Disposable after use.	Is not nearly as reliable as other barrier methods. Allergy to spermicide common.	Must be bought from a chemist.
Easy to obtain and use. Can protect against some sexually transmitted diseases (including AIDS) and may protect women from cervical cancer.	Must be put on before genital contact at height of love-making; new one must be used for each act. May slip off; some men claim loss of sensitivity. Must be carefully removed so that no sperm enters woman.	Male takes responsibility. Some couples experience reduced pleasure using a sheath.
Easy to take. Can reduce menstrual flow and period pain. Does not interfere with love-making.	Major and minor side-effects. Should not be taken by women over 35, smokers or those with family or personal histories of high blood pressure, heart attacks or strokes.	High-dose pill may be used for 'morning-after' contraception. Should be discontinued 3 months prior to conception; not advised if breastfeeding.
Easy to take. Fewer clotting and high blood pressure side-effects so more suitable for older women. Can be used while breastfeeding.	Menstrual cycle may become irregular, with breakthrough bleeding and some missed periods. Easy to forget to take at same time every day.	If pregnancy does occur it may be ectopic. Irregular periods a major disadvantage.
No pills to remember to take. Does not interfere with love-making. May be used when other methods are unsuitable.	Periods may be disturbed for about 6 months after injection; fertility may not return for 8–10 months.	A controversial method. If it is offered to you, make sure the doctor explains the side-effects fully.
Once inserted, can be forgotten. Effective immediately. More suitable for women who have had a baby.	Body may expel it. Will not suit all women, particularly those who have not had babies. Sometimes periods heavier or longer; may cause anaemia, period pain and spotting. Greater chance of pelvic infection and infertility. Ectopic pregnancy and miscarriage risk if pregnant when using the IUD.	Never used after pelvic infection, ectopic pregnancy or infertility. Now banned in USA because of litigation and because manufacturers were unable to obtain insurance cover.
Effective immediately. Suitable for women who have decided that their families are complete.	Must be considered irreversible. Sometimes heavier periods are noticed. May fail; ectopic pregnancy is possible.	Counselling is important before this is undertaken to prevent depression. Partner's consent not needed.
Suitable for couples who have decided that their families are complete. Does not affect a man's potency.	Must be considered irreversible. It can take many months before all sperm are out of the system, so other methods must be used meanwhile.	Counselling is important before this is undertaken. Partner's consent not needed.

Cot death

This term refers to the sudden, unexpected death of a baby – hence its other name, *sudden infant death syndrome* (SIDS). Annually, it affects about 1500 babies up to 18 months old in the United Kingdom.

Just under half of the deaths can be explained, with overwhelming infection being the principal cause. There are many theories about unexplained cot death, which is known to have existed for centuries. One suggests that an inherited disorder might make the breathing centre in the baby's brain unresponsive; another proposes undiagnosed infection because half the babies have a minor cold or snuffles at the time of death. More recently, a theory has been put forward that an enzyme deficiency in the liver makes the baby unable to convert fat into glucose for energy, but this is unlikely to account for many deaths.

It is notable that cot death is rare in countries such as Japan where mothers traditionally sleep with their babies at night for the first year after birth. This would seem to indicate that cot death may be related to the use of cots.
See also LOSS OF A BABY

Coughs *see* COLDS, COUGHS AND RESPIRATORY INFECTIONS
Cracked nipples *see* BREAST PROBLEMS AFTER CHILDBIRTH
Cradle cap *see* SKIN PROBLEMS IN THE BABY

Cramp

The prolonged contraction of a group of muscles produces the severe pain known as cramp. Many women suffer from this during pregnancy, usually in the calves, thighs or buttocks, and also in the neck and lower back. Cramp is more common in hot weather, after intense physical activity and at the end of the day or at night, when the muscles are tired. Postural imbalance contributes to it: for instance, wearing high heels leads to shortened calf muscles, which become susceptible to cramp with the extra load of pregnancy. Although cramp can recur frequently, it is intermittent and usually not serious.

Treatment

In hot weather increasing your salt or calcium intake may cure the cramp; see page 99 for list of calcium-rich foods.

Cramp in the calves can be treated by stretching the affected muscles daily (*see* pages 242-3). Sleeping on a harder bed, perhaps created by placing a board under your mattress, or even on a mattress on the floor, sometimes helps to cure night-time cramps. Homoeopathic remedies, especially tissue salts, may work wonders, while others find osteopathy useful.

Croup *see* COLDS, COUGHS AND RESPIRATORY INFECTIONS IN THE BABY

Cystic fibrosis

This is the most common genetic disease in the United Kingdom. Five per cent of the population are carriers, although only one in every 2000 children are affected.

This is a recessive condition (*see* CHROMOSOMAL AND GENETIC ABNORMALITIES). Out of every four children born to parents who are both carriers, one will develop cystic fibrosis and two others will be carriers. Consequently, if parents are known to be carriers, genetic counselling is essential (*see* CONGENITAL ABNORMALITIES AND GENETIC COUNSELLING). Ante-natal diagnosis is now possible, using gene mapping, a technique of molecular biology.

The disease is characterized by abnormal mucous secre-tion, with thick mucus blocking the outlets of the mucus glands. This leads to respiratory problems including lung infections and intestinal absorption difficulties.

Newborn babies may have an intestinal obstruction called a meconium ileus, or may fail to gain weight. Most of those affected are diagnosed when they are older, when chest infections, impaired intestinal absorption and poor weight gain make the condition apparent. Diagnosis is established by analysing the mineral content of sweat: that of cystic fibrosis sufferers contains extra minerals.

The outlook for babies with cystic fibrosis has improved greatly in recent years. Many children lead full and happy lives well into adulthood.

Cystitis *see* URINARY TRACT AND KIDNEY PROBLEMS IN THE MOTHER
Cysts *see* OVARIAN CYSTS

Cytomegalovirus

Infection with the cytomegalovirus (CMV) is more common in pregnancy than RUBELLA, although it is less well known. Spread from person to person by airborne droplets, it may go unnoticed in a pregnant woman because it may be symptom-free. If infection occurs during pregnancy, the virus may not have any effect on the baby, or it may reduce growth, cause partial deafness and liver enlargement, and damage the brain, eyes and ears.

There is no effective treatment at present although cytomegalovirus can be detected by a blood test.

Deafness

Deafness is rare in infancy, with two in 1000 children born completely deaf and rather more partially deaf. The causes include the mother contracting RUBELLA in the early months of pregnancy and extreme prematurity, but in most cases, congenital deafness is inherited.

Loss of hearing usually leads to late speech development and learning difficulties. The earlier deafness is diagnosed, the sooner special teaching can begin.

Death of a baby *see* COT DEATH, LOSS OF A BABY, MISCARRIAGE, STILLBIRTH AND NEONATAL DEATH
Deep-vein thrombosis *see* VENOUS THROMBOSIS AND PULMONARY EMBOLISM
Dehydration in labour *see* PROLONGED LABOUR: SECOND STAGE
Dental problems *see* TEETH AND GUMS IN PREGNANCY

Depression and stress

The word 'depression' usually describes feelings of sadness and despondency, but depressed people may also feel angry, confused and frustrated. In *post-natal* depression, these feelings occur in women after childbirth. In a supportive environment geared to helping new parents before, during and after a birth, post-natal depression is virtually unknown; in modern society, however, depression is more common.

Predicting post-natal depression

Why some women become depressed and others do not is still unknown. One theory says that it is a hormonal problem, another that the stress of having a baby only causes depression when a tendency towards it already exists. Often the origins of post-natal depression stem from long before the pregnancy. The incidence of emotional difficulties after birth can be greatly reduced when the natural process unfolds without disturbance.

It is not easy to predict which women will become depressed. However, certain stress factors are worth considering in an attempt to prevent post-natal depression.

● The mother's own infancy and childhood, especially if she was emotionally deprived or physically injured, and if her relationship with her own parents is not an easy one.

● Disturbance of the normal physiological events of labour, or trauma caused by unnecessary intervention during birth.

● Fear of hospitals or disappointment stemming from the birth experience, together with a sense of having 'failed'.

● Conflict with the baby's father.

● Loneliness. This is often linked to giving up work and losing both colleagues and career, moving to an area that inadequately caters for mothers and babies, living away from friends and family, and separation from partner.

● Financial problems.

● Conflict between motherhood and the need to pursue other interests and be independent.

● Lack of sleep and tiredness after the birth; lack of help at home, and a feeling of being isolated or neglected; pain from stitches or piles and the loss of sexuality.

● A baby who is difficult to satisfy.

● Abnormality or death of the baby.

Symptoms of post-natal depression

A few days after the birth, it is common for women to feel a bit depressed or weepy. This is the 'low' – the well-known 'baby blues' (p. 176) – following the 'high' of the birth and its immediate aftermath, and such feelings come and go.

In a true depression, however, the mother may experience overwhelming and debilitating listlessness. Simple tasks may be almost impossible, and it may be very hard to cope with the baby and life in general. This may only surface weeks after the birth, and the true depths of post-natal depression may not occur until the baby is three to six months old.

There is a fine line between abnormal depression and the normal emotions of pregnancy, childbirth and early parenthood. To some degree, most of the following emotions are normal at this time, but if they last for weeks, help is needed.

● A woman may feel irritable or bad-tempered, wanting to harm her partner or baby.

● She may feel trapped, despondent and despairing.

● She may feel inadequate and unable to cope.

● She may feel deeply exhausted, weepy and miserable.

● She may suffer from insomnia, phobias or nightmares.

● She may feel guilt, anger or fear.

Treatment

It is important to determine the exact cause of post-natal depression, and the best way of doing so is to have a consultation with a psychotherapist.

Post-natal exhaustion may be eased by vitamin supplements, living in rhythm with the baby and obtaining help with housework. Physical exercise and yoga can be immensely calming and will increase energy. Some women find that progesterone supplements are useful.

If family or friends cannot offer the necessary support, it is worth finding out about local support groups (pp. 227-8). Doctors, health visitors and local clinics may put mothers in similar circumstances in touch with each other. Anti-depressants and admission to hospital are a last resort, but there are mother-and-baby units which allow the mother to recover and care for her baby in a supportive environment.

Dermatitis *see* SKIN PROBLEMS IN THE BABY

Diabetes

Diabetes mellitus is a disorder of sugar metabolism. The pancreas produces the hormone insulin, which is needed for the absorption of glucose from the bloodstream. The pancreas of a diabetic person produces insufficient insulin, or the insulin it does produce does not work properly, and sugar levels in the blood and urine become abnormally high.

Types of diabetes

There are two types of diabetes, depending on whether injections of insulin are needed. *Insulin-dependent* diabetes usually begins before the age of 30 and sufferers need regular doses of insulin to maintain the correct sugar balance. If you have diabetes of this type, you should ideally talk to a specialist before becoming pregnant.

Non-insulin-dependent diabetes usually begins after the age of 50, but the hormonal changes of pregnancy may reveal an underlying predisposition. This 'gestational diabetes' usually disappears within hours of birth.

Symptoms and diagnosis

The high levels of blood sugar (*hyperglycaemia*) lead to excessive thirst, the passing of large quantities of urine and dehydration. Untreated, this may progress to a coma. However, most cases of gestational diabetes are mild, and symptoms may not appear.

Women are routinely screened for diabetes in pregnancy by having their urine tested for sugar. Any woman with a family history of diabetes should automatically have a glucose tolerance test when she becomes pregnant.

Treatment

Many people can keep their diabetes under control simply by reducing the amount of sugar and calories in their diet. Most women with gestational diabetes fall into this category.

Diabetics needing regular injections of insulin require the exact quantities to be carefully worked out. In pregnancy, it is vital that the woman monitors her blood sugar frequently.

A diabetic woman needs extra ante-natal checkups so that any complications can be dealt with as early as possible. If there are none, a normal birth is perfectly feasible, as long as maternal and foetal well-being are carefully monitored.

Any woman who develops gestational diabetes during pregnancy should have an annual glucose tolerance test from then on, even if the symptoms disappear after the birth.

Possible complications for the mother

The better controlled the diabetes, the lower the incidence of complications. The mother may find that an excessive amount of AMNIOTIC FLUID builds up in late pregnancy. There is more of a chance of her having a urinary infection or thrush. Pre-eclampsia is more common and the blood vessels may be affected, causing eye and kidney problems.

Possible complications for the baby

When diabetes is poorly controlled, there is a higher risk of CONGENITAL ABNORMALITY. The baby may also grow very large because high sugar levels crossing the placenta stimulate the baby's pancreas to produce excessive insulin, which in turn stimulates the baby's organs to grow quickly (*see* LARGE BABIES). Paradoxically, a large diabetic baby born at full term may behave like a premature infant, with the typical respiratory problems of prematurity (*see* LOW BIRTH WEIGHT AND PREMATURITY). An early induction of labour is sometimes recommended in case the baby gets so large that birth at full term will be difficult.

However, if blood sugar levels are stable and foetal well-being is good in late pregnancy, this is generally not necessary. A CAESAREAN SECTION is performed only when the baby is very large or ill. During labour and birth, all babies must be carefully monitored for FOETAL DISTRESS.

For the first days after birth, the baby's blood-sugar levels continue to need careful monitoring, because her pancreas often continues to produce excessive insulin for some weeks.

Diaphragmatic hernia *see* HERNIAS IN THE BABY

Diarrhoea and gastro-enteritis in the baby

In the first few days after birth, a sticky greenish-black substance known as meconium (p. 59) is passed by the baby. This is followed by transitional stools (so called because they are the result of the changeover to ordinary digestion), which may be loose, greenish-brown and full of milk curds. True diarrhoea is the passage of numerous loose and watery stools which are green rather than yellow.

Diarrhoea
Dextrose water occasionally causes diarrhoea in the newborn, especially if large amounts are given to those that are 'small for dates' (*see* LOW BIRTH WEIGHT AND PREMATURITY). Some bottle-fed babies are sensitive to certain types of formula, and finding the right one usually stops the diarrhoea.

If you are breastfeeding, modifying your own diet may stop your baby's diarrhoea. Some infants are sensitive to substances in foods which appear in the breastmilk (p. 204).

Gastro-enteritis
Breastfed babies virtually never develop gastro-enteritis. The mother acts as a filter between her child and the micro-organisms in the environment, and the milk itself contains antibodies.

Acute diarrhoea in a bottle-fed baby, especially if accompanied by vomiting, suggests gastro-enteritis, inflammation of the stomach and intestines. You must get medical help quickly: a small infant will lose fluid from his body very rapidly, causing dehydration and a dangerous reduction in vital minerals. Meanwhile, give the baby boiled spring water and add to it an electrolyte powder (available from chemists) containing salt and other minerals.

It is important to prevent the development of bacteria by carefully sterilizing bottles and all other feeding equipment.

Discharge, vaginal *see* VAGINAL DISCHARGE

Dislocation of the hip

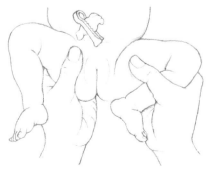

In some newborn babies, the head of the femur, or thigh bone, is distorted, and the hip joint is shallow and therefore unstable. Six times more common in girls, this instability occurs in about one in 1000 births.

Sometimes a dislocated hip is discovered by the doctor during the routine examination of the baby after birth (p. 187) or at the six-week post-natal checkup. Often, however, it is the parents who notice a difference in the shape of the skin folds at the top of one of the baby's thighs, or who feel or hear a click in the hip as they move the legs apart to change a nappy.

Treatment
A newborn is usually treated with a special plastic splint which will hold the joint so that its structures have time to develop. This is washable and removable, and will not distress the baby. Splinting for a few weeks is usually enough to make the joint perfect.

Early diagnosis almost always means that surgery is unnecessary. However, if the child has started to walk before the dislocation is detected, an operation is often needed.

Disproportion *see* LARGE BABIES, PROLONGED LABOUR: FIRST STAGE

Down's syndrome

Down's syndrome (formerly known as *mongolism*) is the most common chromosomal abnormality (*see* CHROMOSOMAL AND GENETIC ABNORMALITIES), and the commonest cause of mental retardation in industrialized countries. It was first described in 1806 by John Down, and is usually caused by the presence of an extra chromosome on chromosome pair no. 21 (hence its alternate name *trisomy 21*). At birth, the distinctive mongoloid features, protruding tongue and single crease on the palms are already evident, and the physical features become more prominent as the child grows.

Down's syndrome is more common in children born to women over 35, who are usually offered ante-natal diagnosis by AMNIOCENTESIS or CHORION BIOPSY. Since most babies are born to women under that age, the majority of Down's babies are not diagnosed before birth.

Down's children are usually very lovable and happy. There are special schools and methods used to improve their intellectual development, but early stimulation is vital. They may have associated heart or abdominal defects, but despite this, the average life expectancy for Down's sufferers has risen to over 30 years.

See also CONGENITAL ABNORMALITIES AND GENETIC COUNSELLING, OLDER MOTHERS

The percentage of Down's syndrome babies increases with the age of the mother, as the following table shows.

Mother's age and Chromosomal abnormality (%)								
35	36	37	38	39	40	41	42	43
1.3	1.4	1.5	1.7	2.1	2.4	2.8	4.0	5.0

Drugs and chemicals

Since 1961, when the relationship between thalidomide and congenital abnormalities was established, pregnant women have been aware of the potential of drugs to affect the unborn baby. Few have been shown to be conclusively harmful, but no drug is safe beyond doubt in the first 12 weeks after conception, when the baby is at his most vulnerable.

Despite this, many women take one or more drugs during pregnancy, the most common being painkillers, anti-nausea drugs, antibiotics and antacids. It follows that relatively few drugs actually cause malformations, and even with high-risk drugs, not every baby is affected.

It is wise to avoid drugs altogether during the first trimester. Care should also be taken later in pregnancy as well as after the birth if you are breastfeeding. If treatment is necessary, the least toxic agent should be taken.

Medicines

All medicines taken in pregnancy should be checked with your midwife or obstetrician. The doses should be kept to a minimum. Breastfeeding women should avoid medicines if possible, as the majority cross into the milk. Homoeopathic remedies can provide safe alternatives in some cases, but they should always be prescribed by a qualified homoeopathic practitioner.

Illegal drugs

Cannabis Laboratory studies on animals have shown that this can cause congenital abnormalities and reduced birth weight, but these effects have not been proved in humans.
Cocaine This is potentially harmful to the baby.
Amphetamines and barbiturates These should be avoided in pregnancy, for fear of possible damage to the baby's nervous system.
LSD If this is taken there is a possibility of damage to the baby's chromosomes. The hallucinogenic effects of the drug may also be experienced by the baby.
Heroin This causes post-natal withdrawal symptoms in the baby, who becomes addicted in the uterus. Long-term behavioural problems are common in those affected in this way. Addicted mothers should not breastfeed.

Chemicals and industrial hazards

The chemical industry has become more aware of possible risks to foetal development among their women employees. Each industry is different, and any health risk needs to be investigated individually. Women exposed to chemicals or employed in the chemical or nuclear industry or in hospital operating theatres are advised to contact the Health and Safety Executive for information about their own industry.
See also ALCOHOL, PAIN RELIEF IN LABOUR, RADIATION, SMOKING IN PREGNANCY

Duchenne muscular dystrophy

This rare disease is a genetic disorder affecting one in 3000 male babies. It causes muscles to become weak, initially in the thighs and pelvis, and later in other parts of the body. The disorder may first be apparent when the child begins to walk, and by the time the child is ten he may be confined to a wheelchair.

In affected families, there is a 50 per cent chance that a boy will have the disease and that a girl will be a carrier because the abnormality is carried in the X chromosome (*see* CHROMOSOMAL AND GENETIC ABNORMALITIES). Carriers can be identified by raised levels of a specific enzyme in their blood, and if a woman with a family history of the disease becomes pregnant, AMNIOCENTESIS or CHORION BIOPSY can be performed to determine whether the child she is carrying is male. If so, a TERMINATION OF PREGNANCY may be offered.
See also CONGENITAL ABNORMALITIES AND GENETIC COUNSELLING

Dyspnoea *see* BREATHLESSNESS

Ear infection in the baby

Ear infections are uncommon in babies under six months, and are very hard to diagnose. If they do occur, they are potentially serious. Protect your baby's ears by keeping her head covered in cold, windy weather.

Infection of the outer ear (*otitis externa*)

Sometimes the delicate membrane lining the canal leading from the outer ear to the eardrum becomes infected. The baby will be in pain and cry, and may rub her ear, which may look red.

Homoeopathic remedies prescribed at the onset of symptoms can be very effective in treating this type of ear infection, but if there is no improvement within 12 hours consult your doctor.

Acute infection of the middle ear (*acute otitis media*)

The Eustachian tubes that run from the middle part of the ear to the back of the throat are short and wide in children and can be easily blocked as a result of a cold. Then the fluid that collects in the middle ear is unable to drain into the throat and becomes the ideal medium for bacteria.

A baby with an acute middle ear infection will seem unwell and may have a high fever. A doctor will look at the eardrum and prescribe antibiotics and decongestants.

Eclampsia *see* FITS IN PREGNANCY

Ectopic pregnancy

In a normal pregnancy, the fertilized egg travels down the Fallopian tube to implant in the uterus. In an ectopic pregnancy, the egg implants in the Fallopian tube. The embryo begins to develop, but the tube cannot stretch and the placental cells burrow through the wall of the tube. The result is internal bleeding into the abdominal cavity. Although rare, ectopic pregnancy is serious because the internal bleeding may cause a life-threatening medical emergency, with immediate resuscitation essential.

Some ectopic pregnancies occur for no apparent reason, but certain factors do increase the risk:
- any previous infection in the Fallopian tubes.
- any surgery on the tubes, including sterilization.
- the presence of an IUD contraceptive device or the use of a progesterone-only contraceptive pill (*see* CONTRACEPTION).

Symptoms

An ectopic pregnancy may initially appear normal, suppressing periods and causing breast changes. On the other hand, there may also be intermittent vaginal bleeding because the placenta fails to produce enough oestrogen.

Sharp pain, usually on one side of the lower abdomen, is a major symptom. It can last for hours or only a few minutes and may stop and start. If internal bleeding continues, the pain spreads over the entire abdomen and worsens. In extreme cases, massive bleeding may cause collapse and shock.

Diagnosis

Pain or a late period when pregnancy is suspected should be reported to your doctor. If the bleeding is slight, diagnosis is often difficult. If an internal examination is inconclusive, an ULTRASOUND SCAN may show that there is no pregnancy in the uterus, and may also reveal a mass in the pelvis. The ultra-sensitive HCG pregnancy test (p. 28) is usually

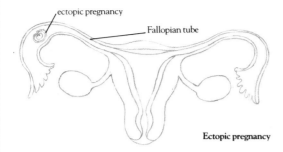

ectopic pregnancy

Fallopian tube

Ectopic pregnancy

positive, and may help to distinguish between ectopic pregnancy and other causes of pelvic pain, such as painful ovulation (pp. 22, 327).

Treatment

An ectopic pregnancy must be surgically removed under a general anaesthetic. Occasionally it is possible to leave the affected Fallopian tube intact, but in most cases the surgeon has to remove this as well. If the remaining tube is normal, it is perfectly possible for a woman who has suffered an ectopic pregnancy to have a normal pregnancy later. However, it may take longer to conceive, because ovulation will sometimes occur on the side without a tube.

See also LOSS OF A BABY

Eczema *see* SKIN CHANGES IN PREGNANCY, SKIN PROBLEMS IN THE BABY

Embolism, pulmonary *see* VENOUS THROMBOSIS AND PULMONARY EMBOLISM

Emotional deprivation *see* LOW WEIGHT GAIN AFTER BIRTH

Entonox *see* PAIN RELIEF IN LABOUR

Epidural anaesthesia *see* PAIN RELIEF IN LABOUR

Epileptic fits *see* FITS IN PREGNANCY

Episiotomy *see* TEARING AND EPISIOTOMY

Erosion of the cervix *see* CERVICAL EROSION

External version *see* BREECH BIRTH

Eyes in pregnancy *see* VISION IN PREGNANCY

Eyes, watering *see* BLOCKED TEAR DUCT IN THE BABY

Face and brow presentation

At the start of labour, the baby's chin is usually tucked into the chest and the top of the head presents. Occasionally the baby extends her head up and back. If the head is halfway back, this is known as a *brow presentation*. Face and brow presentations are rare complications and have to be treated with great skill. A brow presentation can be particularly difficult, and a Caesarean section is usually necessary, unless the baby happens to be small and the pelvic capacity large.

In a face presentation, the baby's head is thrown so far back that its diameter is only slightly larger than in the normal position. This makes vaginal delivery more likely, with the baby being born face instead of crown first, although a Caesarean is still sometimes needed.

Fainting *see* LOW BLOOD PRESSURE AND FAINTING

Fallopian tube infections

The majority of tubal infections, if diagnosed and treated early, do not affect tubal function because the lining is not destroyed. However, if the tubes become completely blocked with scar tissue, the result is infertility. If partly blocked, kinked or distorted, ECTOPIC PREGNANCY may result.

During pregnancy the developing baby and membranes seal off the uterine cavity and prevent micro-organisms from entering. In the first week after childbirth or a MISCARRIAGE, micro-organisms may enter the uterine cavity, travel to the Fallopian tubes and cause the infection known as *salpingitis* or PID (*pelvic inflammatory disease*). Symptoms include an offensive-smelling vaginal discharge, pelvic pain and fever.

In the days before antibiotics, PID was extremely hazardous. Today antibiotics are administered, by intravenous injection if necessary, to destroy the invading organisms. The chances of infection are lessened by antiseptics in labour and complete delivery of the placenta and membranes.

Falls *see* INJURIES TO THE BABY

Fever in the baby

Unlike adults, newborn babies are not able to control their temperature by sweating, and a baby kept too hot in an incubator or overdressed in a warm room will experience a rise in body temperature. This is also a sign of illness or infection. If a baby has a high temperature, keep her cool. Undress her and sponge her all over with cool (not cold) water, allowing this to evaporate.

A feverish baby may be successfully treated by a homoeopath, who should be consulted as soon as the symptoms arise. If HOMOEOPATHY does not work within 12 hours, take medical advice; antibiotics may be necessary if there is a specific bacterial infection.

Some babies may experience febrile convulsions – fits brought on by fever. These are very frightening for parents, although they stop when the temperature comes down and are not usually a sign of anything serious. However, for safety's sake, urgent medical attention is essential. First-aid measures consist of cooling the baby by removing her clothing and sponging her with tepid water.

It should be remembered that fever alone is not a symptom on which to base a diagnosis. Babies can be quite ill and have a very low temperature, and can also feel quite hot for no reason at all. It is better to judge the well-being of your child by considering all aspects of her health, especially feeding. If she is unwell, medical advice is essential.

Fibroids

Fibroids are thickened muscle fibres in the muscle tissues of the uterine wall. They are usually benign (i.e. non-cancerous), there may be one or many and they may be as small as a pea or larger than an orange. They may be on the outer surface of the uterus, within the uterine wall or on the inside of the uterus. Large fibroids on the outer wall of the uterus are almost never a problem. However, those on the inner wall are rather more likely to cause trouble:

* they may block the Fallopian tubes, preventing conception.

* they may become large enough to cause MISCARRIAGE or stimulate premature labour.

* they may swell and degenerate during pregnancy, causing pain and fever.

* rarely, they may block the passage of the baby at birth.

* after the birth, large fibroids may cause bleeding or fever.

Fibroids cannot be treated during pregnancy; bedrest is the only remedy for pain. Post-natally, they usually shrink back but may need to be removed surgically.

Fingers, numb and painful, *see* NUMB AND PAINFUL FINGERS IN PREGNANCY

Fits in pregnancy

Fortunately, fits (convulsions) are extremely rare during pregnancy. There are two possible reasons for them, both serious: epilepsy and eclampsia.

Epilepsy

Women with epilepsy may continue to be susceptible to fits during pregnancy, and for this reason should take medical advice before conceiving. The drug treatment that controls the epilepsy needs to be carefully monitored before and throughout pregnancy: the doses must be high enough to prevent fits, but low enough to reduce the risk of the baby developing a CONGENITAL ABNORMALITY.

If a fit occurs, medical help must be obtained at once, and the woman protected from injury. There is no need to restrain her or put anything in her mouth. After the fit, she should be laid on her side, with any tight clothing at the neck loosened. She must be able to breathe freely, so if she vomits, any obstruction must be removed from her mouth.

Eclampsia

Pre-eclampsia is characterized by high blood pressure, swelling of the body tissues (see OEDEMA) and protein in the urine (see HIGH BLOOD PRESSURE AND PRE-ECLAMPSIA). When the swelling affects the brain, it may cause convulsions and is known as *eclampsia*.

Prevention by treating the pre-eclampsia is vital: eclamptic fits are extremely dangerous because the brain swelling, combined with the convulsions, can lead to a reduced oxygen supply for both mother and baby and may even be fatal.

The immediate action if a fit occurs is the same as for an epileptic fit (see above). As well as administering suitable drugs to control the fits and giving artificial respiration, hospital staff may deliver the baby by CAESAREAN SECTION to save the lives of both baby and mother.

Fluid retention see OEDEMA
Foetal alcohol syndrome see ALCOHOL

Foetal distress

A baby's metabolism is adapted to deal with labour. During contractions, the blood vessels in the uterine wall are constricted and the placental blood flow is reduced, but the baby is able to use the reserve of oxygen in the pool of blood in the placenta.

If the baby's oxygen level becomes low, he is able to change to a different type of metabolism, called *anaerobic* ('without oxygen'). He survives by deriving energy from glucose, which comes from the reserves of sugar that his body has accumulated over the months. In this way, babies are able to manage without oxygen for up to ten minutes, much longer than adults. This is a natural protective mechanism.

If, however, the flow of blood from the placenta to the baby is reduced for a relatively long time, not enough oxygen reaches his brain. This is known as foetal distress, which in severe cases can lead to brain damage and even death. Acute foetal distress is a rare but serious event.

Causes

The reasons for foetal distress are not always clear, but certain factors make it more likely:

Babies that are severely 'small for dates' (see LOW BIRTH WEIGHT AND PREMATURITY) or are malnourished with low sugar reserves may be unable to cope with labour.

If a woman lies on her back during labour, the blood flow to the placenta may be reduced. This is sometimes exacerbated by an epidural anaesthetic (see PAIN RELIEF IN LABOUR), which can cause blood to pool in the lower limbs.

If the umbilical cord is around the baby's neck, it may tighten as the head descends and reduce the flow of oxygen.

Rarely, there is a PLACENTAL ABRUPTION, when the placenta shears off the uterine wall.

Symptoms

It is known that certain changes in the baby's heart rate are significant indicators of foetal distress. These changes are detected by FOETAL-HEART MONITORING, and may be confirmed by measuring the oxygen in a sample of the baby's blood taken from the scalp.

MECONIUM STAINING OF AMNIOTIC FLUID occurs when the baby empties his bowels before birth, and can sometimes be a sign of foetal distress.

Prevention

Foetal distress can be reduced if the predisposing factors are eliminated. 'Small-for-dates' babies should be diagnosed ante-natally and carefully monitored.

Treatment during and after labour

Sometimes a simple change of the mother's posture or some inhaled oxygen may be enough to alter an abnormal foetal heart pattern.

If true foetal distress is present early in labour and the birth is still far away, the baby should be delivered quickly by CAESAREAN SECTION. If the mother is already in the second stage, labour should be shortened by the adoption of an upright position and an episiotomy. The mother should not hold her breath while pushing.

Babies with foetal distress require extra attention after birth. They may need RESUSCITATION, and if their sugar stores are low early feeding is essential. A full paediatric examination will reveal whether the reduced oxygen supply will have any long-term effects.

Foetal-heart monitoring

The sound of the baby's heart beating regularly indicates that she is alive and well. An abnormal pattern can be a sign of FOETAL DISTRESS.

The simplest way of monitoring the foetal heartbeat is for the midwife to place her ear on your abdomen, near where the baby's heart is lying. An ear trumpet or stethoscope is often used. In the last 20 years, increasingly sophisticated types of electronic foetal-heart monitor have been developed. While they can be life-saving in high-risk births, like all machines they can malfunction and give a false record of the heart rate, and this may lead to action when there is no problem. Despite this, the rising use of obstetric intervention that requires careful monitoring has made continuous electronic monitors a popular choice among obstetricians.

Hand-held electronic monitors

These portable instruments, which are the size of a telephone, are ideal for an active birth, as they can be used with the mother standing, squatting or kneeling. A simple transducer using ultrasound is held against the mother's abdomen near the baby's chest, and the magnified sound of the baby's heartbeat can be heard.

Continuous electronic monitoring

Larger electronic monitors (also using ULTRASOUND) print out a graph of the heartbeat, as well as the mother's uterine activity. They have the advantage of providing a continuous record of the baby's heart rate. There are two basic types:

Strap on the mother's abdomen If this is used, the mother may be made to lie down, making an active birth impossible. Many women find these monitors uncomfortable, and this can increase pain and disturb the flow of labour.

One solution is to have the monitor attached while the mother is in a kneeling position on the bed, supported by cushions. Another is to use this type of monitor, but to hold it by hand.

Clip on the baby's scalp This method involves clipping an electrode to the baby's scalp, with a wire running out through the cervix to the machine. Before the clip can be applied, the membranes of the amniotic sac have to be ruptured; the clip itself may be painful or uncomfortable for the baby and may cause a sore on the baby's scalp. The monitor can be used with the mother in an upright position.

This type was designed to monitor the most vulnerable babies, and is the most accurate. Used routinely, the disadvantages and risks probably outweigh the advantages, but for a baby truly at risk the careful observation it provides can prevent the need for a CAESAREAN SECTION.

There are also some scalp monitors that use radio waves rather than wires, and which allow the mother complete mobility. These will be used increasingly in the future.

When monitoring is done

Pregnancy The baby's well-being can be checked by monitoring the foetal heart regularly in problem pregnancies, as often as circumstances require.

First stage of labour In normal labour, intermittent monitoring every 30–60 minutes is adequate. Continuous recording is used in high-risk pregnancies or if the woman has an epidural anaesthetic or an induction.

Second stage of labour The general rule is to monitor regularly unless the second stage is very short or obviously progressing well.

Heart rate: The foetal heart rate is faster than an adult's. The average is 140 beats per minute within a normal range of 110 to 170 beats. A fast rate may be a sign of distress or maternal fever. A slow rate may also be a sign of distress.

Variation: Within the average, it is normal for the foetal heart rate to vary by ten beats per minute. Variation of under five beats per minute indicates that the baby is either asleep or in distress.

Acceleration: During foetal movements, the rate should speed up by 10–20 beats a minute. This is a sign of a healthy baby. A lack of acceleration may be the earliest sign of foetal distress.

Deceleration (dips): When the rate drops at the beginning of a contraction and rises at the end (Type I dip), this is usually caused by pressure on the baby's head and is not a sign of distress. When the rate drops to below 100 beats per minute soon after a contraction (Type II dip), there is a significant risk of foetal distress. If dips are not related to contractions, there is usually foetal distress.

Foetoscopy and foetal surgery

Foetoscopy enables the foetus, placenta and umbilical cord to be seen. Guided by ULTRASOUND, a thin instrument called a *foetoscope* is inserted through the mother's abdominal wall into the uterine cavity under a local anaesthetic. The foetoscope is fitted with a fibre-optic light source, and sometimes has surgical attachments so that blood samples, biopsies (tissue samples) or minor surgery can be undertaken.

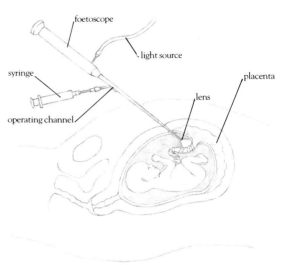

Foetoscopy

foetoscope

light source

syringe

placenta

lens

operating channel

Risks of foetoscopy

Detailed ultrasound scanning before the foetoscope is introduced into the abdomen is the key to success. However, miscarriage occurs in five to ten per cent of cases – a risk ten times higher than with amniocentesis – so foetoscopy is only used when the likelihood of congenital abnormality is greater than five per cent.

Uses of foetoscopy

A sample of foetal blood may be taken from the blood vessels running along the umbilical cord from the placenta. This is done if there is a suspicion of haemophilia, sickle cell disease, thalassaemia or an inborn error of metabolism, as well as in foetal viral infection.

If there is an obstruction to the flow or urine from the bladder, this can now be treated before birth by the insertion of a catheter through the baby's abdominal wall which will drain the urine. This can sometimes prevent a lethal build-up of pressure and the destruction of the foetal kidneys.

The advantage of foetal surgery is that wounds will heal completely with virtually no scarring. This branch of medical science is still in its infancy, and developments in the next decade will be of great interest.

Foetal blood transfusion for rhesus disease and bone marrow transplants for sickle cell disease, thalassaemia and immuno-deficiency are also theoretically possible.

See also URINARY TRACT AND KIDNEY PROBLEMS IN THE BABY

Food allergies *see* ALLERGIES AND HYPERSENSITIVITY

Forceps delivery and vacuum extraction

The introduction of forceps was a milestone in the history of obstetrics. Invented in about 1600, they provided the first mechanical assistance in childbirth. Consisting of two metal blades applied to either side of the baby's head, they are used to exert a pull on the baby's head to assist delivery.

In 1957 a Swedish obstetrician invented the vacuum extractor, or *ventouse*, in which a cup connected to a vacuum pump is attached to the baby's scalp. A vacuum is created so that the cup remains attached to the scalp by suction, upon which the pull is applied. For historical reasons, forceps tend to be used in Britain and the United States, while northern and central Europe favour the vacuum extractor. Safety is comparable, although vacuum extraction is more comfortable for the mother.

Avoiding for forceps or vacuum extraction

Forceps or vacuum extraction are used in up to 20 per cent of births. A large number of these interventions are avoidable: some are the result of the arbitrary time limits set by obstetricians; the increased use of epidural anaesthesia (*see* PAIN RELIEF IN LABOUR) is responsible for others.

You can help by making sure that you are well nourished throughout pregnancy and physically fit, and by avoiding epidural anaesthesia. Once the second stage starts, it is best to remain upright, using the supported squatting position, to obtain the maximum help from gravity.

When an assisted delivery is necessary

If the baby's head is difficult to deliver, the second stage may be prolonged. If the head is large in relation to the mother's pelvis, or if the baby is in an *occipito posterior* position (p. 325), contractions often slow down and an assisted delivery may be necessary. Forceps or vacuum extraction are used to correct the abnormal position and to provide the additional moderate force needed to deliver the baby. CAESAREAN SECTION is safer than a traumatic forceps delivery. If the baby is BREECH, forceps are sometimes used to ease the birth of the head, especially if an epidural has also been given. An active breech birth does not usually require forceps.

Assisted delivery is more common when epidural anaesthesia has been used, because it slows down contractions, removes the natural urge to bear down and push, and relaxes the pelvic-floor muscles so that the baby's head is not encouraged to rotate in the second stage.

If the baby suffers severe FOETAL DISTRESS in the second stage of labour, forceps or vacuum extraction can be a life-saver in achieving rapid delivery.

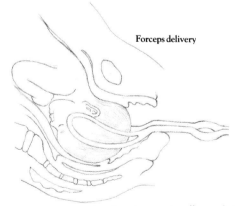

Forceps delivery

Forceps or vacuum extraction is occasionally used to protect the mother. Women who have severe HIGH BLOOD PRESSURE, lung or HEART DISEASE may be advised not to bear down, and an assisted delivery may be called for.

Conditions for a forceps or vacuum delivery The cervix must be fully dilated and the bladder empty. The head must be engaged in the mother's pelvis; if the head is still high a Caesarean will be necessary.

Sometimes a forceps or a vacuum delivery is performed when the baby's head has 'crowned' but the mother is too anaesthetized or tired to push her out. This is known as a 'lift-out' delivery, needing only a local anaesthetic to numb the birth outlet. Occasionally the baby is lodged a little further up the pelvic cavity, especially if she is in an occipito posterior position. When forceps or vacuum extraction are used, this is known as a 'mid-cavity' delivery, usually requiring an epidural or caudal anaesthetic. The other common reason for a mid-cavity delivery is when the epidural reduces the mother's urge to bear down.

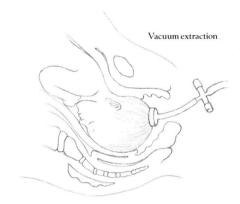

Vacuum extraction

What happens during an assisted delivery The mother is asked to lie on her back with her legs supported by stirrups. You can request that your partner stay with you throughout, although some men may not wish to witness an assisted delivery and the episiotomy that is sometimes done; a compromise might be for your partner to sit next to you at the top end of the delivery table, while a screen blocks off the view of the birth.

In a forceps delivery, the blades are inserted into the vagina to cradle either side of the baby's head. Holding them together at the handle, the obstetrician applies a pull during two or three contractions to rotate the head or to help the baby out. In between contractions, the pressure is relieved.

In a vacuum delivery, the cup is inserted into the vagina and fitted on to the baby's scalp. It takes five minutes for suction between the two to build up. Traction is then applied during a contraction, to help the head to descend. An episiotomy is not always needed because, unlike forceps, the suction cap does not take up any space along the sides of the vagina.

If the baby is in an occipito posterior position, a mid-cavity delivery will include rotation of the baby's head. This can be done manually by the obstetrician, or with a vacuum cup or specially shaped Kiellands forceps. After rotation, the mother's bearing down may be enough to deliver the baby, with minimal help from the obstetrician.

What assisted delivery is like for the baby

During a forceps delivery, the baby will feel the blades along the side of her head and the pulling force of the forceps during two or three contractions, for a minute at a time, and may experience a strong tug or even some pain in her head and neck. She may be born with marks on her cheeks and ears, which will disappear within a few days.

In a vacuum delivery, the baby may feel the suction on her scalp, and it may or may not be painful. Like forceps, the pulling force is exerted for a minute at a time. She may be born with a round, swollen, red area on the crown of her head, which will take a few days to subside.

A skilled obstetrician, aware of the possible effects on the baby, will sensitively apply the minimum of force to assist the birth. Most babies make a rapid recovery after an assisted birth, but because they may have a sore head and feel irritable, they need to be handled very gently during the first few days. This usually subsides quickly, especially with the help of close body contact and massage (*see* Part V).

The mother's reactions
Women often feel sore and bruised, especially after a forceps delivery. Episiotomy, stitches and pelvic pain are more common with these procedures.

If you know that your baby might not have been safely delivered without help, you will probably feel relief and gratitude. If the forceps were skilfully used, you may not have much pain or too great a sense of invasion. If, however, you feel some disappointment at not having achieved a natural birth, you should let the feelings surface, accepting that you are entitled to be disappointed if you wanted something that did not happen.

Your emotions will need to be understood and resolved after the birth. You could begin by talking to the midwife who takes care of you post-natally, as well as the doctor who performed the procedure. Usually the anger resolves in a few weeks, but if it continues and is a source of post-natal DEPRESSION AND STRESS, you should consider expert counselling. Otherwise your enjoyment of your baby's first few months may be affected.

Repeat forceps or vacuum deliveries
Forceps are most commonly used for a first baby, subsequent deliveries usually being quicker and easier, even if the baby is larger. If you are keen to avoid a second assisted delivery, follow the suggestions above.

If forceps were used because your first baby was in an occipito posterior position, subsequent babies may not be. Even if the next one is, your cervix will probably dilate and the pelvic tissues open more readily, and the second stage will be easier.

If the reason for assisted delivery was the size or shape of your pelvis, a repeat forceps birth or a Caesarean section is possible. However, each baby is an individual, and the second may be smaller or in a better position.

Foreskin narrowing *see* CIRCUMCISION
Gas-and-air *see* PAIN RELIEF IN LABOUR
Gastro-enteritis *see* DIARRHOEA AND GASTRO-ENTERITIS IN THE BABY
General anaesthesia *see* PAIN RELIEF IN LABOUR
Genetic counselling *see* CONGENITAL ABNORMALITIES AND GENETIC COUNSELLING
Genital herpes *see* VAGINAL INFECTIONS
German measles *see* RUBELLA IN PREGNANCY
Gingivitis *see* TEETH AND GUMS IN PREGNANCY
Gonorrhoea *see* VAGINAL INFECTIONS

Haemophilia
This is an inherited blood disorder caused by the absence of a vital blood-clotting substance known as *Factor VIII*. Women are carriers, and male babies have a one in two chance of being affected because the abnormal gene is on the male X chromosome (*see also* CHROMOSOMAL AND GENETIC ABNORMALITIES).

In haemophilia, the blood either fails to clot or takes a long time to do so; bleeding can also occur spontaneously, especially in the joints, causing them to swell painfully. The condition is treated with injections of Factor VIII, which is obtained from donated human blood; large quantities of highly purified Factor VIII obtained through genetic engineering will soon be available. If the disease is well controlled, disability is not severe.

Family history will lead to the condition being suspected, and the mother's blood can be tested for abnormality. If she is found to be a carrier, AMNIOCENTESIS at 16 weeks (or, possibly, chorion biopsy at 9 weeks) can be used to determine the sex of the foetus. If the child is male, FOETOSCOPY can be used to sample the foetal blood and test for clotting factors. Some parents whose babies are at risk of haemophilia may opt for testing in pregnancy, while others may prefer to accept the risk, rather than choosing a TERMINATION OF PREGNANCY. *See also* CONGENITAL ABNORMALITIES AND GENETIC COUNSELLING

Haemorrhage *see* BLEEDING, PLACENTAL ABRUPTION, PLACENTA PRAEVIA
Haemorrhoids *see* PILES
Hare lip *see* CLEFT PALATE AND HARE LIP
Headache *see* PAIN IN PREGNANCY AND AFTER CHILDBIRTH
Head injury *see* BIRTH INJURIES TO THE BABY

Heartburn
The valve between the oesophagus (gullet) and stomach is softened by hormonal secretions during pregnancy. As a result, gastric acid may escape upward into the oesophagus, where it can irritate the sensitive lining and cause pain.

Self-help
Avoid pressure on the abdomen, especially that caused by corsets or constricting clothing. Exercises that stretch the trunk and relax the digestive system (*see* Part V) will help. Try raising the head of your bed on two bricks and sleeping on pillows so that you remain semi-upright.

Avoid irritating the stomach. Meals should be frequent and small to reduce gastric acid, and it makes sense to avoid alcohol, highly spiced or fried foods, chemical additives and any other substances that disagree with you.

Heartburn may be relieved by alkaline foods that will neutralize the acid, such as yogurt, milk, or commercial antacids. Other women find that neutralizing the acid in this way causes the stomach to overreact and produce even more, so they benefit from taking mildly acidic foods, such as fruit juice or tomatoes.

Heartburn that is not relieved by any of the above suggestions may need further investigation.

Heart disease in the baby *see* CONGENITAL HEART DISEASE

Heart disease in the mother
With the virtual disappearance of rheumatic fever, heart disease under the age of 50 has become rare. Most pregnant women who have heart problems were born with them.

If a murmur is found when the heart is examined during pregnancy, it is usually an 'innocent flow' murmur caused by the increased blood flow through the mother's heart, in which case it disappears after the birth. However, if heart disease is present, the increased cardiac and circulatory work of pregnancy carries with it a greater risk of heart failure.

Women with a major heart problem should give birth in a hospital with specialized facilities. The load on the heart is greatest in late pregnancy and, particularly, after the third stage of labour, when the uterus contracts and shrinks and extra blood enters the mother's circulation. Prolonged bedrest during pregnancy may be necessary, as well as drugs to boost heart function.

The birth itself should be gentle, with minimal straining in labour. To avoid any extra load on the heart, drugs to enhance uterine contractions (oxytocin or ergometrine) should not be used. The mother needs to be monitored intensively for 24 hours after the birth.

Hernias in the baby

A weakness in part of a muscular wall (usually the abdominal wall) which allows some of its contents to protrude is called a *hernia*. There are several types, depending on the site.

The most common variety found in babies is the *umbilical hernia*, in which the naval protrudes, especially when the baby cries. Not painful and rarely serious, it usually disappears within five years, although it may need surgery if it is still present by the time the child is a teenager.

An *inguinal hernia* involves the inguinal canal in the groin, where a swelling may be seen or felt when the baby cries. This type needs prompt surgery because part of the bowel may become trapped, leading to 'strangulation'. In boys, the testes should be checked because sometimes this hernia is associated with UNDESCENDED TESTES.

A *diaphragmatic hernia* is caused by an undeveloped diaphragm, which allows the abdominal contents to protrude into the chest cavity. This can cause breathing difficulties in newborn babies, and requires surgery to repair the diaphragm.

Herpes *see* VAGINAL INFECTIONS

High blood pressure and pre-eclampsia

Blood pressure measurements, part of every ante-natal checkup, are necessary because high blood pressure (*hypertension*) may be associated with risks to the baby, to the mother or to both.

Causes

High blood pressure on its own may occur during pregnancy in women who are already hypertensive, or in those, mainly women in their 30s with a relevant family history, who have an underlying predisposition towards developing it in later life. Mildly elevated blood pressure (under 150/100 mm of mercury) poses only a minimal risk to mother and baby; all that is needed are frequent checks to ensure that pre-eclampsia (*see below*) does not develop.

Very rarely, high blood pressure is caused by a kidney disorder. Pregnancy increases the workload for the damaged kidneys, which may further raise blood pressure.

Pre-eclampsia is peculiar to pregnancy, and is characterized by high blood pressure, fluid retention (*see* OEDEMA) and protein in the urine. If untreated, it may progress to life-threatening eclampsia, which causes convulsions and may damage the mother's heart, kidneys, liver and blood-clotting system (*see* FITS IN PREGNANCY). There is also a risk to the baby, as very high blood pressure can cause placental insufficiency (*see* LOW BIRTH WEIGHT AND PREMATURITY).

Why pre-eclampsia occurs is unknown, although it may be caused by the mother's immune system reacting inappropriately to the baby or to the placenta. It is more common in twin pregnancies and in women whose diets are inadequate. It usually occurs in a first pregnancy, disappearing completely within a few weeks of the birth, and does not usually recur in subsequent pregnancies.

Symptoms and diagnosis

A blood pressure reading higher than 140/90 is abnormal, while levels in excess of 160/110 are very serious. On its own, oedema is not significant, but if there is high blood pressure as well, oedema, especially of the hands and face, is a symptom of established pre-eclampsia. Protein in the urine suggests pre-eclampsia only when other possible reasons for it (such as urinary infection or vaginal secretions in the urine sample) have been excluded.

Treatment

Diet It is sensible to help prevent high blood pressure by eating a good diet without excess salt, although once pre-eclampsia is present an adequate salt intake is important.

Bedrest One of the main treatments for pre-eclampsia, bedrest ensures the best use of the available blood flow to the placenta.

Anti-hypertensives Yoga, meditation, acupuncture and homoeopathy may all be effective in bringing blood pressure down, even when anti-hypertensive drugs are also needed.

The latter are used long-term by women with underlying hypertension discovered before or during early pregnancy. They may also become necessary when there is an acute blood pressure problem in late pregnancy or during labour. They are powerful agents and need to be skilfully administered, but fortunately have few effects on the baby. Mother and baby need frequent monitoring to ensure correct dosages are correct.

Acute severe pre-eclampsia is treated with an intravenous drip and anti-hypertensive drugs, and anti-convulsant drugs may also be given. However, alternatives should be tried because anti-convulsants are potentially addictive for the mother, and premature babies exposed to them may be ill for weeks after birth until they have completely excreted them.

Early birth If severe hypertension is causing placental insufficiency, the baby must be delivered, usually by CAESAREAN SECTION, even as early as 28–32 weeks. If the mother develops eclampsia or is at high risk of it, delivery must be immediate and also usually by Caesarean section. If hypertension is less severe, labour may be INDUCED, but this requires intensive maternal and FOETAL-HEART MONITORING (*see also* p. 318) to ensure the baby's well-being. Induction is not necessary if blood pressure is only mildly elevated (under 140/100 mm) and there is no protein in the urine.

Labour Dangerously high blood pressure in labour is often treated with epidural anaesthesia, which reduces blood pressure with few effects on the baby. Of the drugs used to enhance uterine contractions, Syntocinon should be employed with caution because, in high doses, it may elevate blood pressure, and ergometrine (p. 333) should also be avoided for the same reason.

After the birth Blood pressure checks will be continued to make sure that post-partum eclampsia is prevented. If high blood pressure persists for six weeks, post-natal investigations may be undertaken to detect any underlying hypertension or kidney disease. The baby must be carefully examined at birth and receive appropriate treatment if she is premature or small-for-dates.

Hip, dislocated *see* DISLOCATION OF THE HIP

Homoeopathy

In 1796, a German doctor, Samuel Hahnemann, discovered a new method of curing the sick, which he called *homoeopathy* (from the Greek words meaning 'similar suffering'). Whereas the orthodox medical approach to, say, a case of insomnia would be to give a drug to induce artificial sleep, the homoeopathic way is to give a minute dose of a substance that in large doses would cause sleeplessness in a healthy person. Surprisingly, this may enable the sufferer to sleep naturally.

Homoeopathic remedies may work by stimulating the body's own healing power. This power is very great and the body is often able to cure itself unaided, but when the healing process is blocked, faulty or slow, a homoeopathic remedy can act as a stimulus.

When to use homoeopathic remedies

Pregnancy They can be useful in treating nausea, vomiting and other digestive disorders, respiratory and urinary problems, anaemia, high blood pressure and a variety of other conditions common in pregnancy. Certain remedies may promote iron absorption; others may be helpful in preparing for labour and birth.

Labour Remedies can be taken in labour for pain relief, to stimulate contractions and to relieve exhaustion. If complications arise, homoeopathic remedies can be used to aid healing and recovery, and they can be invaluable in relieving discomfort after surgery or intervention.

After the birth There are also a number of common preparations that can be used post-natally to excellent effect: calendula tincture, to clean the baby's cord and to apply to the mother's stitches; calendula cream, for sore nipples; hypercal cream, for nappy rash and burn ointment.

How to use homoeopathic remedies

Not all preparations are safe, and some should not be used unless specifically prescribed. It is therefore always best to consult a homoeopath, who will prescribe the right remedies as well as advising you about self-help and which remedies you can keep at home for first aid and general care and where you can obtain them. To find a homoeopath, contact the British Homoeopathic Association (p. 347).

You should avoid coffee, peppermint, eucalyptus, camphor and menthol while taking any homoeopathic remedy, as they have an antidote effect.

Hyaline membrane disease *see* BREATHING PROBLEMS IN THE BABY
Hydrocephaly *see* NEURAL TUBE DEFECTS
Hyperemesis *see* VOMITING IN PREGNANCY
Hyperglycaemia *see* DIABETES
Hypersensitivity *see* ALLERGIES AND HYPERSENSITIVITY
Hypertension *see* HIGH BLOOD PRESSURE AND PRE-ECLAMPSIA
Hypnosis *see* PAIN RELIEF IN LABOUR
Hypoglycaemia *see* DIABETES
Hypospadias *see* URINARY TRACT AND KIDNEY PROBLEMS IN THE BABY
Hypotension *see* LOW BLOOD PRESSURE AND FAINTING

Hypothermia in the baby

If an infant's temperature drops below 35°C (95°F) for longer than an hour, he is said to be suffering from *hypothermia* – a subnormal body temperature – which causes all the vital functions of the body to slow down. Severe hypothermia may be very serious for a newborn baby, especially if he is ill or premature. Hypothermia is less common later on because the body is better able to regulate its temperature and the baby has a smaller area of skin in relation to the size of his body. Babies who are gradually acclimatized to cooler temperatures over several months withstand them well.

Symptoms

If an inadequately dressed baby has been left for a long time in a poorly heated room in cold weather, his skin will feel cool to the touch, on the trunk as well as the limbs. He will probably not have the energy to cry, and will lie motionless. The slow circulation of blood in the skin may give him a superficially pink and healthy look, but this can disguise a dangerously slow heart and breathing rate.

Treatment

The best place for a newborn baby is on or right next to his mother's body, which is at the perfect temperature for him. Positioned like this, he cannot become chilled.

Premature infants lose heat from the skin particularly fast, and RESUSCITATION after birth, if needed, should be done under an overhead radiant heater. Any baby who has been chilled for only a short period can safely be warmed by body contact with his mother. However, if the chilling has been prolonged, or if the baby's temperature has dropped below 32°C (89.6°F), slow warming in a special-care baby unit for 24 hours or more may be necessary.

Illness in babies

If your baby is merely off-colour or slightly ill, it is usually possible to look after her properly at home. It is important for all sick babies to be held a lot and to be close to their mothers. Constant holding may be tiring for you, but your warmth and contact with your body will be the best medicine for your child. It is encouraging to bear in mind that a young baby's self-healing capacity is very efficient and recovery is usually rapid. If she needs hospital care, you have the right to stay with her and most hospitals welcome parents.

Surgery

Some babies need surgery soon after birth, and this may come as a shock to parents who may wonder how their tiny baby will survive. It is reassuring to know that surgical and anaesthetic techniques have improved enormously so that, now, even open heart surgery is possible on the first day of life. Non-urgent surgery is postponed until the baby is older.

Special-care baby units (SCBUs)

A sick baby may need to be cared for in a special-care baby unit. The hi-tech machinery found there may be disturbing at first: tiny babies always look vulnerable, and in this context even more so. Generally the staff want parents to stay as long as they wish, and mothers are encouraged to express milk or breastfeed if possible as the baby benefits from the antibodies and nutritional quality of the milk, and this will help establish the breastfeeding relationship later on. Hiring or buying an electric breast pump (p. 205) may be a good idea. However, should your baby be fed formula, loving contact while feeding is beneficial.

The more time parents spend touching, cuddling and caring for their child, the better it is for all of them. If the baby is in an incubator and cannot be held, your presence is still important, and you may be able to touch and stroke her or participate in her care.

It can be difficult to be separated from your newborn baby, but it is not always possible to remain with her all the time, especially if there are other children at home.

The very sick baby

If your baby is very ill, it is best to make the most of your time together if you possibly can. Many people are afraid of bonding with a baby they may lose, but in fact, bonding may

make separation by death easier. Special counselling and support groups are available to help parents with seriously ill babies (p. 347).
See also LOSS OF A BABY

Incompetent cervix *see* CERVICAL INCOMPETENCE
Incontinence *see* URINARY INCONTINENCE
Indigestion *see* HEARTBURN

Induced labour

The vast majority of women begin labour spontaneously when their babies are mature and ready to be born. When labour is initiated before it begins spontaneously, this is known as *induction*.

Few issues in obstetrics arouse greater passion than induction, which has been described as 'the most predictable way of creating abnormal labour and the need for operative delivery'. In the late 1960s, as sophisticated and safe methods of stimulating contractions to induce labour were developed, induction rates rose and the associated Caesarean rate rose too.

Why labour may be induced

When the risks to the baby of remaining inside the uterus are greater than the risks of induction, it may be necessary to deliver the baby before term. If the baby is already at risk, it must be decided whether induction or a Caesarean section would be to the mother's and baby's best advantage.

The following are the most valid reasons for induction:

Placental insufficiency If a baby is not receiving enough nourishment through the placenta to meet her needs (*see* LOW BIRTH WEIGHT AND PREMATURITY and POSTMATURITY), induction is a common solution, although it requires very careful monitoring. A Caesarean section might be safer.

Multiple pregnancy Induction may be necessary if one child is receiving less nourishment than the other(s) (*see* TWINS).

Diabetes Improved methods of diabetic control now mean that even severely insulin-dependent women can often go into labour spontaneously at term.

Congenital abnormality Very rarely, induction is done because the baby is abnormal or has died.

High-risk mothers Induction is more common in a number of well-defined high-risk groups: malnourished women, smokers and women with HIGH BLOOD PRESSURE.

The disadvantages of induction (*see below*) are numerous and considerable. To avoid unnecessary inductions, each case should be individually assessed. With careful monitoring techniques, intervention can be reserved for those who really need it.

In addition to the relatively valid reasons for induction listed above, there are others that are far more questionable:

Disproportion Occasionally an induction is proposed before the expected delivery date because a previous baby is too large for the mother's pelvis (*see* LARGE BABIES), but the risks of induction outweigh any potential benefit.

Breech presentation A BREECH BIRTH is not a valid reason for induction.

'Small-for-dates' babies Small size on its own is not an indication for induction. This is only necessary if there is also a significant risk of placental insufficiency.

Postmaturity If birth has not occurred within a week or two of the expected due date, induction is unnecessary if mother and baby show no problems. It should only be done if tests indicate placental insufficiency.

Convenience Induction of labour for the convenience of birth attendants cannot be justified; induction for the convenience of parents should be carefully considered in light of the possible risks to the baby.

Ways of inducing labour

Sexual intercourse Human semen contains significant quantities of prostaglandin (*see below*), which stimulates uterine activity and helps the cervix to ripen. Intercourse at the end of pregnancy may bring on labour if the birth is imminent. There is no danger of it stimulating labour prematurely.

Acupuncture If the cervix is ripe and labour is imminent, acupuncture may be able to stimulate the uterus to contract. Although this technique is often effective and without side-effects, it cannot be relied upon if the need for induction is urgent.

Castor oil, hot bath and/or enema These old-fashioned and ineffective ways of starting labour are rarely used now. The diarrhoea caused by the castor oil is unpleasant and may cause dehydration.

Stretching the cervix and 'sweeping' the membranes This technique has been used for centuries. During a vaginal examination, the midwife may insert her finger through the opening of the cervix and 'sweep' the membranes of the amniotic sac by gently massaging the cervix. This causes the secretion of prostaglandin by its inner lining which, as long as the cervix is ripe, may stimulate labour.

Artificial rupture of the membranes (ARM) This method – also known as *amniotomy* and 'breaking the waters' – can be a potent way of starting labour within a few hours in women who have had previous children and whose cervix is extremely ripe. The procedure itself – the insertion of a plastic instrument resembling a crochet hook through the cervix to puncture the membranes – is uncomfortable, but if skilfully done it is not painful as long as the cervix is slightly dilated. ARM makes infection in the uterus possible, so birth must occur within 24 hours.

Prostaglandin The discovery of synthetic prostaglandin similar to that found in the lining of the uterus represented a major breakthrough for induction, and is its least invasive form. It is usually introduced into the vagina or cervix in the form of pessaries or a cream, inserted at 6–12-hourly intervals. This method is preferable as it leaves the woman free to walk about, and it does not involve breaking the waters.

The pessaries can ripen the cervix over 24–48 hours, and this frequently stimulates labour. In most cases, labour begins after two doses, but if the cervix is unripe it may take longer.

With prostaglandin, the mother is less likely to have an over-stimulated uterus or a failed induction than if Syntocinon (*see below*) is used. However, because of the risk of over-stimulation, prostaglandin should not be given to a woman whose cervix is already partly dilated.

If it is found that prostaglandin on its own is not sufficient, Syntocinon may be given or the membranes may be ruptured. If these fail too, a Caesarean section will be needed, so there must be a good reason for inducing labour in the first place.

Syntocinon This powerful stimulator of uterine activity is a synthetic hormone similar to the oxytocin (p. 135) produced by the pituitary glands of both mother and baby. It can be used to accelerate or augment a labour that is proceeding slowly as well as for induction.

It is usually given by means of an intravenous drip. This generally restricts the woman's movement, although mobile drips are available. The drip will be kept in throughout labour (to ensure that contractions continue) until well after the birth.

Syntocinon usually begins to work almost immediately,

and although the speed of the drip is adjustable, the contractions are likely to be longer, more intense and more painful and with shorter intervals between them than in a spontaneous labour. The strength of the contractions and the foetal heart will be monitored continuously to detect any signs of overstimulation or foetal distress.

On its own, Syntocinon is not always reliable in starting labour, and so it is usually combined with artificial rupture of the membranes. However, there is a failure rate of between 10 and 20 per cent with this combined method, and in these cases, a Caesarean section will then be needed.

Disadvantages for the mother
As well as restricted mobility because of the intravenous drip, induction has a number of other disadvantages for the mother.

● *Intense contractions* With Syntocinon, days of pre-labour uterine activity may be condensed into a few hours. The pain may be greater from the start, and with no natural build-up there may be no time for the mother to adjust.

● *Over-stimulation of the uterus* In this, uterine activity becomes uncoordinated and the cervix fails to dilate. In extreme cases, the uterine muscle may go into spasm, with FOETAL DISTRESS (*see below*), and the uterus itself may rupture.

● *Caesarean section* The chances of a Caesarean section are much increased.

● *Side-effects* In large doses, Syntocinon may cause OEDEMA and HIGH BLOOD PRESSURE. Prostaglandin can irritate the smooth muscle of the bowel, causing vomiting, diarrhoea or migraine, and the pessaries may cause vaginal irritation.

● *Post-partum haemorrhage* This is more likely because an overstimulated uterus reacts less effectively to natural oxytocin or the similar drugs used in the third stage of labour to deliver the placenta and membranes.

● *Emotional problems* When labour is induced and actively managed by medical staff, control passes away from the mother. If she feels that the induction was unnecessary she may feel angry, resentful and violated. While induction can be a positive experience, many women find it an intrusive event and need to come to terms with their feelings afterwards.

Complications for the baby
● *Prematurity* Because there is a chance that the baby may be born prematurely – especially if dates are wrong – induction should only be done if the risks of continuing the pregnancy are greater than the risks of prematurity.

● *Foetal distress* The increased strength and duration of contractions in an induced labour will reduce blood flow to the placenta, possibly resulting in distress and a Caesarean section. This can be made worse if the woman is in a reclining position because of continuous monitoring or an epidural.

● *Problems after birth* Breathing difficulties are more common when labour is induced, especially if the baby is premature with immature lungs. Syntocinon has also been linked with an increased risk of jaundice.

Infant death *see* LOSS OF A BABY
Infection, vaginal, *see* VAGINAL INFECTION
Inguinal hernia *see* HERNIAS IN THE BABY
Inherited disorders *see* CHROMOSOMAL AND GENETIC ABNORMALITIES, CONGENITAL ABNORMALITIES AND GENETIC COUNSELLING

Injuries to the baby
No matter how careful you are with your baby, accidents can happen. As long as you avoid leaving your baby unsupervised on a bed or table, falls in early infancy are unlikely. Nevertheless, tiny babies do sometimes fall or are dropped, and the result could be anything from a minor bump to a major injury. Various aspects of safety in and outside the home are outlined on page 221.

Bruises, cuts, sprains and fractures
The most common injury is a bruise, which will eventually fade on its own. If the skin is torn, pressure may have to be applied before bleeding will stop. A cut needs to be cleaned with warm water or a mild antiseptic, and may need to be stitched if it is large or gaping.

A twisting force on a baby's loose and flexible joints can cause strains and sprains, and severe force may cause a broken bone. Sprains and fractures are rare in infancy, and bones knit quickly and easily. If the affected area looks deformed, seems very painful and has restricted movement, take your baby to the doctor.

Head injuries
Head injuries caused by a fall are potentially very serious. Fortunately, the bones of an infant's skull are not yet fused, and it is able to absorb considerable force without damage. Copious bleeding occurs if the scalp is cut, but this does not necessarily mean that the injury is serious. If you suspect a serious head injury, especially if a child is or has been unconscious, skilled emergency treatment is vital. Stay calm, breathe deeply, hold the baby and phone for an ambulance, or take the child to the nearest hospital casualty department.

Non-accidental injuries
If the baby is injured by an adult, help should be sought urgently. Baby battering is very serious and unfortunately common. Parents who injure their children usually cannot help it, so it is important not to let guilt or shame prevent them from approaching a doctor or other supportive agency (p. 347); without help, the injuries may get more serious.

Insomnia *see* TIREDNESS AND INSOMNIA
Insufficient milk *see* BREAST PROBLEMS AFTER CHILDBIRTH

Inverted nipples
As pregnancy advances the nipples tend to project more, and once your baby begins to suckle he will probably draw the nipples out. However, if yours do not rise above skin level, you may have inverted nipples. To check, place your thumb and forefinger on either side of each nipple at the base and gently press them together. If your nipples protrude they are not inverted, but if they shrink back into the breasts they are.

To reduce breastfeeding problems, it is worth encouraging the nipples to protrude during pregnancy. Place your thumbs on either side of one nipple, at the edge of the areola. Press in firmly and pull your thumbs away from each other to stretch the nipple. Then place your thumbs above and below it and pull away again. Repeat several times on each nipple. With daily practice, this should loosen any tightness and draw them out. If you do find that you have inverted nipples, it is advisable to contact a breastfeeding counsellor (p. 347) before your baby is born. There is always a possibility you may have feeding problems.

Itching *see* SKIN CHANGES IN PREGNANCY

Jaundice

One of the functions of the liver is to break down haemoglobin derived from red blood cells when their three-month lifespan is over. One breakdown product is brownish-yellow *bilirubin*, which is formed in the liver and excreted in bile.

If the baby's liver is not mature at birth or excess red cells break down, the bile is not excreted efficiently and bilirubin may spill into the bloodstream. This causes the baby's skin and eyes to turn yellow, a symptom known as jaundice. It is common and usually clears up within a few days, but rarely, the bilirubin may continue to build up. The major danger of excessively high levels is that some of it may be deposited in the brain (*kernicterus*), leading to brain damage.

Neonatal physiological jaundice

Mild jaundice is more common in premature babies, whose liver cells cannot excrete bilirubin. If a baby is bruised at birth, severe jaundice may result from red cells absorbed from the bruise. The condition becomes obvious on the second or third day after birth and the level of bilirubin can be measured by testing a small sample of blood from the baby's heel.

Neonatal jaundice usually peaks by the fourth day, after which the liver is able to deal with the bilirubin. Generally no special treatment is needed. If bilirubin levels continue to rise, the baby is given phototherapy – ultraviolet light treatment. In sunny weather, minor rises in bilirubin levels are well treated by exposing the baby to the ultraviolet rays in sunlight. Otherwise, it is given to the baby in a cot or incubator, where she lies naked apart from pads to protect her eyes.

Phototherapy alters the bilirubin in the blood beneath the skin, allowing it to bypass the liver and be excreted by the kidneys; urine production is encouraged by giving the baby extra fluid. Phototherapy is given when bilirubin levels are very high, although for premature babies phototherapy is necessary at lower levels.

Phototherapy may be given in the mother's room, so that separation of mother and baby is minimal. This allows the mother to hold and feed the baby when necessary, and to place her under the lights when she is relaxed or asleep. The yellowish skin colour may last for weeks without danger, as long as the baby's bilirubin levels are kept at a low level in the first week.

Rhesus and ABO incompatibility jaundice

In some babies the red blood cells are broken down by antibodies to the child's rhesus factor produced by the mother or, if the mother's blood type is Type O, to the baby's A, B or AB blood group. In this case phototherapy may be needed earlier and for longer. The antibodies will disappear in a few days, and once the initial stress is over, the baby's red cells no longer break down.

Other types of jaundice

Very rarely indeed, there may be a maldevelopment of the liver or the system of bile ducts leading from it, or an enzyme defect in the liver cells. Treatment will again involve phototherapy, but the outlook depends on the underlying cause of the problem.

Kidney problems *see* URINARY TRACT AND KIDNEY PROBLEMS IN THE BABY; URINARY TRACT AND KIDNEY PROBLEMS IN THE MOTHER

Large babies

Adequate maternal nutrition has brought about an increase in the birth weight of babies born in Britain. Usually the baby's weight, and thus his size, are perfect for the mother, but occasionally there is a problem.

Mothers with DIABETES often have large babies who behave like premature babies. The major problem with a large baby in labour is *disproportion* between the baby's size and the mother's pelvis. This may lead to difficulty in labour and the need for an assisted delivery or CAESAREAN SECTION. Sometimes the baby's head is born but the birth of the shoulders is delayed, a rare but important emergency complication of labour. This can usually be avoided if the mother uses upright postures during labour. Post-natally, most large babies usually thrive.

Let-down failure *see* BREAST PROBLEMS AFTER CHILDBIRTH

Loss of a baby

The death of an unborn baby or of a child in the first months of life can be emotionally devastating, straining the resources and reserves of parents to their limits.

In some families, particularly those belonging to cultures in which death and dying are considered part of life, a death may be accepted by the parents relatively quickly and smoothly. In others, the loss of a baby may have profound long-term effects, and unless it is well handled, it may occasionally lead to great emotional disturbances in other members of the family.

The first day

The usual reaction to death is a great sense of shock, which can be incapacitating in its intensity, and there may be an emotional numbness. Events may overtake the parents and push the reality into the background.

If you have had a late MISCARRIAGE or a STILLBIRTH, you will have been through labour, and there may be post-natal discomforts to cope with as well. If you have lost a child through COT DEATH, dealing with bureaucracy can be painful and trying, requiring you to communicate and answer questions at a time when you may be least inclined to do so.

It may help you to see and touch your baby as soon as you can after the death. Giving the child a name will increase the sense that she was a real person, and will make it easier to grieve. You may find it especially difficult if you have lost a baby before, or had trouble conceiving the child who has just died. For some families, a baptism, a prayer from a priest, vicar or rabbi and a religious funeral are important events.

Certain arrangements will be necessary, although sometimes distasteful. A post-mortem may be required to establish the exact cause of death (although parents may have the option of not having one), and a funeral may have to be organized.

A woman in hospital may be separated from other new mothers, but the sounds of other newborn babies may still be audible, and this can seem intolerable. Because of their own embarrassment, medical helpers and friends may avoid you or not know how to talk to you. Talking to a counsellor may be a great relief.

The first week

This usually passes in a vague haze. If you have just given birth, there may be stitches to attend to and you will have milk coming into your breasts. If necessary a drug can be given to dry this up. Post-natal discomfort and breasts full of milk without a baby can be extremely upsetting.

Seeing the baby and attending the funeral if physically possible are key elements of the mourning process. Women who are unable to do this often cannot accept the death as a reality and may take longer to recover. Emotionally they may expect the baby to appear, although rationally they know this to be impossible. Asking bereaved parents to participate may seem very cruel at the time, but it is worth while in the long term. Funerals can be arranged even for babies born before 28 weeks' gestation.

The first six weeks

On the surface, the first week may appear the most difficult, but problems often intensify as time passes. Anger and resentment are often intense, and the feeling of deprivation may become more powerful. Many women find it difficult to watch healthy babies and children, and may even be unable to shop or walk in the street for fear of seeing a baby or pregnant woman. Some feel shame or acute pain that they do not have their own baby, and violent feelings are common.

Many women experience obsessive thoughts – *'If only I had done this . . . If only that had not happened . . .'* – which dominate their days and nights. Guilt may lead to blame, with the parents accusing each other, or the family blaming the hospital doctors. Even a young child may unconsciously blame himself for the death of a sibling; it will help if he clearly understands the reasons for the death.

The practical events set in motion by the death will continue. You may be awaiting the results of tests determining the cause of death, and you will want to discuss with your doctor what happened and what measures to take next time. (You may find it helpful to have a list of prepared questions for this meeting.) About this time, you may be expected to return to work, where you will have to face colleagues and friends. Re-adjusting to work when you had planned to take time off after the birth may be especially difficult.

The next few months

The process of coming to terms with your loss continues, but by now you are probably receiving far less special attention. This is the time when many suppressed physical symptoms may emerge – e.g. pain, headache, lethargy. You may not feel motivated to exercise every day, but this can be a helpful way of dealing with stress and releasing tension.

These months are difficult because, although others expect you to be 'getting over it', your feelings are still likely to be acute at times. Grief may come in waves, receding only to return with surprising intensity some time later, and this may continue for a year or two. Anniversaries of the baby's birth and death may be especially upsetting and occasions for grieving over the years.

The parents' relationship

Relations between parents may be strained following a death. Many seek help from a professional counsellor or therapist, or from support groups. Your family doctor or hospital will be able to help you get in touch with an appropriate group (*see also* p. 347).

Problems may arise because men are not expected to show their grief and respond to loss in the same way as women. However, the death of a child is usually felt as acutely by fathers as by mothers, and they may need as much love and support as their partners, even though they may feel that they cannot ask for it as openly.

When a death occurs in a family, an unconscious process may take place in which, as well as self-blame, each family member blames one or more of the others as they all struggle to understand and accept what has happened. Apparently unrelated arguments may stem from grief at the death, and one partner may think that frequent signs of grief in the other are a weakness when, in fact, this may be indicative of long-term strength. Counselling can be helpful in bringing these feelings to the surface so that they can be dealt with, and it may be vital to seek medical advice about the cause of death to end this 'blame sequence'.

Other children

The loss of a baby is part of your family life, and your other children may be as upset as you are. Even very young children will 'know' that something is wrong and react accordingly. Older children may have had conflicting emotions about the arrival of the new baby, so they may now feel an unconscious responsibility for the death.

No matter how difficult it is for you, your children need to be reassured that you love them. Tell them honestly what happened and how you feel. By allowing them to tell you how they feel and letting them ask questions, you will discover how much reassurance they need. They should be encouraged to express their feelings through play; drawing and painting are particularly therapeutic. If you find that you need time after the death before you can face your other children, make sure that those caring for them emphasize how much you still love and want them, even though at the moment you are sad about what has happened.

Planning the next pregnancy

Before embarking on another pregnancy, it is important for you to realize how long the process of mourning can continue. Many people may encourage you to 'get over' your sorrow by having another baby quickly. This may upset you because the child you have lost cannot simply be replaced by another. It is best to allow time to mourn. If the process is abruptly interrupted by a new pregnancy, you may suffer depression after the new birth, even if everything is fine.

During the next pregnancy, it is natural to be more worried and anxious than usual. Such fears are deep-seated, and you and everyone around you will be relieved when your next baby is born healthy.

See also CONGENITAL ABNORMALITIES AND GENETIC COUNSELLING, ILLNESS IN BABIES

Common reactions to bereavement

The manifestations of grief are varied, and the following are some very common reactions to bereavement. Accepting that these are all usual may help you to come to terms with the death.

● *Shock* may only last a few minutes, or it may continue for days, weeks and months. Discovering that your baby is abnormal, dying or dead can be devastating. For some parents, the shock is so traumatic that it takes them years to recover.

● *Denial* may precede shock, taking the form of 'This can't be happening to me'. The need to deny the death may be intense.

● *Anger* may seem a strange reaction to the death of someone you love, but many people react angrily, rather like children when something they are enjoying is taken away. Allow yourself to express anger and do not feel that you must hide it, even if you are shocked to find yourself hating the dead child for deserting you. The sooner this emotion is released, the more quickly it will fade.

● *Guilt* is a common reaction to the death of someone close. You may feel that you lost your baby because of something you did or did not do. Many women who lose babies, including those who have had a termination, have a deep sense of guilt which may block other feelings.

● *Sadness and weeping* are the classic signs of mourning, and may continue for weeks, months or even years. With time, loss does become easier to bear, but it is important to allow grief to emerge, to be expressed rather than suppressed.

● *Depression* may be a major factor in mourning, and it too may last for months or years. In men and women with an underlying tendency towards it, the loss of a baby may be catastrophic. It may manifest itself as dependence on alcohol, tranquillizers or other drugs, and psychotherapy is essential.

● *Physical symptoms* may be intense, and can include headaches, chest, abdominal or back pain, or intestinal or bladder problems. Miscarriage is sometimes followed by nausea until the time when the baby would have been born. Your doctor should check all physical symptoms, but you should bear in mind their possible relationship to the death.

Low birth weight and prematurity

There are two main reasons for low birth weight, that is, below 2.5 kg (5 ½ lb). Some babies grow more slowly than normal and are known as 'small for dates'; others develop normally but are born early – this is *prematurity*; or a baby may be both.

The vast majority of babies of low birth weight have developed properly and are no cause for concern. However, very tiny babies, particularly those in the premature group whose organs are too immature for life outside the uterus, are often very tender and fragile, needing intensive help, love and support to attain their full potential. Advances in neonatal care have improved the outlook for tiny babies, but being born very small can still be a problem.

'Small-for-dates' babies

A baby is considered to be 'small for dates' if his weight at birth is in the lowest five per cent of the range of 'normal' birth weights, after allowances have been made for sex and ethnic origin and for the mother's height and weight.

One reason why a baby may be small for dates is *placental insufficiency*, when the blood supply to the placenta is inadequate. This may occur without obvious cause or may be associated with HIGH BLOOD PRESSURE in the mother. It is also relatively common in multiple pregnancies to find one twin deprived of placental blood flow (*see* TWINS).

As the placental flow decreases, the baby's head and brain continue to grow while the other organs slow down – a phenomenon known as the 'brain-sparing effect'. Four-fifths of all babies who are under-sized at birth belong to this category, and are called 'asymmetrical small-for-dates babies'. They are likely to have reduced sugar stores and may be prone to FOETAL DISTRESS during labour. However, if labour is normal and feeding begins soon after birth, these babies catch up rapidly with normal physical and intellectual development.

The remaining small-for-dates babies are known as 'symmetrical' as, from early pregnancy on, all parts of them are consistently small. Often there is no obvious reason for their impaired growth, although this is sometimes associated with infections such as RUBELLA, CYTOMEGALOVIRUS and TOXO-PLASMOSIS, CONGENITAL ABNORMALITIES, maternal starvation or addiction to DRUGS such as heroin, ALCOHOL or cigarettes (*see* SMOKING IN PREGNANCY). Symmetrical small-for-dates babies may sometimes be born with disability, but the majority are small babies from small mothers and are perfectly fit and well; placental function is normal and foetal distress in labour is uncommon.

Diagnosis During an ante-natal checkup, examination of the mother's abdomen combined with measuring the height of her uterus can detect up to 75 per cent of all small-for-dates babies. If there is doubt about the date of conception, an ULTRASOUND SCAN performed in the first half of pregnancy may help to confirm the approximate age of the baby. In the majority of cases when a baby is thought to be small for dates, he is normal but the dates are wrong, conception having occurred later than the mother thought.

If a woman has any of the predisposing factors she may be the first to become suspicious. Some mothers feel that their baby is growing too slowly or that foetal movements are fewer. In most instances, such fears are unfounded, but they always warrant investigation.

Treatment Once the diagnosis of small for dates has been confirmed, it is important to keep a careful check on the baby, and additional ante-natal care is usual. Improved maternal nutrition is essential, and zinc supplements may encourage foetal growth. Bedrest and treatment for high blood pressure if it is present may improve the placental flow.

Symmetrical babies usually withstand labour very well, and induction is rarely necessary. However, a small minority of asymmetrical small-for-dates babies may be safer outside the uterus if bedrest does not improve growth and the placental flow becomes critically reduced. The key test is a count of the baby's movements and monitoring the heartbeat for signs of foetal distress. If growth ceases, or if there are signs of distress, an early birth is essential, either by a carefully monitored induction or by elective CAESAREAN SECTION. Birth under 32 weeks may be preceded by giving the mother cortisone in an attempt to help the baby's lungs mature.

Some asymmetrical babies have low sugar reserves and may become distressed. Careful monitoring during labour is vital, while the mother's use of upright positions ensure the best possible blood flow to the placenta. If foetal distress is present, an emergency Caesarean section may be needed.

After birth, warmth is critical as a premature baby may lose heat rapidly and have few fat reserves for insulation and heat production. Close body contact with the mother is ideal, supplemented by an overhead heater.

The baby should be breastfed as soon as possible and frequently thereafter, because reduced sugar stores increase the risk of low blood sugar, which may cause brain damage – the most serious complication affecting small-for-dates babies post-natally. If, despite frequent feeds, there are still signs of low sugar (e.g. irritability or floppiness), the blood sugar levels must be measured and concentrated dextrose (sugar) water given to the baby.

The baby will also need to be examined fully to determine exactly why he was small for dates and to exclude any underlying problem. Asymmetrical babies usually gain weight rapidly and catch up within a few months. If there is no obvious reason for a symmetrical baby's smallness, he will probably develop normally, but may remain short.

Many women with small-for-dates babies are very worried when they are told before the birth. This anxiety is natural and unavoidable.

Premature babies

Most premature births are unpredictable and can occur unexpectedly in any pregnancy. A baby is deemed to be premature if he is born after the 24th week and before the 36th week of pregnancy. Approximately three to five per cent of babies are premature.

Poor nutrition and poor housing are the most important predisposing factors, and premature babies are also more common in women with cervical incompetence and in twin pregnancies. In medical conditions such as severe high blood pressure, the obstetrician may recommend delivering the baby early, because the risks of prematurity may be fewer than the risks of the baby staying in the uterus. In addition, PREMATURE RUPTURE OF THE MEMBRANES may precede the onset of labour by days or even weeks, with the possibility of some infection developing that may necessitate immediate delivery.

Delaying labour Once true labour has been confirmed – i.e. contractions are associated with dilation of the cervix – drugs may be given to try and stop it. These can have side-effects in both mother and baby which are sometimes serious, so the risks need to be weighed carefully.

Most commonly, drugs are used to postpone labour for 24 to 36 hours if the pregnancy has lasted less than 32 weeks. During this time, cortisone injections can be given to the mother in an attempt (not always successful) to stimulate foetal lung development and reduce post-natal breathing problems.

Managing premature labour It might seem sensible to rupture the membranes to provide continuous monitoring, but, in fact, intact membranes lessen the pressure of the baby's head on the cervix as it dilates, reducing the risk of head injury during the birth. A premature baby's skull is softer and more prone to bruising and moulding than that of a full-term baby.

PAIN RELIEF should probably be limited to gas-and-air or epidural anaesthesia. Anything else may cause severe problems in the baby – for instance, pethidine injections or tranquillizers may take weeks to be cleared from the circulation of the newborn.

CAESAREAN SECTION is only necessary in a minority of premature births and, if possible, should be performed under epidural rather than general anaesthesia to protect the baby. In premature BREECH BIRTHS, a Caesarean section may be the gentlest for the baby.

Post-natal treatment Like small-for-dates babies, premature infants need to be kept very warm and fed frequently (*see above*). If a baby is too tiny to suck, it can be fed expressed breastmilk via a tube until the sucking reflex develops.

The major problem facing premature babies is an immature breathing system, and those born before 32 weeks often develop respiratory distress. The treatment is to give oxygen to the baby in an incubator. In severe cases, the baby is artificially ventilated: a tube placed in his windpipe is connected to a machine that blows air into the lungs under mild pressure. Babies on such ventilators require intensive monitoring and need to be in special-care baby units.

Tiny premature babies, especiallly those on ventilators, are at risk of internal bleeding because their blood-clotting system is not fully developed. Modern monitoring systems help to reduce the risk of damage, but cannot entirely prevent it.

Premature babies are particularly prone to infection, and they also require expert nutritional care. Breastmilk is essential for optimal growth of the brain; if he is separated from his mother, the baby can be fed with expressed breastmilk from either his mother (pp. 204–5) or a milk bank.

The survival rate for premature babies has increased dramatically in the last ten years, and today 70 per cent of those born before 32 weeks survive, and 90 per cent after 32 weeks. A small minority of these survivors suffer some physical and/or mental handicap; at highest risk are very tiny babies, those needing ventilation and those suffering from internal bleeding.

Emotional reactions The birth of a premature child can come as a shock to both parents, who may not yet be ready, psychologically and practically, to receive their baby. They may feel guilty about the premature birth, as well as real concern about the infant's long-term development.

If a baby is fighting for his life, his parents often feel powerless to help, but the baby will really benefit by your presence: spend as much time with him as you can, and have as much body contact as possible, even if at first this may mean that you can only stroke his body through the holes in an incubator. Simply being there and helping to take care of him will reduce your anxiety and help him to thrive. Recent research has shown that premature babies who are fit enough to be carried by their mothers or a nurse in a sling thrive and gain weight more rapidly. This is known as the 'Kangaroo' method.

Ideally, the incubator should be next to your bed, but this is not always possible: a very small or ill baby will need to be in a special-care baby unit. Sometimes the physical arrangement of a hospital can make things difficult, for example, if the special-care unit is separate from the post-natal ward. The baby's father will be an important go-between.

You will need as much support as you can get; both during the anxious days in hospital and during the perhaps strangely empty or anticlimactic days or weeks at home without your baby. When things seem to be becoming overwhelming, always remember that the majority of premature babies survive to reach normal adulthood.

Going home The recent trend has been to send premature babies home before they have reached the 'normal' birth weight of 2.5 kg (5½ lb), provided they have overcome any breathing or nutritional problems. Many areas have special-care nurses who visit mothers and babies at home, an arrangement that is usually preferable to a mother having to travel long distances each day to see and feed her baby.

When your baby comes home, try to spend as much time with him as you can, even sharing a bed at night, to make up for the time apart. Body contact, loving care and pleasant experiences later on will compensate for the difficulties some premature babies encounter at first. *See also* ILLNESS IN BABIES, LOSS OF A BABY.

Low blood pressure and fainting

Low blood pressure (*hypotension*) is usually a sign of good health and fitness and is, on the whole, desirable during pregnancy. However, if it drops very suddenly or becomes very low, it can cause dizziness and faintness.

Certain causes of low blood pressure are serious – for instance, blood loss may lower blood pressure, which is an early sign of shock. More commonly, susceptible women will find that simply lying on their back for a while lowers blood pressure enough to cause faintness when they get up. This type of *postural low blood pressure* – feeling faint or dizzy after getting up suddenly or after standing for long periods – is more likely in pregnancy, particularly if you have varicose veins or are taking anti-hypertensive drugs, and it will worsen during late pregnancy. Extreme heat and drinking alcohol will exacerbate the problem.

If you feel faint, sit down quickly; otherwise you might fall heavily and injure yourself. Apart from this, postural low blood pressure has no damaging effects. To avoid it, regularly contract and relax your leg and buttock muscles like a pump, to get the blood flowing back to your brain. Lying on your side instead of your back in bed (so that the heavy uterus does not press down on the large blood vessels) will prevent you feeling faint when you get up.

There is no risk to the baby unless the fall in blood pressure is extreme.

Low temperature *see* HYPOTHERMIA IN THE BABY

Low weight gain after birth

It is generally obvious if a baby has gained very little weight after birth, and frequent weighing is only necessary if the gain is grossly below normal. Most babies with low weight gain are merely of small build and not undernourished.

Feeding can be the problem. Some babies react adversely to certain brands of formula, and an alternative needs to be found. Some mothers may only produce a small volume of breastmilk, or there may be a delay in the let-down reflex so that the baby is only getting the foremilk (*see* BREAST PROBLEMS AFTER CHILDBIRTH). Sometimes infection in the urine or bowel, THRUSH or NAPPY RASH prevent the baby from thriving.

If a baby's need for affection and stimulation is not satisfied, he may fail to thrive, and physical, emotional and intellectual development may all be disturbed. Such babies lack close contact, love and security, and the feeding relationship between mother and child is abnormal or absent.

If you are concerned that your baby may be underweight, visit your local clinic or doctor, where your baby will be given a thorough medical investigation, if the cause of the problem is in failure to establish breastfeeding correctly. Often, early difficulties can be overcome, with perseverance.

Low weight gain in pregnancy *see* WEIGHT GAIN IN PREGNANCY
Mastitis *see* BREAST PROBLEMS AFTER CHILDBIRTH
Maternal age *see* OLDER MOTHERS, YOUNG MOTHERS

Meconium staining of amniotic fluid

Meconium is the sticky, greenish-black substance normally passed from a baby's bowels during the first day or two after birth. Sometimes, however, the baby passes meconium while still in the uterus, and this then stains the amniotic fluid. The most common reason for this is foetal maturity: if the baby is ready to be born, she may have a chance bowel action, but this is nothing to worry about. In about ten per cent of cases, however, the passage of meconium is a sign of FOETAL DISTRESS.

There is no justification for artificially rupturing the membranes to test the amniotic fluid, as meconium on its own does not indicate definite foetal distress. If thick meconium is present, FOETAL-HEART MONITORING is used to confirm the diagnosis.

There is a further problem with thick meconium if it is sucked into the baby's lungs at birth (*see* BREATHING PROBLEMS IN THE BABY).

Megacolon *see* CONSTIPATION IN THE BABY
Migraine *see* PAIN IN PREGNANCY AND AFTER CHILDBIRTH

Miscarriage

A pregnancy that ends spontaneously before the 28th week is called a miscarriage or, in medical terminology, a *spontaneous abortion*.

Only about 25 per cent of all conceptions culminate in the birth of a live child. Many fertilized eggs do not implant in the uterus, and the woman is not even aware that she has conceived. Some miscarriages occur slightly later, giving rise to a delayed or slightly heavier period. Obvious, recognized miscarriages occur in approximately 15 per cent of all pregnancies. Knowing these statistics will probably not prevent the shock of a miscarriage, but may help to place it in perspective.

Causes

A miscarriage that occurs during the first ten weeks of pregnancy is most likely caused by the abnormal development of the embryo. Correct embryonic development depends on the state of both the egg and the sperm, so developmental anomalies are as likely to come from the man as the woman. Because early miscarriage is nature's way of filtering out abnormalities, it is just as well that there is no treatment that will artificially prolong early pregnancy.

Some miscarriages may be caused by a low production of progesterone, but the case for this has not been proved conclusively. This hormone is normally produced by the ovaries for the first few weeks of pregnancy and then by the placenta. Doctors have been known to prescribe progesterone supplements for women whose output is low, but this is generally inadvisable, as synthetic progesterone may adversely affect the developing sex organs of the baby, and it has not been shown to reduce the number of miscarriages.

Miscarriage in mid-pregnancy may be the result of CERVICAL INCOMPETENCE, in which case a stitch can be inserted in subsequent pregnancies to keep the cervix closed.

Symptoms and diagnosis

The main symptom of a miscarriage is vaginal BLEEDING. If this is painless, you may be having a 'threatened miscarriage': the chances are high that the baby is alive and that the pregnancy will continue to term. Slight spotting in early pregnancy can often be dealt with by bedrest for a day or two until it stops.

After a threatened miscarriage, there is no extra likelihood of the baby being abnormal. The bleeding always involves the maternal blood, from the uterus.

If bleeding is associated with cramp-like abdominal pain and/or the passage of blood clots, miscarriage is usually inevitable. The more severe the pain, the more likely the miscarriage. In these circumstances, a gentle vaginal examination is performed to confirm the diagnosis.

The standard way of checking used to be a pregnancy test, but this is no longer done because, in some cases, the placenta may function even though the embryo is no longer alive, with the result that the pregnancy test is falsely positive.

This is true in an embryonic pregnancy, or 'missed abortion'. This occurs when the embryo dies early in pregnancy but the placenta continues to grow and produce amniotic fluid, so that miscarriage does not immediately occur. Pregnancy may continue for as long as 14 weeks, with placental hormones keeping pregnancy tests positive, even though there is no baby. An ULTRASOUND SCAN will reveal the absence of an embryo; miscarriage always occurs eventually.

If a scan reveals the presence of an embryo, its heartbeat is seen, movements are present and there is no obvious congenital abnormality, then the mother will be reassured that the pregnancy is highly likely to continue.

Treatment

If a threatened miscarriage has occurred but not settled down, the doctor's advice will probably be to take it easy at home and cut down on work. There is no evidence that strict bedrest prevents miscarriages.

If a scan confirms that the baby is not alive, the treatment will probably be admission to hospital where surgical dilation and curettage of the uterus (D&C) will be performed under anaesthetic. Even if a miscarriage has already occurred, the doctor may want to ensure that it is complete by performing a D&C, because any fragments of membranes or placenta remaining in the uterus could cause infection.

In very early pregnancy (before eight weeks), curettage is usually unnecessary. In these circumstances, it may be preferable to wait for the inevitable miscarriage to occur spontaneously.

Recurrent miscarriages

An incompetent cervix may be suspected if miscarriages occur repeatedly after the 12th week of pregnancy, particularly if they are relatively painless.

New research has revealed that the cause of three or more miscarriages is, in some cases, failure of the immune system of a woman to recognize the presence of the embryo if the father's blood group and tissue type are similar to hers. If current theories are confirmed, it may be possible to prevent this by immunizing a woman before conception with some white blood cells taken from the father – encouraging news for the small number of women who fall into this category.

Emotional reactions

For many women, the emotional trauma of miscarrying can be great. Nevertheless, miscarriage is often underestimated: women are expected to get over it quickly and start again. Women who have had a previous TERMINATION OF PREGNANCY may have deep-seated or unresolved feelings of guilt, and a miscarriage can seem to be a consequence or punishment. Partners may contribute to these guilt feelings, sometimes unintentionally. Infertile women who have taken a long time to conceive may be especially upset if they miscarry.

However early in pregnancy you miscarry, it is important to allow yourself to mourn the loss (see LOSS OF A BABY).

Returning to normal

The later in pregnancy you miscarry, the longer it will take your body to get back to normal. If you lose a baby very late, your breasts may even produce milk. Periods usually return within about six weeks, but in some women it takes longer.

Some women feel the need to conceive again as soon as possible, but it is best (although not essential) to wait for at least three menstrual cycles before trying – waiting is known to reduce the statistical risk of miscarrying again. It is natural that any woman who has miscarried should be anxious about doing so again. However, having had one miscarriage does not necessarily mean that there is any greater chance of having another, although after two the chances do increase slightly.

Mongolism see DOWN'S SYNDROME
Morning sickness see VOMITING IN PREGNANCY
Multiple pregnancy see TWINS
Muscular dystrophy see DUCHENNE MUSCULAR DYSTROPHY

Nappy rash

An angry red rash in the nappy area is extremely common, and babies with sensitive skins are especially prone to it.

The usual cause of nappy rash is ammonia in the urine and enzymes in the faeces combining to irritate the skin. Moist heat sealed in by plastic pants is another culprit, and stiff terry nappies may scratch the skin. Baby products may disturb the skin's oil and chemical balance, lowering resistance to bacteria. Persistent nappy rash may be due to THRUSH, or the baby may be sensitive to a particular type of formula.

Treatment

Help to prevent nappy rash by changing your baby's nappy frequently, and leave it off for some time every day if possible. Do not use soap or baby wipes to clean his bottom; instead, put a few drops of pure oil in the bath water or on a piece of cotton wool. If you use fabric nappies, try disposables to see if they improve matters. Avoid washing fabric nappies with strong detergents (especially biological ones) or using fabric conditioners. If the baby is bottle-fed, a different water or formula may produce less acid in the urine; you should also not give any fruit juice to a baby under three months. If you breastfeed, avoid very acidic food or drink.

At the first signs of redness, change your baby's nappies even more often. After washing him, dry him very gently with a soft towel, using a blotting action (never rub). To dry him really thoroughly, try using a hair dryer set to medium. This will avoid contact with the sore area and will promote rapid healing.

Apply a very light film of zinc or castor oil cream or homoeopathic hypercal cream to the baby's dry skin before putting on a clean nappy. Put him to sleep on his stomach so that urine drains downwards away from the skin. Use one-way nappy liners at night. The worse the rash, the more you should expose your baby's bottom to the air. With a very bad rash, let the baby sleep on a soft absorbent towel without a nappy. Cover the baby and change the towel whenever it has become wet.

Nausea see VOMITING IN PREGNANCY
Neck pain see PAIN IN PREGNANCY AND AFTER CHILDBIRTH
Neonatal herpes see VAGINAL INFECTIONS
Neonatal resuscitation see RESUSCITATION OF THE BABY

Neural tube defects

Four in 1000 babies in Britain are born with a serious defect of the brain or spinal cord caused by abnormal development of the embryonic neural tube. The most common of these are: *anencephaly* (the incomplete formation of the brain and skull); *spina bifida* (the incomplete formation of the vertebrae and/or the spinal cord); and *hydrocephaly* (an excess of cerebro-spinal fluid inside the brain).

The outlook for babies born with one or more of these defects depends on the degree to which they are affected. Isolated hydrocephaly may be treatable, but it can be associated with mental retardation. A child with mild spina bifida, in which the vertebrae are abnormal but the overlying skin and underlying spinal cord are normal, is likely to lead to a relatively normal life. However, open spina bifida, in which the defect is not covered by skin and there is underlying spinal abnormality, is associated with a high degree of mental subnormality and paralysis of the lower limbs and lower trunk, together with incontinence. At least half of those born with this die within the first five years of life, and only a minority are free from major handicap. Anencephalic babies cannot live.

Causes

Anencephaly and spina bifida are relatively common in Britain, especially in Scotland and western areas of Wales and England. The cause is unknown, but there may be a link with mineral and vitamin deficiency.

There is now considerable evidence that vitamins and minerals taken before conception reduce the likelihood of a neural tube defect. This is particularly important where there is a family history of this or a previously affected baby, as the likelihood of having another child with a similar defect rises.

Diagnosis

When you are 16 weeks pregnant, you may be offered a blood test to measure the level of alpha-foetoprotein (AFP) in your blood (p. 86). This test detects 75 per cent of the cases of open spina bifida, but it is not infallible.

For this reason, confirmation is needed. While AMNIOCENTESIS may be carried out to measure AFP in the amniotic fluid, recent improvements in ULTRASOUND SCANNING make this the method of choice. Occasionally, abnormalities in the development of the foetal intestines cause high levels of AFP, and scanning can detect these too. Eventually, ultrasound scans at 16 weeks will probably replace the AFP blood test altogether, because scans can also diagnose hydrocephaly, a defect not diagnosable from the AFP test.

Treatment

Treatment of neural tube defects depends on the severity of the condition. Isolated mild hydrocephaly can be treated by the insertion of a valve to drain the fluid from the brain into the bloodstream. Closed spina bifida needs no treatment.

Open spina bifida represents the biggest dilemma: whether surgery to close the defect will save a life or merely prolong suffering is an immensely difficult decision to make. Closing the skin will not cure the paralysis or the associated mental handicap. As spina bifida sufferers grow older, their emotional problems increase; their incontinence causes many difficulties; and associated hydrocephaly usually becomes worse.

It is in the context of this knowledge that parents have to decide about the future of their affected child, with the help and support of the health-care team. If the decision is not to operate, many families prefer to care for their infants at home.

See also CONGENITAL ABNORMALITIES AND GENETIC COUNSELLING, ILLNESS IN BABIES

Non-accidental injuries *see* INJURIES TO THE BABY

Nosebleeds in pregnancy

During pregnancy the nasal blood vessels dilate, and some women suffer from frequent nosebleeds as a result. A medical check is sensible. If nosebleeds become very frequent and annoying, cautery can be performed to destroy the dilated blood vessels. If your nose is bleeding, sit upright with your head back and apply gentle pressure to the sides of your nose. It is not wise to blow your nose or disturb the scabs.

Numb and painful fingers in pregnancy

Numbness and tingling in the fingers is fairly common during late pregnancy, particularly if there is fluid retention (*see* OEDEMA), and swollen finger joints may ache, especially if rings become tight.

Carpal tunnel syndrome Caused by compression of nerves in the wrist, this is treated by reducing fluid retention, massaging the wrist and sleeping at night with your arm raised on pillows. The following yoga wrist stretch will also help. Kneel on the floor. Place the palms of your hands on the floor, fingers pointing towards your knees, the front of the wrists pointing away. Keep your elbows straight. Slowly move your knees back, until you can feel a gentle stretch at the front of your wrists. Repeat for three to five minutes four times a day, including last thing at night.

Any numbness, weakness or tingling in the upper arms should be reported to your doctor, as this may be caused by compressed nerves in the neck, which will also need treatment.

Obesity in the baby

Obesity is caused by an excess food intake or by a metabolism that tends to store food as fat. It is rare in early infancy, but nutritional patterns established early in life have an important bearing on the development of later obesity. In infancy, it is almost impossible for exclusively breastfed babies to become obese, whereas formulas rich in added sugars and other refined nutrients are a potent cause of overweight babies. If your baby is gaining excessively, check with your doctor or health visitor. The formula may need to be changed, or water substituted for one or two feeds a day.

Obesity in pregnancy *see* WEIGHT BEFORE PREGNANCY

Occipito posterior position in labour

A baby in the *occipito posterior* position is head down but facing her mother's navel, with the back of her head towards the mother's spine. You may then feel her kick at the front rather than at the side.

Why some babies are occipito posterior

The most usual reason for an occipito posterior presentation is simply that the baby is more comfortable facing the placenta, which may have implanted on the front wall of the uterus. Sometimes the reason is the shape of the mother's pelvis. Instead of being the usual oval, it may be almost triangular, with the widest space at the back; the angle between the pubic bones at the front is small and cannot be used by the baby's head. Since the diameter of her head is also widest at the back, there is a better fit in the back part of the pelvis. If the pelvic size is ample this may not present a problem, but when the occipito posterior presentation is due to pelvic shape, labour may be prolonged. The baby's head may be *deflexed* with the chin not tucked in. Because of the pressure exerted by the head on the sacrum, labour can be associated with backache and pain in the sacrum, and be long, with uncoordinated uterine activity. If the birth is active, such difficulties are reduced.

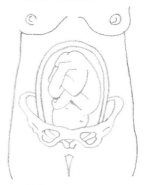

The first stage of labour

If your baby is occipito posterior, you may have backache which continues between contractions.

Once labour is strongly established, experiment with different positions. You might feel comfortable kneeling, to reduce the pressure of the baby's head on the sacrum. Kneeling also encourages rotation, because the heaviest part of the baby's body, the spine, may turn downwards with gravity. Moving and changing position freely, staying upright as much as possible, will help the baby's head to flex and to engage in the pelvis. Circling your hips will also encourage rotation. Immersion in water (p. 151) or massage (*see* Part V) can greatly relax the muscles that surround the pelvis, so increasing pelvic capacity.

The second stage of labour

It is wise to stay upright, using the supported squat (p. 126) to help the pelvis open fully with maximum help from gravity. This increases the chance of an unassisted birth.

If it is impossible to give birth unaided, you will be offered an assisted delivery (*see* FORCEPS DELIVERY AND VACUUM EXTRACTION). A vacuum extractor may be applied to the baby's scalp, encouraging the head to tuck in and then rotate. The obstetrician may turn the head manually, or use Kiellands forceps. This manoeuvre requires epidural anaesthesia and a high degree of obstetric skill. Occasionally, disproportion makes a CAESAREAN SECTION necessary.

Repeat occipito posterior presentations

If the reason for the presentation is disproportion, your next baby is likely to be occipito posterior too. However, the stretching of the tissues and pelvic ligaments that occurs during a first birth usually makes subsequent ones easier.

Oedema

Oedema, a slight puffiness of the feet, legs and fingers, is normal during pregnancy, when some of the increase in fluid in the mother's body enters the soft tissues, causing them to swell. More common in a TWIN pregnancy, in overweight women and in those who gain excessive weight when pregnant, it is also more likely in hot weather and after standing for a long time.

Excessive puffiness extending to the face and neck may indicate pre-eclampsia or, rarely, kidney disease. Fluid retention should be checked medically to exclude these.

For a week after the birth, excess fluid in the body is excreted. While this adjustment takes place, your legs may swell considerably.

Treatment

Oedema can be uncomfortable and is treated by resting during the day with your feet up. If your fingers swell, take off any rings before they get stuck. You may find that wearing support tights reduces swelling. Exercises such as 'legs apart on a wall' (p. 249) will encourage the return of blood (and excess fluid) to the heart. Bear in mind that HOMOEOPATHY can be very affective in correcting fluid balance.

See also VARICOSE VEINS

Older mothers

Statisticians and obstetricians have tended to exaggerate the effects of increasing maternal age on the outcome of pregnancy. Today many women have their first baby when they are over the age of 35, when they may be described medically as *elderly primagravidae*. There is a slight increase in risk to older mothers and their babies, but not a big enough one to warrant excluding such women from normal activity during pregnancy, from active birth or from, in the right circumstances, home birth.

Physical factors

It may take older women longer to conceive – about six to nine months on average for those in their late 30s. This decreased fertility rate occurs even when ovulation is normal, and the reason for it is unknown. Miscarriage rates tend to be higher, as do those of Down's syndrome. Women over 35 are usually offered AMNIOCENTESIS or chorion biopsy to diagnose Down's syndrome. They also have slightly higher incidence of high blood pressure, pre-eclampsia and diabetes.

Despite these risks, childbirth for most fit women in their late 30s and early 40s is usually uncomplicated, and active birth can be the rule rather than the exception. When choosing the place of birth and the attendants, it is helpful to find out about policies and attitudes to your age, if you are over 35.

Social and psychological factors

Parents are usually financially more secure by their 30s, they tend to have realistic needs and expectations and are usually more confident of their ability to respond to change. Women often make the most of the experience of motherhood and are very dedicated.

The post-natal weeks are rarely a problem. On the whole, establishing breastfeeding is straightforward, although older mothers may be more tired and are less resilient about night feeds than young women. The sense of commitment to the new baby is usually intense. Since the children of their friends may be quite grown up, it may be particularly important for older women to join ante-natal and post-natal support groups.

See also CONGENITAL ABNORMALITIES AND GENETIC COUNSELLING, NEURAL TUBE DEFECTS

Oligohydramnios *see* AMNIOTIC FLUID
Otitis externa *see* EAR INFECTION IN THE BABY
Otitis media *see* EAR INFECTION IN THE BABY

Ovarian cysts

The most common type of ovarian cyst is the *corpus luteum*, which develops after ovulation and is essential for the first eight weeks of pregnancy (p. 18). It normally regresses by 16 weeks, and if it fills with fluid it may reach 15 cm (6 in) in diameter; the fluid is then absorbed into the body as the cyst shrinks. Rarely, the *corpus luteum* may rupture and cause internal bleeding resembling an ECTOPIC PREGNANCY. Several other types of benign cysts may be present in the ovary, but malignant tumours are extremely rare.

Symptoms

An ovarian cyst may cause no symptoms, and only be discovered during a routine ante-natal checkup. The main symptom is pain on one side of the lower abdomen, caused by sudden enlargement of the cyst with fluid, by it twisting the affected ovary or rupturing, with internal bleeding. There can also be urinary problems if a large cyst presses on the bladder. Symptoms are usually most acute in the first 12 weeks as the uterus enlarges and expands out of the pelvis.

Treatment

If the cyst has ruptured or twisted, or if it is bigger than 15 cm (6 in) in diameter, this is an acute emergency and an operation is urgently needed. There is a risk of MISCARRIAGE if this is done in the first 12 weeks of pregnancy.

A small cyst or tumour may be left until after the birth. If still present at the six-week post-natal checkup, it may then require surgical removal.

Overactive thyroid *see* THYROID DISORDERS IN MOTHER AND BABY
Overbreathing *see* HYPERVENTILATION
Overheating *see* FEVER IN THE BABY

Pain in pregnancy and after childbirth

It is not surprising that some women feel discomfort and pain during pregnancy and after childbirth, given the relatively dramatic changes the body undergoes. A small minority of the pains indicate a serious problem.

Abdominal pain

Where pain arises Pain may arise from the digestive tract, kidneys, bladder or genital organs, from the muscles or from nerves arising from the spinal column. Pain may also be 'referred' to other parts of the body.

* Pain from the stomach can produce HEARTBURN and discomfort in the upper abdomen.
* If the colon is affected, there may be CONSTIPATION, flatulence ('wind') or lower abdominal discomfort.
* There may be anal pain if the anus is affected.
* Kidney pain is usually felt in the loin area at the back of the upper abdomen.
* Bladder pain is felt in the pubic area, and is often associated with urinary frequency or burning (see URINARY TRACT AND KIDNEY PROBLEMS). In late pregnancy, when the pubic bones widen, pain may occur below the bladder.
* Pain from the cervix feels like a menstrual pain in the lower abdomen, either back or front.
* Uterine pain is cramp-like, as in labour, and usually felt in the front of the lower abdomen. The round ligament of the uterus may pull in the groin.
* The ovaries and Fallopian tubes usually give a low pain beginning on one side of the abdomen.
* Pain arising from the muscles and joints of the spine and pelvis is felt over the affected area, but may also radiate forward into the abdomen or pelvis, or down into the thighs.

Different pain at different times

* *Early pregnancy* Some women experience stomach and intestinal pain associated with nausea (see VOMITING IN PREGNANCY). Lower abdominal discomfort like a period pain is common and, provided there is no bleeding, does not indicate a miscarriage. Sharp severe pain, beginning suddenly, may indicate an ECTOPIC PREGNANCY, especially if felt more on one side; urgent medical help is essential.
* *Late pregnancy* Discomfort often arises from the spine, stomach, bladder or pubic bone. Pain from the uterus may indicate the onset of labour, but if it is continuous or severe it may be the result of internal bleeding requiring urgent medical attention.
* *After the birth* Lower abdominal pain is usually caused by the uterus contracting – 'after-pains' (p. 173) – but it may come from the bladder or vagina following bruising or stitching, or from the spine.

Treatment The vast majority of abdominal aches and pains are an indication of your body accommodating to the pregnancy. If any pain is severe, urgent attention is essential; otherwise, you should mention them at your ante-natal checkups. Treatment will depend upon the diagnosis.

Back and pelvic pain

Back pain is so common in pregnancy as to be almost taken for granted. Yet a healthy pregnancy should and need not involve back pain.

During pregnancy, the ligaments that surround all the joints in the body become soft. The shape of the spinal column alters, and the pelvic joints expand (p. 136). Any underlying imbalance in the mechanics of the spine will be affected during pregnancy, improving or becoming worse.

Pain caused by tension in the muscles surrounding and supporting the spine is common. It is felt as back pain, or if muscle tension is on the front of the spine it is often felt as abdominal pain; tension in the back muscles high in the neck may pull on the skull and cause headache (see below); and tension lower down may give pain in a buttock or thigh.

Back pain may also arise in the kidneys, or a prolapsed ('slipped') disc in the spine may cause numbness or weakness in a leg or foot as well as back pain. These problems need urgent treatment.

Low back pain Most commonly felt in the lumbar region of the lower back – the area most affected by poor posture and muscle weakness – the pain may extend forward into the groin or down into the thighs. It is usually caused by tension and strain in the lumbar ligaments.

Pain felt post-natally is sometimes caused by an injury that occurred during the birth.

Sacroiliac pain Experienced in the buttocks, lower back or hip joints and possibly also running down one leg, this common pain is caused by a 'twist' in the sacrum accentuated by pregnancy. The pain is especially noticeable if you lie on your back, and driving a car can also be very painful. Sometimes the sacrum twists periodically, so that pain is intermittent.

Post-natally, sacroiliac pain usually settles, but in rare cases pain continues or may appear for the first time.

Treatment Always take medical advice on back pain to exclude any serious underlying condition. Regular practice of the stretching exercises in Part V and an awareness of your postural habits will eradicate or improve minor back pain. Pain of a more chronic nature will need medical treatment, physiotherapy and/or osteopathy. Acupuncture can also be effective in reducing muscular tension.

Back pain cannot be dealt with in isolation. The tilt of the pelvis, the angle of the head and neck, the curvature of the spine and the position of the shoulders are all interrelated, and so a comprehensive programme is essential for back pain, in addition to any specific exercises. Swimming is an excellent way of improving muscle tone in a weight- and gravity-free setting.

Your occupation may be adding to the tension, and you should review how you sit and stand.

If pain is really severe, small doses of a mild analgesic (e.g. paracetamol) will probably not harm your baby, but should be avoided in the first ten weeks of pregnancy and during the last month, when they may cause bleeding in the baby.

Corsets are not recommended, and strict bedrest is no longer prescribed, unless the woman has a suspected slipped disc; adequate rest and sleep on a firm bed, on the other hand, are vital.

Headache

During pregnancy, most headaches are caused by tension in the vertebrae of the neck, which is then transmitted to the muscles of the head. This is often felt at the back of the head and over the forehead, and may be more prominent on one side. Other possible reasons for headache include: migraine, which often improves with pregnancy; sinusitis, which is common and very painful; tooth and jaw pain, which can be difficult to diagnose; and pre-eclampsia, which is potentially serious (see HIGH BLOOD PRESSURE AND PRE-ECLAMPSIA).

Treatment See your doctor if you suffer from severe headaches, to exclude anything serious. Migraine can often be helped by identifying and excluding allergens in the diet. The vast majority of headaches in pregnancy arise from the alterations in the normal mechanics of the lumbar spine and pelvis. They are often associated with low back pain, and are treated identically.

See also CRAMP, NUMB AND PAINFUL FINGERS IN PREGNANCY

Pain relief in labour

Pain is an important subject for women approaching childbirth. There are some women for whom one strong contraction is too much, whereas others reach the point of exhaustion and beyond before asking for help. Between these extremes there are many women who would prefer to give birth without drugs or intervention, but who would accept and welcome technology if needed. Given the right environment, enough privacy and positive care, most women find it possible to draw on their own resources to cope with labour (pp. 150–2), but for some people the pain can be intolerable. Understanding a woman's needs in labour and the use of positive breathing, massage and immersion in warm water all help to reduce, release or relieve pain. It is important to recognize when some form of pain relief is required.

Historically, pain relief has always been available during labour, ranging from emotional support and herbal remedies to the sophisticated anaesthetics of today. All the drugs used to relieve pain have some side-effects for mother and baby, all of them crossing the placenta and entering the baby's system in the same concentration as in the mother's blood. To use pain relief most effectively, these side-effects need to be understood. Timing and dosage are also very important, and the extent of cervical dilation should always be checked by vaginal examination. If full dilation is imminent, it may be better to avoid certain types of pain relief that could affect progress of the second stage or the baby's breathing at birth.

Transcutaneous nerve stimulation (TNS)

This modern method of relieving pain has parallels with acupuncture. A battery-operated generator, about the size of a cigarette lighter, is connected by wires to two pads, which are attached with sticking plasters to the skin on either side of the spine. A very low electric current then stimulates the nerve endings in the skin, and this blocks the pain signals coming from the uterus. When the pads are in place, there is a tingling sensation. Some TNS systems have a button that the woman can press during a contraction to increase stimulation. TNS is a safe form of pain relief with no side-effects, but to be effective it needs to be used continuously from early in the first stage of labour. There is only a mild degree of pain relief, which some women may find insufficient for intense pain late in labour; however, many find it helpful.

Hypnosis

When you are hypnotized, you are aware of what is happening but you do not feel it as pain, and in exceptional cases, if a woman responds well to it, even a CAESAREAN SECTION can be done under hypnosis.

If you plan to use hypnosis during labour, preparation should begin in pregnancy, and the hypnotherapist could be present at the birth. (Some doctors and midwives are also hypnotherapists.) You can practise self-hypnosis, either after training by a hypnotherapist or as part of your own intuitive ability. (Some women cannot be hypnotized, however, while most others need several sessions before hypnosis works.)

Hypnosis has no physiological side-effects.

Gas-and-air (Entonox)

This combination of 50 per cent nitrous oxide (laughing gas) and 50 per cent oxygen is inhaled through a rubber mask. This has a valve that opens when you inhale and closes when you exhale. You should begin to inhale the gas just before the start of a contraction; the anaesthetic effect builds up and lasts for 60 seconds, taking the edge off the pain without completely eradicating it. Each breath of gas-and-air may leave you feeling a little 'high' and perhaps a bit dizzy. Once the contraction reaches its peak or you have had enough, you can put down the mask and the effects soon wear off. It has a minimal effect on the baby.

Gas-and-air is best used late in the first stage, during transition, but not in the second stage. It is only useful for a relatively short time – perhaps an hour – because the anaesthetic effect wears off.

There are some disadvantages. The 'high' may leave you feeling confused or out of control. If pain is very intense, the pain relief may be inadequate. Finally, women often focus on breathing the gas-and-air rather than on bearing down during the second stage, and this may affect the expulsive reflex and delay the birth.

Pethidine

This is a powerful narcotic derived from morphine which acts on the nerve cells in the brain and spinal cord to alter the perception of pain: the pain impulses are still present but the sensations are more acceptable.

Pethidine is administered by injection into the thigh or buttock. The dose varies, depending on the woman's size, and may be repeated after four hours. Small doses of 25–50 mg are preferable, and 150 mg is the maximum permissible.

Effects on the mother As well as altering pain perception, pethidine also alters consciousness. Some women feel good, high and floating with minimal pain; others become nervous, afraid, out of control and still aware of pain. Their courage and confidence may disappear, and this can interrupt the rhythm of labour. In very high doses, pethidine may depress breathing, and artificial ventilation may be needed.

Because nausea is a common side-effect, pethidine is often given in combination with Sparine, a powerful tranquillizer that often induces sleepiness. The mother may then be unable to give birth actively and may require intervention.

Effects on the baby Both pethidine and Sparine may cross the placenta and have an adverse effect on the baby, the most dangerous of which is suppression of the baby's breathing reflex at birth. The effect is greater if the baby is small or premature, if the mother receives high doses and if these are given near the time of birth. It is therefore preferable to give a small dose of pethidine (without Sparine) in the first stage of labour, before the cervix has dilated 7 cm. Early in labour, the mother's system helps to clear the pethidine from the baby's, whereas later on the drug is more likely to remain in his bloodstream after birth and take longer to be cleared.

In premature babies, it can take days before the drug is excreted, increasing their need for support systems to help them breathe and feed. The baby may also have sucking difficulties for the first few days after birth, and this may disturb the start of breastfeeding.

For these reasons, many paediatricians prefer women to use other forms of pain relief.

Epidural anaesthesia

This originated in France in 1901, and became popular in Britain recently. A local anaesthetic derived from cocaine is injected into the epidural space in the lower part of the spine, to block the nerve fibres that transmit pain sensation from the uterus. A successful epidural is a highly effective form of pain relief.

In the first stage of labour, pain from uterine contractions may be prevented by a high block, which does not numb the mother's legs; in the second stage, when the pain is felt in the vagina, a lower block is given.

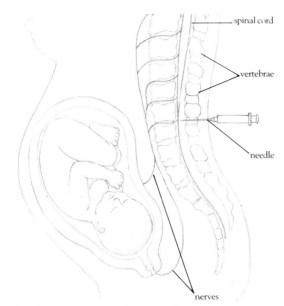

The spinal cord lies within a bony tunnel formed by the protective bones of the spinal column. The cord is covered by a membrane called the dura, and between this and the vertebral bones is the epidural space.

The woman lies on her side, curled up in a foetal position. (If this is uncomfortable, the epidural may be inserted while she is sitting forward on a chair.) The anaesthetist uses a local anaesthetic to numb the skin and the spinal ligaments, and then inserts a needle into the epidural space. A fine cannula, or flexible tube, is threaded down the needle and into the space. The needle is removed and the cannula is taped along the woman's spine to her shoulder, where its end is closed off by means of a sterile filter. Doses of anaesthetic are administered painlessly throughout labour by injection through the filter into the cannula.

Advantages Epidural anaesthesia used during a Caesarean section can enable the mother to remain conscious. It may be very helpful in a PROLONGED LABOUR if pain becomes intolerable or if the mother reaches the point of exhaustion. It may also be used for FORCEPS DELIVERY. An epidural helps to lower blood pressure, so may be beneficial for a mother with pre-eclampsia. It is also useful in premature labour.

Disadvantages Blood pressure may fall as the blood vessels in the lower body dilate and blood pools in them. This may reduce placental flow, resulting in FOETAL DISTRESS. Because of this, every woman having an epidural needs an intravenous drip to top up the volume of her blood. Foetal distress is decreased if the mother lies on her side rather than her back, to reduce pressure on the blood vessels in front of her spine, thus aiding blood circulation in the uterus.

Paralysis of the pelvic muscles removes the natural stimulus for the baby's head to turn in the pelvic canal, and reduces the urge to bear down. Because of this, a forceps delivery or Caesarean section becomes more likely – in some hospitals, up to 40 per cent of epidurals lead to forceps births. If bladder sensation is lost, a catheter has to be inserted to drain it. Rarely, faulty technique results in only partial blockage of sensation, when the whole labour may be felt in one segment of the body or on one side. Occasionally, the affected nerves become weak or tingle; and if the needle penetrates the dura, leakage of spinal fluid can cause severe headaches. If the anaesthetic is accidentally injected into the spinal cord, this may result in paralysis of the respiratory muscles, necessitating artificial ventilation. Epidurals should therefore only be undertaken when ventilation is possible.

When the epidural wears off, the nerves are often very sensitive, and a Caesarean scar or an episiotomy (see TEARS AND EPISIOTOMY) may feel excessively painful for a few hours.

The pain relief gained from an epidural can make birth a positive event, but some women may experience a feeling of deprivation.

Epidural anaesthesia represents a major advance in antenatal care, and is best used selectively, particularly in a long or premature labour, when some form of pain relief may be essential. While the anaesthetic is working, the mother can rest or even sleep; quite often this encourages full dilation. The epidural can then be allowed to wear off at the end of the first stage, and the mother can be helped into an upright position. Working with her contractions and gravity will greatly increase her chances of a spontaneous vaginal birth.

Caudal anaesthesia

Caudal anaesthesia is usually administered in the second stage. It anaesthetizes the vagina and the perineum, and is often the first choice when a forceps delivery or vacuum extraction are needed.

As in epidural anaesthesia, a local anaesthetic is injected into the epidural space, but this time in the sacrum at the base of the spine. A cannula cannot be left in place because the proximity to the anus increases the risk of infection, and so only a single dose for short-term relief can be given.

Pudendal block

Pudendal block has been largely superseded by epidural anaesthesia which offers more complete pain relief, but it may be useful for a low forceps delivery or for an episiotomy. A local anaesthetic is given, via a needle inserted through the vaginal skin, to block the pudendal nerve as it emerges from the side of the pelvic outlet. This removes all sensation from the lower third of the vagina, and from the skin of the labia and the perineum. The main problems are incomplete anaesthesia on one side, and bruising.

Perineal block

This is the most commonly used anaesthesia apart from gas-and-air. An injection, effective within three to four minutes, is used to numb the perineum before an episiotomy is carried out or a tear is repaired. The anaesthetic is injected directly into the area to be stitched, and may sting as it is inserted. The area is then numb for about 90 minutes, long enough for the repair to be done.

General anaesthesia

A general anaesthetic may be needed for Caesarean section, a mid-cavity forceps delivery or removal of a retained placenta. Because it may be needed in an emergency, women are asked to eat little and drink only sips of water during labour. This reduces the risk of the stomach contents being regurgitated into the lungs. To ensure that this does not happen once the mother is anaesthetized, a tube is passed into the airway via the mouth.

Both baby and mother are taken into account when the anaesthetic is given. Sleep is induced with an injection of an appropriate drug, followed by another to induce muscle relaxation which allows the airway tube to be inserted. The mother then inhales further anaesthetic gases to maintain unconsciousness and relaxation. Once the operation is over, the anaesthetic agents are exhaled by the mother, and she slowly recovers consciousness. It may be a while before she is ready to have first contact with her baby. The baby may be sleepy, and some time may pass before he cries. It may occasionally be necessary to resuscitate the baby.

Palpitations

These can be defined as a rapid and sometimes irregular heartbeat which can occur even when you are at rest. They are common and often completely normal during pregnancy because of the increased load on the heart and circulation. They are even more likely in a woman who is suffering from ANAEMIA or is malnourished or unfit. They are also often caused by anxiety and stress. A full medical check to exclude HEART DISEASE and anaemia is recommended.

There is no specific medical treatment for palpitations. You can help to reduce them by paying special attention to nutrition (see Chapter 7), by improving your physical fitness (see Part V) and by practising yoga and meditation to encourage relaxation and lessen anxiety.

Pelvic infection see FALLOPIAN TUBE INFECTIONS
Penis abnormalities see URINARY TRACT AND KIDNEY PROBLEMS IN THE BABY
Perineal block see PAIN RELIEF IN LABOUR
Pethidine see PAIN RELIEF IN LABOUR

Phenylketonuria (PKU)

This inherited condition occurs once in every 15 000 births. An inability to metabolize the amino acid phenylalanine, found in many proteins, causes it to accumulate in the body and damage the brain, leading to severe mental retardation. The disease is caused by a recessive gene, and if both parents are carriers they have a 25 per cent chance of having an affected child (see CHROMOSOMAL AND GENETIC ABNORMALITIES).

There is no ante-natal test for PKU. Screening is done by testing a blood sample taken from the heel of the baby about six days after birth. Treatment consists of placing affected children on a restricted diet until puberty. By then, their brains have developed normally and can no longer be damaged in this way, and their bodies have usually developed the ability to handle the amino acid.

To protect their unborn babies, affected women must return to the diet before starting a pregnancy.
See also CONGENITAL ABNORMALITIES AND GENETIC COUNSELLING

Piles

Also called haemorrhoids, these are distended veins (similar to VARICOSE VEINS) in the anal passage. If the veins near the surface swell, the symptoms are minimal, but if swelling involves the deeper veins, the anal muscle may go into spasm, with bleeding, pain, itching and burning.

Piles are common during pregnancy because of pressure on the veins in the lower part of the body caused by the enlarging uterus. The Western diet with its low fibre content can contribute to their development, when CONSTIPATION leads to straining. Childbirth often makes the problem worse: a prolonged second stage of labour may put a strain on the anal veins; and after the birth, the muscle spasm that may follow stitches (see TEARING AND EPISIOTOMY) further compresses the veins and prevents free drainage of blood. Piles

are usually at their worst in the first two weeks after childbirth.

Symptoms vary from a slight feeling of a lump in the anus to severe pain if the anal muscle is in spasm. Constipated women with piles may notice a little blood on their stools.

Treatment
A good diet in pregnancy helps prevent constipation, so that piles are less likely to develop and more likely to recede. Pelvic-floor exercises (p. 253), concentrating on the anus two or three times a day, will aid the blood flow and help to relieve pressure.

When defecating, relax as much as possible and breathe deeply. Squatting may be the best position. Lubricate the anus with a haemorrhoid cream or pure oil to assist the passage of stools. Should the piles prolapse out of the anus, they can be gently pushed back. If they are painful, it will help to sit on a rubber ring, and to use ice packs to reduce spasm. Very rarely, an operation may be needed, or alternatively the anal canal can be stretched.
See also ANAL FISSURE

Placenta accreta see PROLONGED LABOUR: THIRD STAGE

Placental abruption

More commonly known as 'accidental haemorrhage', placental abruption (*abruptio placentae*) happens when BLEEDING between the placenta and the wall of the uterus causes them to separate before the baby is born. The blood forms a clot between the placenta and the uterine wall, and if there is a great deal of bleeding, some of it may appear in the vagina. The bleeding causes continuous pain, which is difficult to relieve.

Placental abruption can happen at any stage of late pregnancy and, rarely, during labour. It is extremely dangerous for the baby. Any woman who experiences continuous pain with or without vaginal bleeding in late pregnancy should lie down, and an ambulance should be called at once.

Causes
Not much is known about the causes of placental abruption. It is more common in undernourished women deficient in vitamins and minerals, and has been linked to very HIGH BLOOD PRESSURE.

Complications
The shearing off of the placenta reduces the blood flow to it, causing FOETAL DISTRESS and occasionally even the baby's death. Heavy blood loss may cause a fall in maternal blood pressure leading to shock. The clot may use up all the clotting factors in the mother's blood, so that the blood becomes unable to clot, and bleeding increases.

Such serious complications can only be treated in a hospital holding a wide range of blood and blood products, and success depends on prompt arrival in hospital.

Treatment
On arrival, an examination will determine the size of the abruption. If there is little bleeding, and if the baby's heart rate is normal, an ULTRASOUND SCAN is useful to distinguish between abruption and PLACENTA PRAEVIA.

If the abruption is small, bedrest in hospital and FOETAL HEART MONITORING may be the only treatment necessary. A large abruption is an acute emergency, and a CAESAREAN SECTION must be performed to save the baby.

Placental insufficiency *see* LOW BIRTH WEIGHT AND PRE-MATURITY

Placenta praevia

The placenta usually implants in the upper half (segment) of the uterus. If it implants in the lower segment, partly or wholly obstructing the cervical opening, this is known as placenta praevia. Placenta praevia is very rare.

In early pregnancy, an apparently low-lying placenta is quite common, but it usually moves up as pregnancy progresses and the uterus expands. In late pregnancy, BLEEDING may occur. During the last weeks, as the lower segment of the uterus effaces (thins) and the cervix ripens in preparation for labour, the edge of the placenta, unable to stretch, shears off the uterine wall and bleeds.

Symptoms

The first indication of a placenta praevia is usually the painless loss of bright red blood through the vagina. A small amount of bleeding may continue intermittently and then suddenly become very heavy. Occasionally a placenta praevia is not detected until labour begins, when there is sudden haemorrhage. The placenta usually prevents the baby's head from engaging in the pelvis.

Treatment

If your placenta appears low on an early ULTRASOUND SCAN, you will probably be offered a further scan after 32 weeks to check its position. If present, a genuine placenta praevia will then be confirmed, after which you would usually be advised to stay in hospital. Should bleeding occur but you do not want an ultrasound scan, you would have to stay in hospital even if the bleeding stopped, as further bleeding might be torrential. This is the only safe course of action if a scan is not done. Sexual intercourse should be avoided as the pressure could cause further bleeding.

A final internal examination will be done in a hospital operating theatre with full facilities: if there is true placenta praevia, the baby must be delivered by CAESAREAN SECTION.

Because the bleeding associated with placenta praevia is usually painless, women do not always seek medical help if it occurs. However, prompt medical attention is necessary for any kind of bleeding; if placenta praevia is suspected, hospital care is essential.

Pneumonia *see* COLDS, COUGHS AND RESPIRATORY INFECTIONS IN THE BABY
Polyhydramnios *see* AMNIOTIC FLUID

Postmaturity

A baby may be considered postmature if born more than two weeks after the expected date of delivery, and when there is a risk of placental insufficiency with reduced nutrition and oxygen for the baby (*see* LOW BIRTH WEIGHT AND PREMATUR-ITY). The vast majority of babies born late are not postmature and need no treatment; suspected postmaturity is usually the result of the last menstrual period being wrongly dated, or long menstrual cycles with late conception. Occasionally, the onset of labour may be delayed for no obvious reason.

Treatment

There is no risk to the baby unless the mother has HIGH BLOOD PRESSURE, is poorly nourished or smokes or drinks heavily, or unless the baby is 'small for dates'. There may then be more chance of placental insufficiency. Unless there

is a significant risk of this, there is no need to induce labour.

Instead, the mother may be asked to keep a record of foetal movements, and FOETAL HEART MONITORING may be carried out frequently. This system, although requiring patience from parents and midwives, means that induction is very rarely needed for postmaturity.

Post-natal depression *see* DEPRESSION AND STRESS
Post-partum *see* BLEEDING
Pre-eclampsia *see* HIGH BLOOD PRESSURE AND PRE-ECLAMPSIA
Premature babies *see* LOW BIRTH WEIGHT AND PREMATURITY

Premature rupture of the membranes

Leakage of amniotic fluid through the membranes of the amniotic sac which continues for more than 24 hours before the onset of spontaneous labour is called 'premature rupture of the membranes'. Most common around term, it may occur at any time after the 24th week of pregnancy.

If you suspect that your membranes have broken, it is important to have a vaginal examination so that the fluid can be checked. Sometimes leakage is the result of urinary incontinence or mucus from the cervix.

Complications

If your membranes rupture before the 34th week of pregnancy, your doctor will probably try to prolong pregnancy until the baby is more mature. The risks of premature birth are greater than those associated with infection.

Intact membranes form a barrier against infection that may ascend through the cervix. If it does reach the amniotic fluid it can cause respiratory infection in the baby.

Treatment

Once a vaginal examination has confirmed the diagnosis, no further internal examinations should be carried out because they increase the risk of infection. Avoid sexual intercourse.

One school of thought recommends preventive treatment with antibiotics, but other doctors believe that this will just lead to infection by resistant organisms. It is best to delay the use of antibiotics until there are definite signs of infection. Vitamin C and garlic capsules may help to avoid infection.

It is sometimes difficult to diagnose infection in the uterus because it is a 'hidden' site and the usual signs – e.g. high fever or racing pulse – are often absent. A swab taken from the upper vagina can be used to check for organisms. The best way of diagnosing uterine infection is to monitor the odour and colour of the amniotic fluid on sanitary towels. If this changes to a fishy smell and a noticeable colour, infection is present and labour should be induced.

Prickly heat *see* SKIN PROBLEMS IN THE BABY
Prolapse, vaginal, *see* VAGINAL PROLAPSE

Prolapsed umbilical cord

This rare complication of labour only occurs when a loop of umbilical cord is below the baby's head, which has not yet engaged in the pelvis. It is more common if the baby is premature, breech or a transverse lie.

If your waters break and the baby's head is not engaged, contact your midwife or the hospital at once. The cord is only at risk of being compressed (i.e. prolapsed) if the membranes have ruptured, when the descent of the head may compress it and cause FOETAL DISTRESS. If the cord has prolapsed, the mother should stay on all fours to keep the baby's pressure off the cord until a CAESAREAN is done.

Prolonged labour: first stage

It is often difficult to decide exactly when a labour starts, because many women have pre-labour uterine contractions (p. 144) for days before the baby is born. True labour begins when the cervix dilates progressively and contractions are well established.

The first 6 cm of the cervical dilation usually take longer than the final 4 cm, which is the 'active' phase of the first stage. If the rate of progress deviates from what is considered 'normal', labour may be judged to be prolonged.

Since a significant number of women have labour patterns that do not conform to the norm, each labour should be considered individually. Many factors need to be taken into account when deciding whether to wait or take action.

Why some first stages are prolonged

There are many reasons why this stage of labour may take a long time.

The birth environment Labour may be prolonged because the mother is resisting, fighting and working against pain. There are many things that can cause this: not enough privacy, too much distraction, conflict in the woman's relationship with her partner or birth attendants.

Slow uterine activity Slow but progressive dilation with infrequent contractions is called hypotonic, or low-tone, labour. It progresses very slowly, but as long as the mother rests between contractions and takes adequate nourishment, there is no problem.

Uncoordinated uterine activity When contractions are strong and painful, but dilation is very slow, labour is called hypertonic. There may also be pain in between as well as during contractions. A labour of this sort may be linked to disproportion (*see below*).

Malpresentation If an unusual part of the baby's head or body enters the pelvic brim first, labour may be prolonged. The most common variation is known as OCCIPITO POSTERIOR PRESENTATION.

Disproportion If the pelvic cavity is very small or its shape not ideal, or the baby is large, the head may not get through easily. In most prolonged labours, pelvic capacity is adequate, but tension in the ligaments and connective tissues that support the pelvis prevents easy passage. Squatting relaxes the soft tissues and ensures that the pelvis opens to its maximum, increasing its size by 25 per cent. (See LARGE BABIES.)

Coping with a prolonged first stage

First, a diagnosis must be made, to find out if true labour has begun. A full abdominal and vaginal examination will assess uterine activity, the position of the baby and the state of the cervix and the pelvis. Further examinations will probably be done at intervals to determine whether progress is being made. The baby's heartbeat will be monitored at regular intervals.

Self-help A good diet during pregnancy, physical fitness and a positive attitude are all helpful in setting the scene for labour. You will need to take nourishment in early labour to give yourself energy and strength. Immersion in warm water may be the best way of improving progress, and a calm, semi-dark environment without distractions may be helpful. Deep breathing and massage will aid relaxation (*see* Part V).

Changing positions may make a considerable difference. A slow labour with infrequent contractions may respond if you remain upright or squat, whereas very painful uncoordinated labour may be helped if you kneel or lie down, especially in water. If the baby is fine, and your energy and strength hold

out, you can continue unaided just as long as there is some progress, however slow.

Medical help In a slow first stage, artificial rupture of the membranes may be performed to encourage the head to tuck in and descend into the cervix, or the drug Syntocinon may be used to augment uterine contractions (*see* INDUCED LABOUR). The great advantage of the latter is that it may speed up a very slow labour and make a vaginal birth possible. An intravenous drip will prevent dehydration.

A hypertonic labour is often very painful, and PAIN RELIEF may allow the mother to relax. This is sometimes achieved with pethidine, but with epidural anaesthesia dilation can be rapid and progressive.

If labour is excessively prolonged, and it becomes obvious that the contractions are not going to dilate the cervix, the baby has to be delivered by CAESAREAN SECTION.

Prolonged labour: second stage

The length of the second stage varies enormously from woman to woman – from only a few minutes to some hours. The arbitrary time limits so often imposed by obstetricians may not take account of these wide individual variations.

When narrow limits are set – say, 60 minutes for a first birth or 45 minutes for a second – the result is a very high incidence of forceps deliveries and vacuum extraction and fewer normal births. However, as long as the baby and mother are fit and well and the baby's heartbeat is monitored, there is no need for such time limits.

Why some second stages are prolonged

Uterine contractions may be infrequent or lacking in power, and the woman may be tired after a long labour. The reasons for a prolonged first stage of labour often apply here.

If an epidural has been given, or pethidine late in labour (*see* PAIN RELIEF IN LABOUR), the mother may not be able to bear down. If she is also lying down and thus receiving no assistance from gravity, the help she can give will be reduced still further.

It is quite common for progress in the second stage to be held up by the mother's fear – the fear of bursting or tearing, the fear of pain or of actually seeing the baby. Some women are anxious about making a mess as the waters break or their bowels empty during the birth. Others feel deep ambivalence about ending pregnancy and beginning motherhood. These feelings may need to rise to the surface and be expressed before the baby can be born. Sometimes the environment or the birth attendants are the cause of a long second stage, especially if the mother is told to bear down before she feels the urge, or if she has a sense of being watched.

Coping with a prolonged second stage

Self-help Build up your stamina for labour during pregnancy by eating well and making sure you are physically fit. Practising yoga-based exercises and breathing awareness (*see* Part V) will help you to cultivate a relaxed attitude.

During the second stage, try to stay upright, using kneeling, standing or sitting positions, and only using the supported squat at the end (pp. 125-6), so that the expulsive reflex is optimal. Relaxed and confident support from your birth attendants, privacy, peace and calm are essential. The emphasis should be on relaxing and letting go rather than straining to 'push' the baby out. Once the head begins to crown it is time to use a supported squatting position.

Medical help If your labour is very prolonged, you may need extra glucose and/or an intravenous drip to prevent dehydration. A Syntocinon drip can be used to simulate contractions if necessary. If the squatting position is not effective, the baby may need the help of FORCEPS or a vacuum extractor. If his head is not engaged in the pelvis, it is safer to have a CAESAREAN SECTION, even if the cervix is fully dilated.

Prolonged labour: third stage

The third stage of labour begins after the birth of the baby and ends with the delivery of the placenta. There are varying attitudes towards how much time should elapse before the placenta is delivered, and its delivery may be hastened. In this, an oxytocin-like drug – either Syntocinon or ergometrine – is given to make the uterus contract as the baby is being born; the placenta is then expelled within minutes of the birth, with the help of controlled cord traction (p. 168) by the midwife.

In a natural third stage, it may simply be a matter of time before the placenta separates and is expelled, and there is no hurry unless excessive BLEEDING occurs.

Retained placenta

Occasionally the placenta may be partially or completely retained, and intervention may be needed for its delivery.
Placenta accreta This very rare but serious complication occurs when the placenta has rooted itself too deeply in the uterine lining, occasionally penetrating the wall itself. Controlled cord traction cannot deliver such a deeply implanted placenta, so either a general or epidural anaesthetic has to be given, enabling the obstetrician to remove the placenta manually from the wall of the uterus.
Retained fragments Occasionally, a few fragments of the placenta or the amniotic sac are not expelled. If there is no bleeding no action needs to be taken, as small fragments will be expelled spontaneously during the post-natal period. On the other hand, heavy bleeding suggests the presence of larger fragments. It is likely that these will need to be removed surgically.
Premature contraction of the uterus Sometimes the administration of oxytocin-like drugs causes the lower segment of the uterus to clamp down and trap the placenta inside, especially if cord traction is done when the placenta has only partially separated from the uterine lining. In this case the midwife applies continuous controlled cord traction to deliver the placenta. The squatting position will facilitate this. Partial separation of the placenta may cause bleeding, so delivery of the remaining part is urgent. This may need to be done under an anaesthetic as an emergency.

Psoriasis see SKIN CHANGES IN PREGNANCY
Pudendal block see PAIN RELIEF IN LABOUR
Puerperal fever see FALLOPIAN TUBE INFECTIONS
Pulmonary embolism see VENOUS THROMBOSIS AND PULMONARY EMBOLISM
Pyelitis see URINARY TRACT AND KIDNEY PROBLEMS IN THE MOTHER
Pyloric stenosis see VOMITING IN THE BABY

Radiation

Although we are all subject to tiny doses of radiation in our daily life, it is sensible to avoid unnecessary exposure during pregnancy, because radiation can seriously harm a developing baby, especially in the early weeks.

X-rays

Abdominal X-rays in early pregnancy, particularly multiple exposure, may carry a very small risk to the baby, whose ovaries may be damaged or who may develop leukaemia in later life. Diagnostic X-rays in pregnancy have been largely replaced by ULTRASOUND SCANNING, which uses sound waves, not ionizing radiation, and which, thus far, appears far safer for the baby. Even dental X-rays should not be taken in pregnancy unless essential, although no harm is done if your abdomen is screened.

A single X-ray in late pregnancy to check the mother's pelvic size in a case of suspected disproportion (see LARGE BABIES) carries minimal risk to the baby.

Video display units (VDUs)

The increased use of video display units and colour television monitors has led to queries about their safety. Certainly they do emit radiation – in the visible light, ultraviolet, and infra-red wavelengths as well as soft X-rays. The amount of exposure the baby receives depends on how long the operator works at the VDU.

There is no proof that exposure to radiation at these levels has an adverse effect on the developing child, but it is sensible to be cautious. Recently manufactured machines have a much lower output than older ones, and if you spend a great deal of time operating a VDU, it is possible to protect yourself by using a simple radiation shield. This can be quite easily constructed at home, using aluminium foil, which will block out all soft X-rays.

Rashes see SKIN CHANGES IN PREGNANCY, SKIN PROBLEMS IN THE BABY
Respiratory distress syndrome see BREATHING PROBLEMS IN THE BABY
Respiratory infection see COLD, COUGHS AND RESPIRATORY INFECTIONS

Resuscitation of the baby

Even though babies can manage with less oxygen for far longer than adults, a small minority need help with breathing at birth. To minimize this possibility, the umbilical cord should be allowed to continue pulsating to provide additional oxygen until the baby breathes. Any amniotic fluid should be allowed to drain from her airway and if necessary suctioned out gently. She should be kept warm, if possible by close body contact with her mother.

If the baby does not start to breathe, she may be given additional oxygen – by face mask as long as her air passages are clear, or by inserting a tube into the airway to allow the oxygen to be 'pushed in' under gentle pressure. Most babies respond within a few minutes and no longer need the tube; some take longer.

Retained placenta see BLEEDING, PROLONGED LABOUR: THIRD STAGE

Retroverted uterus

A retroverted uterus is one that tilts backwards towards the sacrum instead of forwards.

It normally causes no problems during pregnancy unless it obstructs the outflow of urine as it grows in the pelvis and presses on the bladder (usually at about 12 weeks). To treat this, an obstetrician lifts the uterus manually, if necessary inserting a plastic ring into the vagina for a few days to keep it up. Rarely, a catheter (a thin tube) may be needed to drain the urine. By 14 weeks, when the uterus rises out of the pelvis, the pressure is removed.

A retroverted uterus does not pose any special problem during childbirth or post-natally. Neither is it a cause of MISCARRIAGE, as is sometimes suggested. It may, however, make it difficult to fit a diaphragm for CONTRACEPTION.

Rhesus disease

The blood of 85 per cent of people is Rhesus positive (Rh+), which means that it contains the Rhesus factor, a protein attached to the surface of red blood cells. During pregnancy the blood is tested for the factor, and for any antibodies to it early in pregnancy and again in late pregnancy.

If you are one of the 15 per cent who lack the Rhesus factor – and are therefore Rhesus negative (Rh−) – and if the baby's father is Rh+, a problem could exist.

Cause
When an Rh− woman gives birth to her first Rh+ baby, some of the baby's blood cells may enter her bloodstream. (This can also happen if a woman has a TERMINATION, MISCARRIAGE or AMNIOCENTESIS.) The foetal cells appear 'foreign' to her immune system, causing it to produce anti-Rhesus antibodies. In a subsequent pregnancy, these antibodies cross the placenta into the foetal circulation and, if the second baby is also Rh+, they could damage or even destroy the unborn baby's red blood cells. These form clumps and break down, and the unborn child may then develop ANAEMIA.

Prevention
Fortunately, Rhesus disease is now almost entirely preventable. A sample of cord blood may be taken from the placenta of a baby born to an Rh− woman. If the baby's blood is also Rh−, no action needs to be taken. Otherwise, the mother is simply injected with antibodies called 'anti-D' within 72 hours of the birth (or miscarriage, amniocentesis or termination). The injected antibodies act against the Rh factor and mop up all the foetal Rh+ cells in the mother's bloodstream before they can stimulate the mother into making her own antibodies.

Treatment
In the unlikely event that an Rh− woman has developed antibodies before pregnancy, the baby may be affected. If the concentration of antibodies in the mother's blood is high, the baby is regularly monitored by ULTRASOUND SCAN to see whether there are any signs of cardiac failure (e.g. swollen liver, fluid in the lungs or abdomen). Repeated amniocentesis is also performed to assess the degree of foetal anaemia.

If the baby is severely affected, she may be given a blood transfusion while she is still in the uterus. In less severely affected cases, an early birth induction is the answer, with treatment of the disease by post-natal photo-therapy (see JAUNDICE) or a complete exchange of the baby's blood with that from a donor.

Rubella in pregnancy

Rubella is the viral infection commonly known as German measles. A mild childhood illness, it can have serious effects on an unborn baby if caught by a woman in the first 16 weeks of pregnancy. On average, about 67 children affected by congenital rubella are born in Britain each year, but only half of their mothers developed the characteristic rash or felt ill. The virus is present in the mother's circulation seven days after infection, the rash begins a week after that, and antibodies produced by her against the virus are detectable within another seven days.

Effects
The earlier in pregnancy a woman catches rubella, the more likely the baby is to be seriously affected. The virus does the most damage to the baby during embryonic life – that is, during the first eight weeks of pregnancy – when infection can lead to blindness, deafness, mental retardation or cardiac and abdominal abnormalities, or any combination of these. After the 16th week damage is usually limited to hearing loss. After the 18th week the baby is unlikely to be affected at all.

Prevention
All girls between the ages of 11 and 13 should be immunized against rubella. The vaccine can cause a rash and a flu-like illness with swollen glands, similar to but milder than the full infection. Pregnant women are routinely screened for rubella immunity, but if possible your blood should be screened for rubella antibodies before you conceive: these guarantee lifelong immunity. If you have no antibodies, you can be immunized, but must not get pregnant for three months.

Treatment
If you come into contact with rubella while you are pregnant, or if you develop a suspicious rash, your blood can be tested for antibodies. If antibodies are absent, the test will be repeated two and four weeks later to see whether changes indicate that you were infected.

Because of its drastic effects, if infection is diagnosed in the first 16 weeks of pregnancy, you will probably be offered a TERMINATION. After 18 weeks this is no longer necessary, but the baby's hearing will be carefully checked after birth.
See also CONGENITAL ABNORMALITIES AND GENETIC COUNSELLING

Salpingitis *see* FALLOPIAN TUBE INFECTIONS
Sciatica *see* PAIN IN PREGNANCY AND AFTER CHILDBIRTH

Sickle cell disease and thalassaemia

These are inherited genetic disorders (*see* CHROMOSOMAL AND GENETIC ABNORMALITIES) peculiar to certain ethnic groups: sickle cell disease is primarily found among people of West African origin, thalassaemia among those of Mediterranean and Eastern origin.

In both disorders there is an abnormality in the haemoglobin found in red blood cells. In sickle cell disease this causes the red cells to become sickle-shaped, and they are then prone to block off small blood vessels in various parts of the body, which can be extremely painful. In thalassaemia the walls of the red cells become fragile, leading to a shorter life cycle and over-stimulation of the bone marrow to replace them. In both conditions, there is a chronic, severe ANAEMIA as well as other side-effects. Children affected by either of these diseases may require multiple blood transfusions and intermittent hospital care.

Diagnosis
All high-risk women are tested and carriers detected by analysing their haemoglobin. If both parents are found to be carriers, there is a one in four chance that they will produce an affected child. The mother will then be offered further tests, including foetal blood sampling by FOETOSCOPY or AMNIOCENTESIS or chorion biopsy. If the tests prove positive, the option of a TERMINATION will then be discussed.
See also CONGENITAL ABNORMALITIES AND GENETIC COUNSELLING

Sight in pregnancy *see* VISION IN PREGNANCY

Sinusitis *see* COLDS, COUGHS AND RESPIRATORY INFECTIONS IN PREGNANCY

Size of babies *see* LARGE BABIES, LOW BIRTH WEIGHT AND PREMATURITY

Skin changes in pregnancy

The normal changes to the skin during pregnancy are described on page 41-2. Below are listed some of the more marked alterations.

Pigmentation

Many women find that their skin tans more easily during pregnancy because it produces more pigment. Sunlamps are not recommended during pregnancy because the effects on the baby are not known.

The darkening of the skin directly caused by pregnancy – i.e. *chloasma* (p. 42) – usually fades a few months after the birth, although the skin around the nipples may remain permanently darkened.

Spots and acne

Red spots on the face, chest and arms which blanch when touched are caused by the hormone oestrogen widening the arteries supplying the skin (this also causes the so-called 'glow' of pregnancy). These spots fade post-natally.

Acne may worsen or improve during pregnancy. Long-term antibiotics should be stopped before conception, especially tetracycline drugs.

Itching and rashes

If eczema or psoriasis are present before conception, they frequently improve during pregnancy. The drug etretinate, used in the treatment of psoriasis, should be stopped months before conception, because of possible harm to the baby. Eczema may improve with careful attention to diet.

An infective rash caused by thrush (*see* VAGINAL INFECTIONS) may produce intense itching and redness, particularly over the genital area, thighs and groin. It is easily treated with creams that eradicate the fungal infection.

The skin may also become intensely itchy for no known reason, and this can be hard to treat; it will stop after the birth. Rashes also occur, particularly in the last three months, often spreading over the trunk and limbs and causing itching, discomfort and sleeplessness. These rashes usually disappear within a week or two of the birth. Calamine lotion may help, and wearing loose cotton clothing is sensible.

Skin problems in the baby

In the first days or weeks after birth, a baby's skin may appear spotty or blemished. However, most unsightly marks are perfectly normal and disappear of their own accord. The following skin problems may last longer, be more worrying or need treatment.

Birthmarks and spots

There are many different types of birthmarks. Some disappear over a period of months, and others are permanent. If your baby is born with a birthmark, your doctor will be able to tell you whether it is temporary or not, and whether any treatment is necessary or advisable.

Cradle cap

These harmless conditions are very common in young babies. Glands in their skin overproduce an oil called *sebum*, which collects and forms pimples on the baby's face and scalp. Crusty patches on the scalp (cradle cap) may persist for several months, but will disappear spontaneously in the end.

There is no need to do anything about cradle cap. You may be concerned about its unsightliness, but you should never pick at it. Instead, applying a pure oil may soften the crusts and allow them to be removed; regular gentle brushing of the crusts with a soft baby brush will encourage them to flake off.

Eczema

Also known as dermatitis, this is an inflammation of the skin, which can become dry, rough and sometimes crusty, with redness and itching. It usually affects the face, the backs of the knees and insides of the elbows as well as the hands, scalp and trunk. It is uncommon in babies under three months old.

Since it may be caused by an allergy, breastfeeding for as long as possible before introducing cereals or cows' milk into the baby's diet may help to prevent it, as long as the mother tries to keep allergenic substances out of her own diet.

Prickly heat

The rash known as prickly heat appears when babies are overdressed and hot. It begins as small red areas, most commonly on the neck, chest and upper arms.

The treatment is simple and involves dressing the baby in lighter clothes and cooling the environment if possible.
See also NAPPY RASH, THRUSH IN THE BABY

Small-for-dates babies *see* LOW BIRTH WEIGHT AND PREMATURITY

Smoking in pregnancy

The relationship between cigarette smoking in pregnancy, LOW BIRTH WEIGHT and placental insufficiency has been accepted for many years. Children born to mothers who smoked heavily during pregnancy tend to lag behind in their physical and mental development. The risks are compounded if there are any underlying problems such as HIGH BLOOD PRESSURE or poor nutrition (*see* Chapter 7).

Smoking after the baby is born turns the newborn infant into a passive smoker, with a higher risk of respiratory infections in childhood.

Spastics *see* CEREBRAL PALSY
Special-care baby units *see* ILLNESS IN BABIES
Spina bifida *see* NEURAL TUBE DEFECTS
Spots *see* SKIN CHANGES IN PREGNANCY, SKIN PROBLEMS IN THE BABY

Squinting

Many babies whose eyes are normal appear cross-eyed in the first few weeks of life. These 'false squints' are caused by folds of skin around the eyes and disappear in a few months.

A baby with a true squint has eyes that are permanently unaligned. Initially this causes double vision, but if left untreated, one eye takes over the work of the other to the extent that the vision in the unused eye is suppressed by the brain. Tell your doctor about any suspected squint you may have noticed.

The baby may need a pad over her 'good' eye to force the other to keep working, and when she is older she may be taught eye exercises or have to wear glasses. A few children may be helped by surgery to shorten one of the eye muscles.

'Sticky eye' *see* CONJUNCTIVITIS IN THE BABY

Stillbirth and neonatal death

If a baby is born dead after a pregnancy lasting at least 28 weeks, this is called a stillbirth; a neonatal death is when a baby dies in the first four weeks of life. The two together are perinatal deaths.

When a baby dies before birth, the mother usually knows because of the reduction in foetal movements, even though the baby may still occasionally roll from side to side. Death can be confirmed by FOETAL HEART MONITORING and ULTRASOUND SCANNING. It may be several weeks before labour starts spontaneously. The mother usually has the option of having labour induced after the diagnosis has been confirmed.

Many women prefer to wait for spontaneous labour so that they will have time to begin coming to terms with the death. Some may also want to experience labour rather than having an epidural for PAIN RELIEF, in the belief that going through labour may help them to accept the painful reality of the death. Others may, without hesitation, opt for an immediate induced labour with an epidural. Whatever the choice, care and counselling is essential for both parents before and after delivery. (See also LOSS OF A BABY.)

The majority of neonatal deaths occur within one week of the birth. The baby has usually been very ill and in a special-care baby unit (see ILLNESS IN BABIES).

Causes

Babies with a low birth weight – mainly premature infants (see LOW BIRTH WEIGHT AND PREMATURITY) – and CONGENITAL ABNORMALITIES account for the vast majority of all stillbirths and neonatal deaths. PLACENTAL ABRUPTION and pre-eclampsia (see HIGH BLOOD PRESSURE AND PRE-ECLAMPSIA) are responsible for a small minority of perinatal deaths, as is sudden infant death syndrome (see COT DEATH).

The progressive fall in perinatal death rates has been striking, and as obstetric and neonatal care and the general health of the community all improve, congenital abnormalities will account for most perinatal deaths.

Stress incontinence *see* URINARY INCONTINENCE
Sudden infant death syndrome (SIDS) *see* COT DEATH
Swelling *see* OEDEMA
Syphilis *see* VAGINAL INFECTIONS

Tay Sachs disease

This genetic disorder is found mainly in Ashkenazi Jews, affecting one in 400 children. It is caused by a specific deficiency of the enzyme *hexosaminidase A*, which is involved in fat metabolism. There is no treatment, and those affected do not usually survive longer than four years.

Adult carriers are detected by the measurement of the enzyme in their blood. If both parents are positive, they have a one in four chance of producing an affected baby. AMNIOCENTESIS can identify the disease in the foetus.
See also CHROMOSOMAL AND GENETIC ABNORMALITIES

Tear duct, blocked, *see* BLOCKED TEAR DUCT

Tearing and episiotomy

A tear is a natural hazard of birth. Most tears are minor, involving only the superficial layers of the vagina and labia; they heal easily and are known as 'first-degree tears'. Occasionally, however, more severe 'second-degree tears' occur, involving the underlying muscle.

Episiotomy is a surgical incision beginning on the back wall of the vagina and extending into the skin of the vagina and perineum and the underlying muscles. There are two types of episiotomy: *midline* and *medio-lateral*. The midline cut extends directly backward from the vagina, stopping short of the anus. The medio-lateral starts off like the midline, but then goes backward and to one side to avoid the anus. The midline cut is usually preferable, because it runs between muscles, not through them, and is done as far as possible away from large blood vessels and nerves; it is also less painful while healing. The midline cut may extend into the anus, but a skilled midwife can prevent this type of 'third-degree tear'.

Episiotomy used to be done routinely in some hospitals for all first births, to protect the baby and prevent tears. Tears generally heal better and are less painful than episiotomies. The line of a tear may be more difficult to stitch, but the subsequent ease of healing makes up for this. With the use of upright postures during childbirth, episiotomy is rarely necessary.

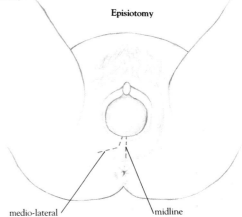

Episiotomy

medio-lateral / \ midline

How to avoid tearing and episiotomy

Preparing in advance Yoga-based stretching exercises, especially squatting, encourage the pelvic ligaments to stretch and the pelvic floor muscles to relax. You can learn to relax and release the perineum at will. Perineal massage (p. 279) in the last month of pregnancy will also help.

Help in labour The birth should not be hurried, while the midwife guides you to release the baby slowly, allowing the tissues time to relax. Spontaneous ejection of the baby will reduce the possibility of a tear.

The most effective way of avoiding a tear is to give birth in an upright position and to wait for the natural expulsive reflex to occur, avoiding strenuous 'pushing'. If you are on your back, the pressure from the baby's head is directed downwards on to the perineum, and the muscles between the vagina and the anus are subjected to maximum tension. The more upright you are, the more the pressure will be brought forward and spread evenly throughout the vagina. Squatting actively relaxes the perineum, so release is optimal. (It is only necessary to adopt this posture when the baby's head has crowned and birth is imminent.)

In the supported squatting position (p. 125-6), tears tend to be superficial, around the vaginal outlet instead of at the back; they are easily stitched and do not cause much post-natal discomfort or pain. Second-degree tears are rare, third-degree even rarer.

If the baby is slow to emerge, supporting the perineum with warm compresses will bring blood to the tissues, helping them to expand and stretch; this is also very soothing. After the birth of the baby's head, gentle delivery of the shoulders prevents tearing.

How episiotomy is done

Episiotomies were traditionally performed with the woman reclining, but kneeling on all fours is better for mother and baby, as well as giving ideal access to birth attendants.

A local anaesthetic is injected to numb the area, and the cut is done during a contraction.

When episiotomy is necessary

If the vaginal outlet is tight an episiotomy may be needed. It may also be required if forceps are needed to deliver the baby. The size of the episiotomy can be kept to a minimum by removing the forceps when the head crowns, so that you can give birth by your own efforts. (Vacuum extractors need less space and do not stretch the vagina as much.)

There is some disagreement as to whether an episiotomy should be routine in a premature birth to protect the baby's head. Although almost always unnecessary, if there is any delay and the head is under pressure, an episiotomy is done.

One argument often used in favour of episiotomy is that it prevents excessive stretching, and reduces later VAGINAL PROLAPSE. Vaginal prolapse has become much less common in the last 40 years, but there is no evidence to prove that episiotomy is the reason for this.

Repairing tears and episiotomies

An episiotomy or tear is stitched by the doctor or midwife, often with the mother lying on her back with her legs in stirrups. Her head and neck should be comfortably supported by pillows, and she may like to hold her baby.

Stitching is tedious, but should not be painful if a local anaesthetic is given. The best time to be stitched is after you have had a chance to see and touch your baby, but before the area feels tender. First, the local anaesthetic is injected into the area to be stitched. Then the vaginal skin, then the torn muscle and finally the external skin are stitched. Usually dissolvable thread is used, and the stitches do not need to be removed. (Painful stitches can be cut at four days, and may be soothed by a herbal bath.)

The immediate post-natal period

Discomfort and some pain are usual in the first day or two, but pain can be severe, especially with a large medio-lateral episiotomy. Pain-relieving tablets or even an injection may be needed. These should be kept to a minimum, however, as the drug will cross into the breastmilk.

Tears on the front of the labia may cause burning on passing urine, but this can be helped by pouring warm salty water from a large jug over the area at the same time. The burning will cease as the tissues heal.

Sitting on a rubber ring or child's swimming ring will reduce the pressure on the area, and applying ice cubes in a plastic bag to the stitches can be very soothing. Calendula tincture will promote healing (see HOMOEOPATHY).

If you have PILES, perhaps brought on by the efforts of labour, these may increase the pain. Women are often afraid of opening their bowels after childbirth for fear that the stitches may burst. This never happens, but you may feel happier if you lubricate the anus with olive oil or a proprietary haemorrhoid cream.

A large episiotomy sometimes causes muscle spasm and urine retention (see URINARY TRACT AND KIDNEY PROBLEMS IN THE MOTHER).

Immediately after childbirth, you should wash and bathe your vaginal area twice a day, and keep the perineum dry, since wetness delays healing. If patting dry with a towel causes pain, use a hair dryer instead. Doing pelvic-floor exercises will encourage blood flow and healing.

You should wait until healing is complete before making love. Gentle penetration is sensible at first; the outer area is usually the most tender, particularly at the back of the vaginal entrance. First lubricate the whole area thoroughly with a pure oil. Initially, avoid lying flat on your back with your partner on top, as this position puts the most pressure on the stitch line. More comfortable alternatives are for the woman to be on top or for the couple to lie side by side.

Post-natal complications

Pain from stitches will normally disappear within ten days after the birth. Any pain that goes on for longer needs to be investigated. A common reason is a local reaction to the stitches causing tenderness, particularly at the vaginal entrance, which resolves with time.

Infection along the stitch line is a rare complication, more likely after a medio-lateral episiotomy because swollen, bruised muscles encourage bacteria. It is treated with antibiotics. Alternatively, a herbal compress can be made with slippery elm, golden seal and comfrey root (1 tsp of each rolled in gauze and steeped in boiling water). Apply while warm three times daily.

Very occasionally, the wound opens up. It usually heals by itself, but the cut may need to be thoroughly cleaned and then restitched.

Deep-seated pain often arises from the lower spine and sacrum, which has twisted during the birth. The sacrum then pulls the underlying muscles and ligaments attached to it, to create tension and pain at the episiotomy site. This may also make intercourse painful. This pain may be relieved by osteopathic manipulation or yoga exercises for the lower spine.

If the birth was unsatisfactory, painful stitches may be the focus of psychological pain and anger. Many women feel especially violated if they believe that an episiotomy was unnecessary. Sometimes these feelings may not surface at the time, because of the joy of having a new baby, but emerge months or even years later.

Very rarely indeed, stitching makes the vaginal outlet too tight for penetration during sexual intercourse, and restitching is needed. Usually, however, when couples think they have this problem, enlightened counselling is the real solution. Women may feel invaded by the birth to the extent that they can no longer relax their vaginal muscles to allow penetration, so great is their need to hold themselves in and regain privacy. A man may have found it upsetting to watch an episiotomy or see his partner being stitched. This can alter his sexual behaviour for months. He may be afraid of injuring his partner.

Conclusions

Whether to risk tearing or to have an episiotomy 'just in case' is very controversial. A few women have an enormous fear of tearing and request an episiotomy in advance; others cannot bear the idea under any circumstances, and prefer to tear if they cannot manage otherwise. The routine use of episiotomy, with all the complications of a surgical procedure, is now the main cause of, rather than the prevention against, vaginal scar formation, pain and discomfort. With the increase in active birth, the number of episiotomies is dropping.

Tears in labour see BIRTH INJURIES TO THE MOTHER, TEARING AND EPISIOTOMY

Teeth and gums in pregnancy

All pregnant women should have routine dental checkups. Injections of local anaesthetic are not harmful, nor are well-screened X-rays (although these should still be done only when absolutely essential).

Gum disease is also common during pregnancy. The gums tend to swell and trap particles of undigested food, giving rise to the gum infection known as gingivitis. If your gums are swollen, sensitive and bleed during brushing, your dentist will advise you. Do not eat between meals, and avoid sweets, biscuits and other foods containing sugar. You should brush your teeth carefully with a soft brush daily, paying special attention to the area where teeth meet gums. Use dental floss once a day to keep the spaces between the teeth clean.

Good dental care continues to be important post-natally.

Termination of pregnancy

Commonly known as abortion, this is not available on demand in Britain. It can only be done if there is a risk to the mother's life, a risk of severe physical or mental abnormality in the baby or a risk to the physical or mental health of the mother or her existing children.

A termination form must be completed by two medical practitioners, after both of them have seen and examined the mother, but many women require further counselling. It may be difficult for a woman to decide to have a termination, particularly if the baby is wanted but abnormal, or when the mother's circumstances make it impossible for her to take care of a baby. The decision to terminate often involves the parents in great conflict and guilt.

What happens

Vaginal termination in the first 12 to 14 weeks of pregnancy is usually done under a general anaesthetic. The cervix is dilated and suction is used to remove the contents of the uterus (i.e. the foetus, placenta and membranes). The woman may come in to hospital just for the day or stay overnight. This is a minor operation, but the emotional consequences may be profound, even when the woman is quite sure that she is making the right decision.

Prostaglandin termination, done after 14 weeks, consists of inserting a fine catheter (tube) into the cervix and slowly giving prostaglandin to ripen the cervix and achieve INDUCED LABOUR; pessaries may be used instead. It may also be necessary to give the drug Syntocinon to stimulate contractions.

The woman has a mini-labour, which often takes many hours to start and may then last for as long as 12 hours. It may be very painful, but anaesthesia can be used.

After termination

Some women feel relieved; others need to grieve. The grieving is important, as is the need to resolve any feelings of guilt (see LOSS OF A BABY). Counselling may be necessary, to include contraceptive advice, or advice about the possibility of future foetal abnormalities (see CONGENITAL ABNORMALITIES AND GENETIC COUNSELLING).

Rarely, termination may be followed by CERVICAL INCOMPETENCE, pelvic infection (see FALLOPIAN TUBE INFECTIONS), and prompt medical treatment is essential if there is a fever. It is sensible to wait for three months after a termination before becoming pregnant again.

See also DEPRESSION AND STRESS

Thalassaemia see SICKLE CELL DISEASE AND THALASSAEMIA
Thrombosis see VENOUS THROMBOSIS AND PULMONARY EMBOLISM

Thrush in the baby

A baby may catch the fungal infection known as *thrush* while being born, if the mother's vagina is infected. Occasionally, the fungus is present on the mother's skin, and the baby is infected during breastfeeding.

The most common site for thrush in babies is the mouth. The tongue and larynx become red, and white flakes appear on the tongue. Unlike milk spots, which they resemble, the flakes cannot be wiped off. The baby may also have feeding difficulties. Other common sites for thrush are the thighs and buttocks, when it can be confused with NAPPY RASH.

If thrush on the skin is mild, washing it several times a day with a solution of one teaspoon bicarbonate of soda to a cup of previously boiled water is often enough to relieve it. Otherwise, treatment is mainly by antifungal drugs, either in a liquid for the mouth or ointment for the skin.

Thrush on the nipples see BREAST PROBLEMS AFTER CHILDBIRTH
Thrush in pregnancy see VAGINAL INFECTIONS

Thyroid disorders in mother and baby

Thyroid gland problems are unusual in pregnant women. Most are present before conception.

Problems in pregnancy

Symptoms of an overactive thyroid may include weight loss, hyperactivity, excess hunger, aggression and an inability to sleep. The baby may also be affected, because the hormone causing your thyroid to become overstimulated can cross the placenta and overstimulate your baby's thyroid for up to six weeks after birth. Both of you may need drug treatment.

An underactive thyroid causes weight gain, lethargy, sleepiness and OEDEMA. It is treated with tablets containing the thyroid hormone thyroxine.

Problems in the newborn

One in 5000 babies is born with an underactive thyroid. There is usually no family history, and the condition is usually detected by a routine test on the sixth day of life, when a blood sample is taken from the baby's heel.

If untreated, thyroid underactivity (cretinism) leads to MENTAL RETARDATION. This can be avoided by giving an affected baby thyroxine daily. In view of the ease of diagnosis and treatment, it is now thought that every newborn should be screened.

See also CONGENITAL ABNORMALITIES AND GENETIC COUNSELLING

Tiredness and insomnia

While some women have boundless energy during pregnancy, others experience fatigue, lack of energy, weakness or insomnia, especially during the first and last trimesters.

Causes

There are many reasons for tiredness during pregnancy. Hormonal changes undoubtedly affect energy levels. Nausea, VOMITING and HEARTBURN may all affect food intake and can drastically reduce the energy available. Dietary deficiencies and eating too many refined foods also cause fatigue, and the effects of poor nutrition are often felt after the birth, when the baby's demands make food preparation difficult, and breastfeeding uses up reserves of calories and nutrients. Your diet during pregnancy and after the birth is vitally important (*see* Chapter 7).

Adequate sleep is essential. Your sleep pattern may alter for physical reasons: you may need to urinate at intervals during the night, you may be uncomfortable or breathless, you may have backache or cramp. Chronic back pain or headaches will certainly make you feel drained during the day and prevent you from sleeping at night. Too little exercise often causes listlessness; your body needs it to promote energy, help you sleep and improve well-being (*see* Part V).

Your sleep pattern may also change for emotional reasons: you may be plagued by bad dreams (pp. 67-8), or lie awake worrying. Anxiety may manifest itself as insomnia and low energy.

After the birth, it may take weeks before the sleep patterns of mother and baby correspond. The demands of a new baby are often exhausting, and an early return to work can increase the strain. Tiredness may also be a symptom of DEPRESSION.

Treatment and self-help

If you feel excessively tired and weak, see your doctor. Very occasionally, extreme weakness, especially accompanied by breathlessness, is a sign of ANAEMIA or other serious problems.

Otherwise, start by trying to accept the pregnancy and flow with its new demands, welcoming your altered body rhythms. Do everything you can to make sure you get enough rest, dealing with any backache, breathlessness or heartburn. If your bladder needs emptying several times a night, reduce your fluid intake after 4 p.m., and have a medical check to exclude the possibility of infection. Exercise (particularly yoga) and massage last thing at night will encourage sleep; deep breathing practised daily may also help. Also try to sort out any emotional problems, getting specialist help if necessary. If after all this you are still unable to get a good night's sleep, perhaps you could try to rest two or three times a day instead of for one long stretch at night.

Pay attention to your diet. Take exercise and practise yoga, and you may well feel quite revitalized. Acupuncture and massage are potent ways of stimulating energy flow.

After the birth, some tiredness is inevitable. Try to delegate as much shopping and housework as possible. Keep the baby close to you at night so that you can feed without getting up or having to wake up completely. Accept that you are going to be led by your baby's rhythms for some time to come: the quicker you adjust to this and get used to attending to yourself and your own needs whenever the baby is asleep, the sooner you will overcome tiredness. Exercise is as important now as it was before the birth.

Toxaemia of pregnancy *see* HIGH BLOOD PRESSURE AND PRE-ECLAMPSIA

Toxoplasmosis

Infection with the parasite toxoplasma occurs through eating or handling undercooked meat or, rarely, from contact with infected cats' faeces. Most women infected during pregnancy have no symptoms, and the baby is unharmed. Affected babies may have only very mild symptoms, but in its severe form, toxoplasmosis can cause mental retardation, blindness and DEAFNESS. There is no known treatment or vaccine for toxoplasmosis, which is diagnosed by testing for antibodies in the mother's blood. Close contact with cats' faeces and raw meat should be avoided during pregnancy.

Transcutaneous nerve stimulation (TNS) *see* PAIN RELIEF IN LABOUR

Transverse lie

Very rarely, at the end of pregnancy the baby lies sideways in the uterus, with either a hand, a shoulder or the umbilical cord nearest the cervix. If this is diagnosed in advance, a gentle massage, or *external version* (*see* BREECH BIRTH), may help the baby to turn. If the transverse lie cannot be corrected and labour has started, a CAESAREAN SECTION is necessary. If your waters break, you need to be examined to make sure that the umbilical cord has not become compressed, threatening the oxygen supply to the baby (*see* PROLAPSED UMBILICAL CORD). If you are at home, it is wise to lie down and have someone call an ambulance.

Trichomonas *see* VAGINAL INFECTIONS

Twins

Approximately 6000 pairs of twins are born in Britain each year – about one in every 100 births.

A third of all twins are identical. This means that a single egg is fertilized by a single sperm, and shortly afterwards splits into two separate embryos which share one placenta. Both babies are the same sex, and have the same genetic makeup, resulting in identical features and blood groups. Identical twins occur at a constant rate around the world.

Non-identical twins are from two eggs, each fertilized by separate sperm, with the result that the twins are no more

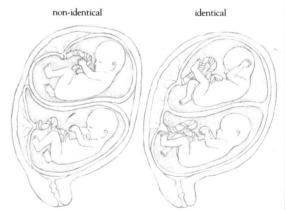

non-identical   identical

alike than ordinary siblings. Each twin is nourished by his or her own placenta. Your chances of having non-identical twins increase if you are over 35, have more than four other children, are of African racial origin, are a non-identical twin yourself or part of a family with a history of non-identical twins, or are taking fertility drugs.

Diagnosis

Twins may be suspected if the uterus is large for the duration of the pregnancy, or if two babies can be felt by the midwife, obstetrician or mother. In the past, it was quite common for twins not to be diagnosed until labour, but the widespread use of ULTRASOUND SCANNING has made this very rare now.

Preparing for birth

Regular ante-natal care is particularly important in a twin pregnancy because the changes in your body are greater than with a single baby, and there is more risk of disorders.

Whereas, with one baby, the uterus reaches the mother's ribcage by week 36, with twins this happens four weeks earlier, and the sheer size of the enlarging uterus causes extra minor discomforts. Attention to posture (see Part V) is especially important because of the added weight on the spine; yoga and exercise can reduce backache and strain (see PAIN IN PREGNANCY). You should rest as often as you can between normal activities.

Diet needs special attention to reduce the incidence of ANAEMIA and to keep both you and the babies in peak condition. Multivitamins, iron and other mineral supplements, particularly zinc, should be taken daily, while alcohol and cigarettes should be avoided. There is no need to 'eat for three': excessive weight will merely reduce your mobility further.

The average length of a twin pregnancy is 37 weeks, compared with 40 for a single birth. Premature labour is more common, and there is a higher chance of twins being affected by hydramnios (i.e. excessive AMNIOTIC FLUID) and pre-eclampsia, with diminished placental flow producing babies who are small for dates. One twin sometimes takes the lion's share of placental nourishment, leaving the second twin undernourished and underweight, but after birth, the smaller one usually catches up with the other.

Planning for life after the birth

It is essential to organize your life so that you will have help after the birth. You will need assistance with housework if you are to get enough rest. You may be eligible for a home help. There is also a greater financial commitment with twins than with one baby, and you should plan for this.

Try to meet other parents with twins, spending time with them in their own homes to see at first hand what life with twins is like. If you are lucky, there may be a 'twins club' in your area (p. 347).

Labour and birth

The principles of active birth apply equally to having twins. An upright position is ideal to prevent a reduction in the oxygen supplied by the placenta. Midwives and obstetricians will be doubly vigilant to ensure that both babies are well. Epidural anaesthesia may be useful if obstetric intervention is predicted for the second twin.

In twin births, the first stage is usually of normal length. The second stage is in two parts: birth of the first twin with clamping of one umbilical cord, followed by birth of the second twin. In the third stage, both placentas, if there are two, are delivered together.

There is a higher incidence of breech presentation with twins. Most twin breech babies can both be born vaginally as the babies tend not to be very large – the average twin weighs 2.5 kg (5½ lb) compared with the average weight of a single baby of 3.4 kg (7½ lb) – and disproportion (see LARGE BABIES) is rare. A more important potential problem is the birth of a very small BREECH baby.

After the birth of the first twin, the doctor will pay careful attention to the well-being and position of the second. If the foetal heart rate is normal, and if the baby is a head or a breech presentation, it is safe to wait for uterine contractions to begin again, as they will naturally after a short interval. If there is any bleeding or any problem with the second twin, the birth will be speeded up by stimulating contractions or rupturing the membranes.

During the third stage, the large placental surface area means that there is a higher risk of bleeding, but placental separation is usually efficient, and the bleeding easily controlled.

Examination of the babies and the placenta at birth is usually enough to establish whether the twins are identical or not. If the babies are of opposite sexes, or if there are two placentas with double membranes, the twins cannot be identical. Very occasionally, it is necessary to test the babies' blood groups.

The first few weeks

Most mothers have both babies with them after the birth, and are able to bond with them and establish breastfeeding without difficulty. The more the babies feed, the more milk is produced, and two babies provide twice the stimulation; what matters is confidence. Talking in advance to mothers who have breastfed twins may help. (See also Chapter 15.)

Sometimes women are encouraged to give additional feeds from a bottle. However, this is only ever necessary if you are ill, or if your babies are not gaining enough weight. A sensible approach is to aim for total breastfeeding, but realize that it may be necessary to top up with a bottle.

Because many twins are premature or small for dates, they tend to be admitted to special-care baby units more frequently than single babies (see ILLNESS IN BABIES). This can be a time of great conflict for the mother, who may find herself with one baby in the special-care unit, one with her in the post-natal ward and older children at home waiting for her to come out of hospital, all while her body is recovering from the double pregnancy and birth. The stress of coming to terms with the 'double joy and double trouble' of twins may be intense; many women need especially strong emotional support and counselling at this time, as well as practical help.

Ultrasound scanning

Ultrasound was first developed during World War II, when it was used to detect submarines. It was then found that the same technology could be used to observe the foetus in the uterus and check its development and well-being.

How ultrasound works

A crystal, expanding and contracting in an electric current, produces a beam of sound at a frequency that is higher than the human ear can hear – ultrasound. When the sound waves are directed at a solid object, they bounce back towards the crystal, which then contracts slightly; this is picked up as an electrical signal, which is translated into an image on a television screen. The sound waves bounce back differently from different surfaces and distinguish between bone and muscle in a baby's body. The ultrasound used on pregnant women is of a very low intensity, thus keeping any negative effects to a minimum.

Routine ultrasound examination

A scan will confirm the presence and normal development of the baby and will also show where the placenta has implanted. It is best done between the 16th and 18th weeks of pregnancy, when the various parts of the foetus can be seen clearly.

Ultrasound is widely available and often recommended to pregnant women, and the majority have a scan at some stage of their pregnancy. It can be exciting and reassuring to see your baby moving on the screen, to see his heart beating and to identify parts of his body. However, some women prefer not to have scans because their long-term or subtle effects are still unknown. Avoiding ultrasound for at least the first eight to ten weeks, when the embryo is developing, is a sensible precaution.

What happens in an ultrasound examination

You may be asked to have a full bladder when you go for your scan, because the liquid in the bladder provides a contrast and improves the quality of the image on the screen. You lie down on a couch and the operator applies a thin layer of oil to your abdomen to improve the contact with the ultrasound probe, which is then glided over the abdomen to produce the ultrasound, and the black-and-white image appears on the screen. In most hospitals, mothers can see the screen as they lie on the couch, and the operator explains what appears on it. Sometimes a photo printout of the picture on the screen can be made for you to take home.

The risks of ultrasound

In 1984, when a medical report in the United States suggested that ultrasound waves damage chromosomes in dividing cells, a committee was set up by the Royal College of Obstetricians and Gynaecologists in London to examine these findings. The committee concluded that, at the intensity currently used, ultrasound scanning is probably safe.

The extremely short pulses of sound – 1000 pulses per second, each last only one-millionth of a second – have never been shown to cause heating or bubbles in the tissues of human foetuses. Certain studies on animal foetuses have indicated that ultrasound can cause abnormalities or reduced growth (depending on the stage of development), but expert opinion attributes this to heating, which does not occur with the low-intensity ultrasound used in pregnancy. Other studies have shown mainly negative results.

It will be several decades before any more subtle or long-term effects can be accurately assessed. One immediate risk is the error possible when any test is performed. False positives do occur and may lead to mistaken diagnosis and treatment. For this reason, any abnormalities revealed by a scan should be very carefully checked: where the clinical findings of a doctor are at variance with a scan, ultrasound takes second place.

Uses of ultrasound in pregnancy

Ovulation and conception Women who have difficulty in conceiving may be given a scan to measure the developing follicle in the ovary (pp. 17-18), and to time ovulation.

Miscarriage and ectopic pregnancy Sometimes a scan may be used to detect whether there is an ECTOPIC PREGNANCY or a MISCARRIAGE. With the latter, doctors can usually tell almost immediately whether a baby is alive or not. However, results are not 100 per cent reliable, and occasionally a normal foetal heartbeat is missed. A repeat scan is essential before a definite diagnosis is made.

Multiple birth A routine scan at 16 weeks can usually diagnose whether a woman is going to have twins.

Gestational age If a woman has irregular menstrual cycles, the exact dating of pregnancy may be difficult. A scan in the first half of pregnancy can allow the length of the baby's body or the size of the head or limbs to be measured, so that conception can be dated to within ten days. Sometimes this is inaccurate if measurements were incorrect. After 20 weeks, scans are unreliable for dating purposes because of the range of sizes of individual babies.

Congenital abnormality By 18 weeks, a scan can detect the majority of cases of NEURAL TUBE DEFECTS. Certain URINARY TRACT abnormalities may be diagnosed from an enlarged bladder or absent kidney, and some gastro-intestinal abnor-

malities may be detectable. A specialized 'sector scanner', capable of looking at small areas in depth, may be used to examine the baby's heart. The majority of CONGENITAL ABNORMALITIES are not detectable by current ultrasound technology.

Amniocentesis and foetoscopy Ultrasound scanning is essential in the performance of both these tests.

Bleeding It is obviously essential to discover the cause of any blood loss during pregnancy. Ultrasound can locate the placenta and exclude PLACENTA PRAEVIA.

Breech presentation A scan can assess in late pregnancy whether the baby is in the normal head-down position or a BREECH.

Foetal well-being If the baby seems to be growing slowly in late pregnancy, ultrasound can be used to monitor its growth. Recent machines have even been used to measure placental blood flow and the output of unborn babies' hearts.

Maternal problems Disorders such as FIBROIDS, pelvic tumours, kidney stones and gallstones may be diagnosed.

Conclusion

Although often invaluable, ultrasound scanning is of doubtful value when used routinely during late pregnancy. As Sally Inch says in *Birthrights: a Parent's Guide to Modern Childbirth (1982)*, 'The techniques which are developed to provide benefits for specific groups of people gradually tend to be used for more and more people, on wider and vaguer indications (on the grounds that what is beneficial for some must be beneficial for all), to the point where people who do not require any treatment at all are being given it. As this latter group will having nothing to gain from the technique, they will be worse off if it carries any risk than they would be if left alone.'

Umbilical hernia *see* HERNIAS IN THE BABY
Underactive thyroid *see* THYROID DISORDERS IN MOTHER AND BABY

Undescended testes

The testes form in the abdomen of a male foetus, normally descending into the scrotum in late pregnancy or shortly after birth. Some baby boys have *retractable testes* – i.e. they retract into the abdomen when exposed to cold. This needs no treatment, as in time the passageway from abdomen to scrotum will narrow spontaneously.

If one or both testes fail to descend at all, the groin should be checked to exclude an inguinal HERNIA, a common association. Surgery to bring the testes down into the scrotum will not be done until the boy is about five years old because the majority will have descended on their own by this time. Left in the abdomen, they may fail to develop their normal fertility.

Urinary incontinence

This is the involuntary passing of urine from the bladder. There are two main types: stress incontinence and urge incontinence. Heavy mucus secretion from the vagina or cervix in pregnancy, or ruptured membranes, may occasionally be mistaken for incontinence.

Stress incontinence

At the outlet of the bladder into the urethra is a valve-like ring of muscle fibres. Normally, as the bladder fills, the natural tone of these fibres keeps the urine in the bladder. If the ring of muscle fibres is lax, any stress that puts pressure on the bladder – e.g. coughing or laughing – will cause urine to leak out.

Stress incontinence may begin during pregnancy, as the hormones relax the muscles. If it occurs in late pregnancy, this may lead to the woman thinking that her waters have broken. Except where the incontinence is caused by a VAGINAL PROLAPSE, it usually disappears after childbirth.

Stress incontinence is more common post-natally, as a result of the pelvic floor stretching during childbirth. Exercising this area (p. 263) during the months after the birth will help to tighten it again.

Urge incontinence

If the bladder wall is irritated by infection, inflammation or bruising at birth, it may become more liable to contract. As urine enters, irritable nerves at the bladder base signal a feeling of fullness and urgency and, in severe cases, uncontrollable contractions of the bladder wall may cause what is known as *urge incontinence*. Bladder infection is a frequent cause. Treatment is with antibiotics if there is infection; otherwise, it is a question of waiting until the bruise disappears.

Other causes

If the bladder outlet and urethra are badly bruised, the muscle fibres may swell and go into spasm. The result is retention of urine, with overflow of the excess. This rare event can occur as a result of epidural anaesthesia, forceps delivery or Caesarean section. Drainage via a catheter – a thin tube attached to a plastic bag – allows the bladder to regain tone and lets the bruising settle.

See also PREMATURE RUPTURE OF THE MEMBRANES, URINARY TRACT AND KIDNEY PROBLEMS IN THE MOTHER

Urinary tract and kidney problems in the baby

Some babies are affected by kidney and urinary problems, which may occur before or after birth. The most common are described below.

Renal agenesis

Very occasionally, the foetal kidneys fail to develop normally. Often the first sign is a lack of AMNIOTIC FLUID, or oligohydramnios, which can be confirmed ante-natally by ULTRASOUND SCANNING.

Renal cysts

An ultrasound scan may indicate the presence of one or more cysts (abnormal fluid-filled swellings) on the kidneys before birth. No obstetric intervention is needed. After birth, the kidneys are studied by X-rays and radio-isotopes, to confirm the nature of the cysts and whether one or both kidneys are involved. The outlook for one cyst is usually good, but it may need to be drained.

Renal obstruction

Sometimes an obstruction in the urinary tract prevents the baby from urinating. This can be detected during pregnancy by a reduction in AMNIOTIC FLUID. If the obstruction is complete, and as long as the kidneys have not been damaged, it may be appropriate to drain the urine while the baby is still in the uterus. This is done by passing a tube through the baby's abdominal wall under ULTRASOUND observation, so that urine drains into the amniotic pool. The tube is removed after birth, and surgery deals with the obstruction.

Hypospadias

Occasionally, in boy babies, the urethra (the tube conducting urine from the bladder along the penis) does not develop properly. The abnormality is obvious at birth: the urethra's opening is at the base of the penis or somewhere along the penile shaft instead of at its end. Sometimes the penis itself is bent. Minor malformations require no treatment, but major anomalies need corrective surgery.

Narrowed foreskin

Obstruction to the flow of urine caused by a narrowed foreskin is uncommon. Fewer than 5 per cent of male children need CIRCUMCISION to improve their urinary flow.

Urinary infection

Infection of the bladder or kidney is difficult to diagnose as the symptoms are often confusing. There may be obvious pus in the urine; on the other hand, the infant may just be off colour, not feeding well and failing to thrive. Diagnosis often depends on being aware of possible causes. A premature baby in hospital is vulnerable to organisms in the urinary tract.

If a urinary infection is suspected, uncontaminated urine has to be collected for analysis – not easy to do with a small baby. If an infection is confirmed, the baby is given antibiotics and the underlying cause is treated.

Urinary tract and kidney problems in the mother

During pregnancy, labour and afterwards, a woman's bladder and kidneys may become susceptible to infection or injury.

Bladder and kidney infection

Cystitis – inflammation of the bladder – causes a burning sensation on urinating and a frequent urge to urinate. *Pyelitis*, a less common but more serious infection of the kidneys, sometimes follows cystitis; it can cause fever and tenderness or pain in the loin area of the lower back.

Because the muscles relax during pregnancy, organisms can enter the bladder to cause cystitis. In some hospitals, urine samples taken from all women in early pregnancy are cultured to check for the presence of certain microbes. If present, antibiotics are given, the aim being to prevent symptoms later in pregnancy.

Rarely, cystitis follows bruising and infection during labour, perhaps after an operative delivery. Infection also becomes more likely if a catheter is needed to drain the bladder.

Bladder injury and urinary retention

Bladder injury during labour is rare. A normal active birth will not injure the bladder, and neither will forceps deliveries or Caesarean sections, if carefully performed.

The common result of bruising is pain and muscle spasm, which may cause retention of urine. During a long labour the baby's head may press on the base of the bladder and bruise it; this may also happen in a difficult forceps or Caesarean delivery. Post-natally, pain in the perineum may cause spasm and urinary retention.

Treatment is with painkillers and by draining the bladder with a catheter.

Kidney disease

It is rare to develop kidney disease for the first time in pregnancy. If you already have kidney disease, take medical advice before becoming pregnant. If you have never had a urine test or had your blood pressure taken before, kidney disease may be first diagnosed during pregnancy screening.

One of the signs of kidney disease is HIGH BLOOD PRESSURE that becomes worse as pregnancy progresses: both mother and baby are at risk from pre-eclampsia and eclampsia and the mother's kidney problems may be worsened.

Vacuum extraction *see* FORCEPS DELIVERY AND VACUUM EXTRACTION
Vaginal bleeding *see* BLEEDING

Vaginal infections

Thrush (candidiasis or moniliasis)

As in the mouth and intestines, microbes live in the healthy vagina. As the vaginal secretions alter in acidity and sugar content during pregnancy, the fungus *Candida albicans* may multiply, resulting in a thrush infection. Almost every woman experiences thrush at some time, and it is particularly common during pregnancy. Diabetes also makes the vaginal environment more sugary and thrush thrives in the presence of sugar.

Symptoms and treatment There may be no symptoms, but usually the skin around the vagina and anus itches and looks red and sore, and there are characteristic milky-white flakes in the vagina.

Because the fungus prefers a sugary environment, thrush may be responsive to diet: cutting down on refined foods in favour of slow-burning ones can alleviate symptoms. Eating live yogurt may be an effective form of self-help, because this contains micro-organisms known as *lactobacilli*, normally present in the bowel and vagina, which actually destroy the fungus and form a natural barrier against re-infection. (Inserting live yoghurt into the vagina is not recommended during pregnancy.) Another effective form of self-help is to add bicarbonate of soda to your bath water: this will help to reduce acidity.

Medical treatment comes in the form of an anti-fungal ointment, liquid or pessary. At the end of pregnancy, treatment minimizes infection being passed to the baby during birth (*see* THRUSH IN THE BABY).

It is also possible to pass thrush to a sexual partner. To eradicate the infection, both partners may need treatment, with the man applying anti-fungal cream to his penis.

Trichomoniasis

This infection is usually transmitted through sexual contact. Symptoms are vaginal soreness and itchiness and a characteristic yellow, frothy discharge; discomfort occasionally spreads to the urethra and bladder. Treatment is in the form of an antibiotic called metronidazole, which usually clears up the infection within a day or two. Metronidazole should be avoided in early pregnancy, and alcohol must be avoided while taking it. Both sexual partners are usually treated. Trichomoniasis does not usually affect the baby.

Herpes

The *herpes simplex* virus is very common. There are two types: type A causes cold sores and mouth blisters; type B, spread by sexual contact, causes genital herpes. The type A virus can also be transmitted to the genitals by oral sex. Primary attacks of genital herpes are very rare during pregnancy because women generally do not have sex with new partners at this time.

The type B virus invades the skin and causes pain in the affected area, followed by blisters and then ulcers, all of which can take from ten days to three weeks to heal. The virus then lies dormant in the underlying nerves for weeks or months, eventually reactivating to cause another attack in the same area. The first attack is usually the most severe, later ones tending to occur less frequently as times goes on. An antiviral agent, acyclovir, reduces the length of each attack, but does not reduce their number.

The vagina of an affected woman should be screened weekly after 36 weeks of pregnancy for the infection – by vaginal examination and viral culture. If the herpes is dormant and the culture negative, there is no risk to the baby, and labour can proceed normally. If the mother is having an attack with open ulcers, the baby is at risk of catching herpes during labour by inhaling or swallowing infected vaginal secretions, so birth is always by CAESAREAN SECTION.

Very few babies in Britain are born with congenital herpes. If a baby is thought to have been infected, acyclovir is given for one week to prevent infection. Neonatal herpes may damage any organ, including the brain, eyes, skin, bowel, liver, kidneys and heart.

Women with genital herpes should have regular CERVICAL SMEARS for life because of an association between the herpes virus and pre-cancerous cells in the cervix.

Gonorrhoea

This sexually transmitted infection may produce a white vaginal discharge, vaginal irritation, the urethral and bladder symptoms of cystitis (*see* URINARY TRACT AND KIDNEY PROBLEMS IN THE MOTHER) or post-natal pelvic infection (*see* FALLOPIAN TUBE INFECTIONS). Many women show no symptoms, so a woman may be a carrier for years without knowing it. During pregnancy, the infection cannot enter the uterus, but the baby may become infected during birth with an eye infection causing severe CONJUNCTIVITIS which may cause blindness. Treatment is with antibiotics.

Chlamydia trachomatis

Like gonorrhoea, this rare infection may be present without producing symptoms, although sometimes it does cause vaginal discharge or urinary frequency. It does not usually harm the mother, but if the baby catches it during birth, she may develop an eye infection or, very rarely, pneumonia.

An affected baby shows signs of 'sticky eye' (conjunctivitis) between 4 and 20 days after the birth, and of nasal infection or pneumonia between one and three months after. The condition usually responds to the antibiotic erythromycin.

Syphilis

The syphilis microbe is transmitted by sexual intercourse, but only a few cases of infection during pregnancy occur in Britain each year. Now rare, syphilis has three stages.

In the primary stage, a small sore usually develops on the labia, vagina or cervix. This is painless and may last for three weeks. Weeks or even months later, the secondary stage begins: microbes in the bloodstream cause fever, a general feeling of illness, swollen glands and a painless skin rash. The tertiary stage may not occur for years, but when it does, it can cause blindness, insanity, heart and liver disorders and other serious problems.

Because the primary stage can pass unnoticed, a routine blood test for syphilis is done at an early ante-natal checkup; if this is positive, more accurate tests are performed. At the primary and secondary stages, high doses of antibiotics can usually halt the infection.

Congenital syphilis is now very rare, in Britain only affecting eight babies a year. These may have severe

CONGENITAL ABNORMALITIES. However, treatment early in pregnancy usually prevents foetal damage.

Vaginal prolapse

Vaginal prolapse occurs when the supporting ligaments and muscles stretch and the vaginal walls drop below their normal limits, sometimes taking with them the uterus, bladder or rectum. It is a hernia of the vagina, which becomes more likely if there is a hereditary predisposition, poor nutrition, obesity, or excessive pressure during childbirth.

Symptoms
You may feel as if something is coming down the vagina, together with an ache in your lower back caused by tension on the ligaments. You may need to urinate frequently, be unable to empty your bladder or bowels easily or even be incontinent. You may feel that your vagina is loose, with reduced sensation during intercourse.

Treatment
The main problem in pregnancy is leaking urine, which is difficult to treat, but after the birth, this usually decreases over a few months. If there is pre-existing vaginal prolapse during labour, it may be necessary to do an episiotomy (see TEARING AND EPISIOTOMY) so that the pressure of the baby's head in the second stage is reduced to a minimum.

Post-natal exercises can very effectively help to tighten the muscles and regain lost tone (see Part V), and these may be all that is needed. Very rarely, a ring may have to be inserted into the vagina post-natally to hold the cervix in place.

Ideally, any surgery required is only done after the childbearing years are over. If a prolapse repair operation is followed by another pregnancy, the cervix has to be very carefully monitored, to ensure that there is no CERVICAL INCOMPETENCE, and the baby will have to be born by CAESAREAN SECTION to avoid injury to the vaginal supports.

Varicose veins

Pregnancy puts extra stress on the veins especially in the lower half of the body. The volume of blood increases, stretching the walls and the valves in the veins. This may cause blood to pool in the lower limbs, and the result is painful, swollen varicose veins. Most common in the legs, in pregnancy they also frequently affect the labia, when they are called vulval varicosities, and the anus, when they are known as PILES, or haemorrhoids.

There is an hereditary tendency to develop varicose veins, but they are also far more likely in women whose occupations involve standing still for long periods. They also occur more often in women who are expecting twins.

Treatment
Vulval varicosities always disappear completely after pregnancy. Unfortunately, varicose veins in the legs do not always return to normal, so they should be treated as soon as they develop.

Wear good-quality support tights. Lie down with your legs up frequently during the day. Raise the foot of your bed by about 15 cm (6 in) and exercise every day – all the stretching exercises in Part V improve circulation.

After the birth, continue to wear support tights until your veins have returned to normal; any post-natal pain or redness should be treated as VENOUS THROMBOSIS. There is surgical treatment for varicose veins, but it is usually not done until the childbearing years are over.

Venous thrombosis and pulmonary embolism

Developing a blood clot in a vein – venous thrombosis – is an uncommon but potentially extremely serious complication of pregnancy. From conception until after childbirth, the mother's blood-clotting system is very active: it is nature's way of preventing bleeding, but increases the risk of venous thrombosis, particularly in the week after the birth.

A clot can destroy one of the valves that makes a vein function properly and so cause severe VARICOSE VEINS. It is even more dangerous if one is dislodged from a vein wall and travels through the bloodstream to the right side of the heart, where it may block the flow of blood to the lungs. This is a pulmonary embolus, which is extremely rare but may be fatal.

Risk factors include:
- existing large varicose veins;
- confinement to bed for long periods during pregnancy;
- CAESAREAN SECTION or a large episiotòmy (see TEARING AND EPISIOTOMY);
- previous venous thrombosis;
- overweight and smoking.

To minimize the risk of venous thrombosis, look after any existing varicose veins. The more gentle and less traumatic the birth and the sooner you are mobile, the less likely is post-natal thrombosis.

Symptoms
In superficial vein thrombosis, the affected vein under the skin feels hot, red and tender, and the leg may become painful and swollen. In deep thrombosis the leg may become unnaturally white. Half of all clots cause no leg changes, however. The clot may be hidden in one of the pelvic veins, so that the first sign is a pulmonary embolus. Symptoms of this are sudden chest pain, shortness of breath and, occasionally, coughing blood.

Treatment
Superficial leg thrombosis carries minimal risk of an embolus, so it may simply be treated with local decongestants, bandages and support. A deep vein thrombosis will need treatment with anticoagulants (drugs which thin the blood), possibly for some months. One of the most common – *heparin* – is relatively safe during pregnancy because it does not cross the placenta; another drug, *warfarin,* should be avoided. Should a large clot occur in deep vein, another pregnancy would be discouraged, and the contraceptive pill should definitely be avoided. An embolus is treated with intravenous anticoagulants, and surgery may be needed to remove the clot.

Ventouse *see* FORCEPS DELIVERY AND VACUUM EXTRACTION

Vision in pregnancy

Vision may alter in pregnancy, especially in the last three months. The changes are caused by fluid retention (see OEDEMA) in the tissues of the eyes. After the birth, you will probably find that your sight returns to normal, so it is unwise to buy new glasses or contact lenses while pregnant.

Blurred vision or seeing flashing lights are symptoms to be taken seriously. Either symptom may indicate severe pre-eclampsia, especially if you also have HIGH BLOOD PRESSURE and protein in your urine. You should seek urgent medical advice.

Visual display units *see* RADIATION

Vomiting in the baby

Very young babies often bring up small amounts of milk shortly after a feed. Known as posseting, this is quite normal.

There are many possible causes of true vomiting in infancy. Some are rare and serious, others common and transient. All babies vomit occasionally, and many vomit easily or for no apparent reason. Most vomiting needs no treatment. However, if the vomiting is projectile (*see below*), acute or persistent, if it is associated with DIARRHOEA, if the baby is not gaining weight or looks obviously ill and dehydrated, medical help should be sought urgently.

Pyloric stenosis

A few babies are born with a narrowed (stenosed) exit from their stomach – i.e. the *pylorus*. This condition, more common in boys, produces a distinctive type of vomiting when the baby is under four weeks old: he brings up most of his feed with great force, so that it may spurt several feet across the room. This *projectile vomiting* may occur after every feed; the baby is also likely to have CONSTIPATION, and fails to thrive.

Pyloric stenosis needs urgent treatment. An antispasmodic drug, given by mouth, is effective only if the stenosis and spasm are mild. If they are severe, the baby must have an abdominal operation to widen the pyloric canal under general anaesthesia.

Vomiting in pregnancy

Nausea and vomiting are two of the most common symptoms of pregnancy, although many women do not experience either at any time during pregnancy. Others find that nausea, which may lead to vomiting, begins at or even before the first missed period. Vomiting – commonly called 'morning sickness' – usually stops by the 12th to 14th week, but it may go on longer, especially with TWINS, and may recur in the last few weeks before birth.

Causes

There is no simple explanation for nausea and vomiting in pregnancy. The hormonal changes of early pregnancy are partly to blame, pressure on the stomach from the uterus is a factor in late pregnancy, and vomiting is often worse with twins. Long-term tension in the diaphragm and abdominal muscles can lead to vomiting when stomach function alters, as it does in pregnancy. Sometimes nausea and loss of appetite occur because of an inadequate B vitamin and mineral intake; eating foods rich in these nutrients (pp. 98-9) for a few days can cause the appetite to return and vomiting to diminish. The most severe vomiting, known as hyperemesis, usually occurs in women who generally respond to stress by developing abdominal symptoms.

Treatment

Most cases of vomiting during pregnancy do not need medical investigation. The baby, who is using the nutritional stores that you built up before the start of pregnancy, is usually unaffected. In fact, women who lose weight in early pregnancy usually gain it back later, some even putting on excessive weight as if in compensation.

If you find nausea and vomiting very debilitating there are a number of things you can do for yourself. Many women find deep breathing and yoga effective treatments for nausea. They also help to reduce any anxiety that may be partly responsible. Attention to posture may also help: sleep propped up, and sit on hard, upright chairs to stop yourself from slouching.

Watch your diet carefully. Avoid refined, fried and spicy foods and alcohol, and eat little and often. If you suffer from nausea in the morning, keep some food by your bed and have a light snack before getting up. If vomiting is severe, eat whatever you can for a few weeks.

Homoeopathic remedies are often successful, and acupuncture can provide real relief from severe vomiting, although usually only temporarily. Yoga and exercises that stretch the abdominal muscles and relieve tension are both excellent (*see* Part V). Tea made from fresh ginger may be helpful.

Anti-emetic drugs to relieve vomiting are now not often given, but if nothing else helps your vomiting, you may be offered one. There is minimal risk to the baby, especially after ten weeks.

In extreme cases of hyperemesis, admission to hospital (where an intravenous drip can be given) can be life-saving. The causes of hyperemesis should be treated with psychotherapy. Often these are deeply subconscious, and only an experienced therapist can help get to the root of the problem. *See also* HEARTBURN

Vulval varicosities *see* VARICOSE VEINS
Watering eyes *see* BLOCKED TEAR DUCT IN THE BABY

Weight before pregnancy

The overweight woman

Conception problems are not usually associated with being overweight, but obese women are at higher risk of HEARTBURN arising from pressure on the stomach, VARICOSE VEINS, TIREDNESS and BREATHLESSNESS, and may also find it harder to sleep comfortably. In addition, they may suffer from skin irritation caused by friction and perspiration, and this may be exacerbated by thrush (*see* VAGINAL INFECTIONS).

Although many fat people are surprisingly strong and healthy, they tend on the whole to be less physically fit. The added weight causes extra pressure on the back, hips and leg joints, with more likelihood of arthritis. However, many overweight women do not feel uncomfortable during pregnancy, as they are used to the discomforts associated with increased size. In fact, some actually feel happier because pregnant women are supposed to be big. Dieting is not recommended during pregnancy, but careful attention to nutrition (*see* Chapter 7) will reduce excessive WEIGHT GAIN.

Babies born to overweight women tend to be slightly larger than average. In labour, women who are not very fit or mobile may find it hard to move about or change position. Epidural and general anaesthesia (*see* PAIN RELIEF IN LABOUR) are technically more problematical, and FOETAL HEART MONITORING may be more difficult through the thick abdominal wall.

During the post-natal period, the main problems are mobility and skin rashes, but breastfeeding is usually normal. If an overweight woman puts on excess weight during pregnancy, it may take some time to lose it.

The underweight woman

An underweight mother poses a far greater potential problem for the baby than an overweight one. It can be difficult to establish when a woman is underweight: many women are thin but perfectly well nourished, while other, slightly heavier women may be undernourished. Very fit women, particularly athletes, are usually thin but not necessarily underweight. In general, a fit, thin woman eating a well-balanced diet is in good health.

If a woman is grossly undernourished or anorexic, ovulation and menstruation cease. This is nature's way of reducing fertility during periods of starvation, ensuring that babies are only born when there is food. Malnutrition before pregnancy is associated with more miscarriages and 'small-for-dates' babies (see LOW BIRTH WEIGHT).

Starvation before or very early in pregnancy has a far more drastic effect on the baby than starvation in late pregnancy, when he is able to extract the essential nutrients from the mother's blood flowing through the placenta. Women who are underweight at conception should concentrate on increasing the nutritional content of their diet.

A low maternal weight is not associated with particular problems in labour for the mother, but the baby needs to be carefully monitored throughout pregnancy and birth. Post-natal nutrition must be good, to improve the flow of milk.

Weight gain in pregnancy

Every woman should put on weight during pregnancy: if she stays the same, she is losing weight as the baby grows.

The average overall weight gain during pregnancy is 10 kg (22 lb), with a normal range of between 5 kg (11 lb) and 15 kg (34 lb). (See p. 34 for how this extra weight is distributed.) A gain of more than 15 kg may be normal if the baby is very large or if there are twins, and tall women of large build can also be expected to gain more weight.

The average weekly gain is 0.3 kg (10 oz), but because an inaccurate reading, or a full bladder or bowel, can give a false result, the overall trend is more important than any single recording.

Excess weight gain

Each pregnancy should be individually assessed, but in general, a gain of more than 15 kg for the entire pregnancy or over 0.5 kg (1 lb 1 ½ oz) a week is excessive. The major effect of this is that the woman will be overweight after the birth. Rapid weight gain in the last ten weeks may be caused by fluid retention or may be an early sign of pre-eclampsia (see HIGH BLOOD PRESSURE AND PRE-ECLAMPSIA).

If your weight gain is excessive, you need to alter your diet (see Chapter 7). The intake of all refined and 'junk' foods, sweets and fried foods should be reduced. Food fads or cravings (p. 97) may indicate a mineral or vitamin deficiency which may disappear with supplements. The emphasis should be on raw vegetables and fruits. If you are eating too much because this relieves HEARTBURN or VOMITING, antacids may be the answer.

Exercise is another potent way of keeping weight down. Swimming or walking briskly will speed up the body's metabolism and burn more calories, both during pregnancy and post-natally. Breastfeeding will also help you to reduce weight by the baby consuming calories, as long as you control your calorie intake at the same time.

Low weight gain

Weight loss in pregnancy, or a gain of under 5 kg (11 lb), indicates either that the mother is not eating enough so that she is losing weight as the baby grows, or that the baby is not growing properly.

Pregnancy is an inappropriate time to diet, because the baby is making great demands on your body for protein, sugar, fat and essential vitamins and minerals. If you diet, the nutrients that the body cannot store for long may become depleted. The baby is well adapted to obtaining what she needs from the mother's blood, but dieting may make this more difficult.

If it seems possible that the baby might not be growing

adequately, your weight must be carefully assessed over a period of weeks. Do not worry about one low reading; it is the overall trend that counts.

Low weight gain in an underweight woman is far more significant than low gain or weight loss in an obese woman. Action may be needed to improve maternal nutrition; if the baby is 'small for dates' (see LOW BIRTH WEIGHT), the pregnancy needs to be carefully monitored.
See also WEIGHT BEFORE PREGNANCY

Weight of babies see LOW BIRTH WEIGHT AND PREMATURITY, LARGE BABIES, LOW WEIGHT GAIN AFTER BIRTH, OBESITY IN THE BABY

Working mothers

In an ideal world, mother and baby would remain together for most of the baby's first year. Sometimes, however, this is not possible and alternative child-care arrangements must be made. However, unless it is completely unavoidable, no mother should leave a baby under three months old. The best advice is to wait before returning to work for as long after the birth as your circumstances allow.

If you will be returning to work, the time you are able to spend with your baby beforehand is especially important. You need to get to know and enjoy each other, and to form a strong bond.

X-rays see RADIATION

Young mothers

In Britain, nine per cent of all babies are born to teenage girls. Although usually physically fit and healthy, such young mothers often have special needs and difficulties.

Physical factors

Teenage mothers, especially those younger than 15, may not have finished growing. As a result, disproportion and difficult labour are more likely because the mother's pelvis may not yet have reached its full size. Recent growth spurts may have depleted their stores of minerals and vitamins.

Many teenagers also consume many refined 'junk' foods, and there is a relatively high incidence of smoking and drug usage. The likelihood of the baby being 'small for dates' (see LOW BIRTH WEIGHT) is increased, mainly because of maternal diet and housing problems.

Social factors

In some societies, teenage marriage and subsequent pregnancy is the norm, but in the West, pregnancy among teenagers often results in single parenthood and economic deprivation. The major problem facing such girls is how to find an environment in which to care for and nourish the baby. Even stable teenage couples have rarely had time (or opportunity) to save money for their needs and those of their baby.

Fear can be an important feature of teenage pregnancy. A young woman may be frightened of telling her parents, leaving school, going through labour and, above all, caring for a baby. The most difficult time is often after the baby is born, when the mother's friends are all out in the world while she is stuck at home with a young child, perhaps unable to afford even essential items. Health-care services play a vital role in supporting teenage pregnancies, as do some ante-natal teachers and post-natal support groups such as the National Childbirth Trust (see opposite page).

Useful addresses

Action Against Allergy
43 The Downs
London SW20 8HG
(01) 947 5082

Active Birth Centre
see International Centre for
Active Birth

Association of Breast-feeding Mothers
131 Mayow Rd, London
SE26 4HZ
(01) 778 4769

Association for Improvements in the Maternity Services (AIMS)
163 Liverpool Rd, London
N1 0RF
(SAE appreciated)
(01) 278 5628

Association for Post-Natal Illness
7 Gowan Ave
London SW6 6RH
(01) 731 4867

Association of Radical Midwives (ARM)
c/o 8a The Drive
London SW20 8TG
0695 72776

Association for Spina Bifida and Hydrocephalus
22 Upper Woburn Place
London WC1H 0EP
(01) 388 1382

Baby Life Support Systems (BLISS)
44–45 Museum St
London WC1A 1LY
(01) 831 9393: fundraising
and support groups for
parents of babies in
intensive care

British Diabetic Association
10 Queen Anne St
London W1M 0BD
(01) 323 1531

British Epilepsy Association
Anstey House
40 Hanover Square
Leeds LS3 1BE
(0532) 439 393

British Pregnancy Advisory Service
Austy Manor
Wootton Wawen, Solihull
West Midlands B95 6BX
(05642) 3225

Brook Advisory Centres
233 Tottenham Court Rd
London W1 9AE
(01) 323 1522

Caesarean Support Group
81 Elizabeth Way
Cambridge CB4 1BQ
(0223) 314211

Cleft Lip and Palate Association (CLAPA)
1 Eastwood Gardens
Kenton
Newcastle-upon-Tyne
NE3 3DQ
(0632) 859396

Compassionate Friends
6 Denmark St
Bristol BS1 5DQ
(0272) 292778:
for bereaved parents

B.M. Cry-sis
London WC1N 3XX
(01) 404 5011: support for
mothers of crying babies

Down's Children Association
3rd floor, Horne's Premises
4 Oxford St
London W1N 9SL
(01) 580 0511
(24-hour helpline)

Family Planning Association
St Andrew's House
27/35 Mortimer St
London W1N 7RJ
(01) 636 7866

Foresight (Association for the Promotion of Preconceptual Care)
The Old Vicarage
Church Lane
Whitley, Godalming
Surrey GU8 5PM

Gingerbread
35 Wellington St
London WC2E 7BN
(01) 240 0953:
for single parents

In Touch Trust
10 Norman Rd

Sale, Cheshire M33 3DF
(061) 962 4441: central
contact and information
agency on all aspects of
mental handicap, and for
parents of children with a
rare physical and/or mental
disorder

Independent Midwives Association
65 Mount Nod Rd
London SW16 2LP

International Centre for Active Birth
55 Dartmouth Park Road
London NW5 1SL
(01) 267 3006: for classes
in the Balaskas Method of
birth preparation

La Lèche League of Great Britain
Vine Lodge
18 Colney Hatch Lane
London N10 1OU
(01) 883 7801: information
and support for breastfeeding
mothers

Maternity Alliance
15 Britannia Street
London WC1X 9JP

Meet-a-Mum Association (MAMA)
c/o 3 Woodside Ave
London SE25 5DW
(01) 654 3137: self-help
groups for new mothers

Miscarriage Association
18 Stoneybrook Close
West Bretton, Wakefield
W. Yorks WF4 4TP
(0924) 85515

National Association for Parents of Sleepless Children
PO Box 38
Prestwood
Great Missenden
Bucks. HP16 0SZ

National Childbirth Trust
9 Queensborough Terrace
London W2 3TB
(01) 221 3833

National Council for One-Parent Families
255 Kentish Town Rd
London NW5 2LX
(01) 267 1361

National Eczema Society
Tavistock House North
Tavistock Sq
London WC1H 9SR
(01) 388 4097

Nippers (National Information for Parents of Prematures: Education Resources and Support)
c/o The Sam Segal Perinatal
Research Unit, St Mary's
Hospital, Praed St
London W2 1NY
(01) 725 1487

OPUS (Organizations for Parents Under Stress)
106 Godstone Rd
Whyteleaf
Surrey CR3 0EB
(01) 645 0469

Pre-eclamptic Toxaemia Society (PETS)
33 Keswick Ave
Hullbridge, Essex SS3 6JL
(0702) 231689

Pregnancy Advisory Service
13 Charlotte St
London W1P 1HD
(01) 637 8962

Society to Support Home Confinements
Lydgate, Wolsingham
Co. Durham DL13 3HA
(0388) 528044
(after 6pm)

Stillbirth and Neonatal Death Society (SANDS)
Argyle House
29–31 Euston Rd
London NW1 2SD
(01) 833 2851

Twins Clubs Association (Twins and Multiple Births Association)
292 Valley Rd
Lillington, Leamington Spa
Warwicks. CV32 7UE

Ireland
Active Birth Ireland
The Hermitage
Newtown, Mt Kennedy
Co. Wicklow

Dublin Birth Centre
3 South Terrace
Inchicove, Dublin 8
(0001) 717295

INDEX

PHOTOGRAPHIC CREDITS
All photographs were taken
by Anthea Sieveking, with
the exception of the
following:
p. 10 Science Photo Library
p. 45, 48 Lennart Nilsson/A
   Child is Born (Faber &
   Faber)